Hypermobility, Fibromyalgia and Chronic Pain

Commissioning Editor: Rita Demetriou-Swanwick
Development Editor: Veronika Watkins
Project Manager: Kerrie-Anne McKinley/Nancy Arnott
Designer/Design Direction: Kirsteen Wright
Illustration Manager: Gillian Richards
Illustrator: Robert Britton

Hypermobility, Fibromyalgia and Chronic Pain

Edited by

Dr Alan J Hakim MA FRCP
Consultant Physician and Rheumatologist & Director of Strategy & Business Improvement
Whipps Cross University Hospital, London UK

Rosemary Keer MSc MCSP MACP
Specialist Chartered Physiotherapist
Central London Physiotherapy Clinic, Harley Street, London UK

and

Professor Rodney Grahame CBE MD FRCP FACP
Consultant Rheumatologist
University College Hospital, London UK

Foreword by
Professor Peter Beighton OMB MD PhD FRCP FRSSA
Emeritus Professor of Human Genetics
Faculty of Health Sciences
University of Cape Town, Capetown, South Africa

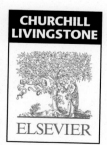

CHURCHILL
LIVINGSTONE

ELSEVIER

EDINBURGH LONDON NEW YORK OXFORD PHILADELPHIA ST LOUIS SYDNEY TORONTO 2010

CHURCHILL
LIVINGSTONE
ELSEVIER

ISBN 978-0-7020-3005-5

British Library Cataloguing in Publication Data
A catalogue record for this book is available from the British Library

Library of Congress Cataloging in Publication Data
A catalog record for this book is available from the Library of Congress

Contents

Contributors

Professor Qasim Aziz PhD FRCP
Consultant Gastroenterologist & Director of
Neurogastroenterology, St Bartholomew's and
the London School of Medicine and Dentistry, &
Queen Mary, University of London,
London UK

Mr Marcus JK Bankes BSc FRCS (Orth)
Consultant Orthopaedic Surgeon, Guy's &
St Thomas' NHS Foundation Trust, London UK

Professor Howard A Bird MD FRCP
Professor of Pharmacological Rheumatology &
Honorary Consultant Rheumatologist, University
of Leeds & Leeds Teaching Hospitals NHS Trust,
Leeds UK

Dr Jaime F Bravo MD
Professor of Medicine, University of Chile Medical
School, and Consultant Rheumatologist, San Juan
de Dios Hospital, Santiago, Chile

Lynn Bryden MSC MCSP MACP
Specialist Physiotherapist, Health Physiotherapy
and The Royal Free Hospital, London UK

Dr Anthony Bulbena MD MSc (Cantab) PhD
Professor of Psychiatry, Universidad Autònoma
de Barcelona. Head of the Institut d'Atenció
Psiquiàtrica Salut Mental i Toxicomanies (IAPS),
Neuropsychopharmacology Group. IMIM-Hospital
del Mar. Barcelona, Spain

Katherine Butler B.Ap.Sc (OT) AHT(BAHT) A.Mus.A(Flute)
Clinical Specialist in Hand Therapy, London Hand
Therapy, London UK

Dr José Alexandre Crippa MD PhD
Coordinator of Psychiatry-Liaison. Departamento
de Neuropsiquiatria e Psicologia Médica
Faculdade de Medicina de Ribeirao Preto,
Universidade de São Paulo, Brazil

Dr H Clare Daniel BSc (Hons) DClinPsy
Consultant Clinical Psychologist, The National
Hospital for Neurology and Neurosurgery,
Queen Square, London UK

Mr Rohit Dhawan MRCS
Research Fellow in Orthopaedics, University
College London Hospitals, London UK

Dr Adam D Farmer MB BS BSc MRCP
Clinical Research Fellow in Gastroenterology,
The Wingate Institute of Neurogastroenterology,
St Bartholomew's and the London School of
Medicine and Dentistry, and Queen Mary,
University of London, London UK

Dr Peter W Ferrell MB ChB
Senior House Officer in Orthopaedic Surgery,
Ninewells Hospital, Dundee UK

Professor William R Ferrell MB ChB PhD FRCP (Glas)
Professor of Clinical Physiology, Western
Infirmary, Glasgow UK

Mr Marc George MBBS FRCS (Trauma & Orthopaedics)
Consultant Orthopaedic Surgeon, Guy's &
St Thomas' NHS Foundation Trust, London UK

Professor Rodney Grahame CBE MD FRCP FACP
Consultant Rheumatologist, University College
Hospital, London UK

Sarah Gurley-Green MA
Writer & Former Chairperson of the
Hypermobility Syndrome Association (HMSA),
Boston USA

Mr Fares Haddad BSc MCh (Orth) FRCS (Orth) FFSEM
Consultant Orthopaedic Surgeon, University
College London Hospitals, London UK
Director of the Institute of Sport, Exercise and
Health, UCL, London, UK

Dr Alan J Hakim MA FRCP
Consultant Physician and Rheumatologist &
Director of Strategy and Business Improvement,
Whipps Cross University Hospital, London UK

Dr Nathan Hasson MB ChB FRCPCH
Consultant Paediatric Rheumatologist,
The Portland Hospital, London UK

Dr Andrew J Holman MD
Associate Clinical Professor of Medicine,
University of Washington, Seattle & Consultant
Rheumatologist, Pacific Rheumatology Associates,
Renton, USA

Mr Colin Hopper MBBS BDS (Lond) FDSRCS (Eng)
FRCS (Ed) MD (Lond)
Consultant in Oral and Maxillofacial Surgery,
UCL Eastman Dental Hospital and Institute and
University College London Hospitals,
London UK

Anju Jaggi BSc (Hons) MCSP
Clinical Physiotherapy Specialist, Royal National
Orthopaedic Hospital Trust, London UK

Mr Waseem Jerjes MSc (OMFS) PhD (Surg) MD
Senior Clinical Research Associate, UCL Medical
School, London UK

Rosemary Keer MSc MCSP MACP
Specialist Chartered Physiotherapist, Central
London Physiotherapy Clinic, Harley Street,
London UK

Mr Simon M Lambert BSc FRCS FRCSEd (Orth)
Consultant Orthopaedic Surgeon & Honorary
Senior Lecturer, Royal National Orthopaedic
Hospital Trust, London UK

Susan M Maillard MSCP
Chartered Physiotherapist, Great Ormond Street
Hospital, London UK

Dr Fransiska Malfait MD PhD
Research Fellow, Centre for Medical Genetics,
Ghent University Hospital, Belgium

Dr Rocío Martín-Santos MD PhD
Head of Section of Hospitalitzation. Institute of
Neuroscience, Department of Psychiatry.
Hospital Clínic. IDIBAPS. CIBERSAM, Barcelona &
Neuropsychopharmacology Group.
IMIM-Hospital del Mar. Barcelona, Spain

Mr Ron S McCulloch BSc FCPodS
Consultant Podiatric Surgeon, Homerton
University Hospital & The London Podiatry
Centre, London UK

Alison Middleditch MCSP
Chartered Physiotherapist, Physiotherapy Clinic,
Coulsdon, Surrey UK

Professor Anne De Paepe MD PhD
Professor, Head of Department, Centre for Medical
Genetics, Ghent University Hospital, Belgium

Julie Payne B.Occ Therapy, MSc
Occupational Therapist, Great Ormond Street
Hospital, London UK

Professor Anisur Rahman PhD FRCP
Consultant Rheumatologist, University College
London and University College Hospital,
London UK

Dr Anthony Redmond PhD
Arthritis Research Campaign Senior Lecturer,
Institute for Molecular Medicine, University
of Leeds, Leeds UK

Dr Anshoo Sahota MB FRCP
Consultant Dermatologist, Whipps Cross
University Hospital, London UK

Prof Gonzalo Sanhueza MD
Professor of Medicine, Universidad del Desarrollo.
Clinica Alemana. Santiago Chile

Dr Maliha Shaikh MBBS MRCP
Clinical Research Fellow in Rheumatology,
Addenbrooke's, Cambridge University
Hospitals, Cambridge UK

Dr Nicholas Shenker PhD MRCP
Consultant Rheumatologist,
Addenbrooke's, Cambridge University Hospitals,
Cambridge UK

Jane Simmonds BPE BAppSc (physio) PGDip Man Ther
MA MCSP MMACP MACPSM
Programme Leader MSc in Sport and Exercise
Rehabilitation, University of Hertfordshire,
Hatfield UK, and Clinical Specialist in
Hypermobility Syndrome, Hospital of St John and
St Elizabeth, London UK

Kaye Walls MSc MCSP MMACP
Physiotherapist Clinical Specialist,
University College Hospital, London UK

Foreword

The association of joint hypermobility with a wide range of clinical manifestations has received general acceptance. The Editors and co-authors of this text have been primarily responsible for the formulation of this concept and for its integration into clinical practice. It is fitting and appropriate that the Editors have now encapsulated current knowledge of hypermobility and related conditions in this comprehensive monograph.

Hypermobility first attracted serious medical attention in the 1960's when lax joints were recognized as symptomatic components of a few rare genetic connective tissue disorders, notably the Ehlers-Danlos syndrome. Families with gross articular hypermobility, in the absence of any other primary manifestations were also identified at this time. It emerged, however, that the vast majority of hypermobile persons were sporadic, without affected relatives; the syndrome status of these individuals remains unresolved.

In the rheumatological context the diagnosis "hypermobility syndrome" was applied to loose jointed persons in whom muscle pains of uncertain pathogenesis were troublesome. The term "Joint Hypermobility Syndrome" JHS was subsequently introduced to denote articular laxity which produced untoward symptoms, especially limb pain and articular instability, but including manifestations in other systems.

In 2003 Professor Grahame and Rosemary Keer published a book entitled "Hypermobility Syndrome, Recognition and Management for Physiotherapists" based on a decade of experience in a JHS clinic. This book provided impetus for the recognition of the clinical importance of the JHS and constituted the first overview of the disorder. Together with Dr Alan Hakim, these authors have now produced the definitive work on the JHS. This monograph embraces many aspects of current understanding of the condition, ranging from manifestations, through pathogenesis to management. The fact that more than 30 experts in different fields have made contributions emphasises the complexity and the extensive ramifications of the syndrome.

This magisterial monograph will constitute the foundation upon which many future developments in the understanding of the JHS will be based, and represents eloquent testimony to the endeavours of the Editors and colleagues in this field.

Emeritus Professor
Peter Beighton, OMB, MD., Ph.D., F.R.C.P., F.R.S.S.A.
University of Capetown
Easter 2010

Preface

This book will be of interest to a wide range of health professionals, both generalist and specialist, as well as to patients, their families and carers. Physicians dealing with fatigue syndromes, pain specialists, rheumatologists and orthopaedic surgeons, acute physicians and general surgeons, occupational therapists and physiotherapists, clinical psychologists and podiatrists, osteopaths and many more beside will find its content absorbing. This is not surprising as there is hardly a single specialty of medicine that is not touched in some way by hypermobility. The book encourages the reader to consider the possibility of joint hypermobility syndrome (JHS), identify it clinically, understand its co-morbidities, and manage it appropriately. Hopefully, it may also influence those in authority – health and social care budget holders and health care insurers – of the need to provide appropriate resources for the care of people with JHS.

JHS is common and yet it is often over-looked or neglected. The syndrome is associated with a number of co-morbidities that include fatigue, chronic pain, autonomic disturbance and anxiety disorders. There is much in common with the underlying pathophysiology and management of fibromyalgia, chronic fatigue syndrome, and complex regional and chronic widespread pain.

Over the last 10–15 years clinicians and scientists from different fields of interest in rheumatology, chronic pain, rehabilitation, anxiety, neurology, gastroenterology, genetics and surgery have come together to work in the field of hypermobility syndromes having become aware of the associations and the need for a multispecialty and multidisciplinary approach to understanding the condition and its management. This book has given us the opportunity to draw together this expertise with contributions from a broad group of internationally recognized authors.

With regard to practical management we have taken and expanded the original and extremely successful text by Keer and Grahame *Hypermobility Syndrome: Recognition and Management for Physiotherapists* (Butterworth Heineman, London, First Edition, 2003). As with the first book, we hope that both clinicians and therapists will benefit from a work that brings together all the latest literature and hands-on practical experience. We also hope the 'lay' person will be able to utilize the book.

With regard to the 'science' we have taken the opportunity to explore the epidemiology, nosology and genetics of the hereditary disorders of connective tissue, the association between JHS, fibromyalgia and chronic widespread pain, neurophysiology and pain pathways, gastrointestinal disorders, and disorders of autonomic function, again bringing together a literature that is totally up to date. We very much hope that all parties will find this aspect of the book both intellectually stimulating and of educational value.

We start with the Prologue. Written by Sarah Gurley-Green, former Chairperson of the Hypermobility Syndrome Association, the prologue is a synthesis of the patients' experience of chronic pain in JHS. We commend this to our readers for its insight.

The book is then split into two sections.

Section One deals with the clinical manifestations of JHS and fibromyalgia, their epidemiology and pathophysiology.

Section Two covers clinical management. Here the reader will find chapters covering pharmacotherapeutics, psychotherapy and physical therapies that address the needs of patients from childhood to adulthood.

There is still a great need for better recognition and understanding of JHS, its associations, and their management. We hope that this book will support all health professionals in achieving this goal, by stimulating interest, encouraging debate, advancing knowledge of therapies, and engaging in further research.

Alan Hakim
Rosemary Keer
Rodney Grahame
London 2010

Prologue

Sarah Gurley-Green

XIX.
THE MYSTERY OF PAIN.
PAIN has an element of blank ;
*   It cannot recollect*
When it began, or if there were
A day when it was not.

It has no future but itself,
Its infinite realms contain
Its past, enlightened to perceive
New periods of pain.

Emily Dickenson (Todd ML &
Higginson TW 1890)

Although few among us can hope to convey the experience of pain with the spare beauty of Emily Dickinson, many patients have turned to poetry as a heuristic and cathartic means of expression, moreover, studies have shown significant clinical improvements for many patients (Smyth et al 1999, Broderick et al 2005).

Dickinson had Bright's disease and suffered greatly from severe physical pain and oedema. Her poem hints at the dark and deep place where one goes when in pain, without time, lost to anything or anyone except pain. Pain is an intimate companion, it curls deeply and silently, familiar yet unwelcome. Pain sometimes whispers calling one away from family and friends, but often shouts, blocking out all else that once was important. Like a spoiled child, it will not be ignored, drawing you in, you turn away from all else until it alone has all your attention. Pain is isolating in part because it is difficult to communicate the experience in words.

"Describe your pain? He said.
Rate it from one to ten? He said.
Eleven, I said.

Where is your pain? He said.
Where is it focused? He said.
All over, I said.

What is it like? He said.
Sharp, dull, twinges? He said.
All and more, I said.

It can't be all, he said.
It can't be all over, he said.
It is in your head, he said.

How do I explain? I said.
Climb in and feel, I should have said.
Something beyond words, I should have said.

He said, I said.
Words were said.
But who understood what was said?"

He Said, I Said. By Graham Venn
Member of the Hypermobility Syndrome
Association (HMSA)

A salient fact about pain is that its only true measurement is the patient's own reporting. At the current time, there is no method to independently measure the quality, or severity of pain, or categorize pain except to rely on the patient's ability to do so effectively and then be able to communicate well.

Suffering '…is really a manifestation not of pain itself but of the losses that occur when pain persists. It is the loss of function that causes suffering.' (Silver 2004). One is able to cope with the sensation of pain, as a pure feeling, like true pleasure, it may even be sought after by some as a sensory experience. However, it is the unpredictability of this sensation that is so damaging; the seemingly random way it tears away at the fabric of the life one tries to create. Over time the tyranny of pain as it capriciously rends career and family life apart, leaves one victim to one's own body.

The Medical community is now recognizing the importance of acute pain; indeed, it is now considered the 'fifth' vital sign after temperature, pulse, respiration, and blood pressure (Silver 2004). But some like Arthur Kleinman have a more nuanced understanding of the situation for patients: 'We [doctors] are unwilling to take the meaning of the pain as seriously as we take its biology' (Kleinman 1988).

In the past the testimony of the patient was the basis of the diagnosis. With the rise of diagnostic tools, there has arguably been a trend towards relying more on the 'test result' than a focus on the patient themselves (Couser 1997) or some meaningful evaluation of the significance of the illness upon their life. The result is a disenfranchisement and objectification of the patient and transference of the clinician from healer to technician; thinking of the illness not the ill. For patients the purpose of the interview may seem to be 'how quickly can one run some tests, start a treatment, or decide what specialist to pass the query on to'. A study in the 1980s, found the average time between the opening of the patient's disclosure of medical experience and the doctor's first interruption was 18 seconds (Charon 2006); universally the health system is under even more strain now than ever before and as such this finding is unlikely to have changed over time. For a chronic pain patient the journey may be years before their story is actually heard.

"I'm clear as crystal,
to me it's become apparent
That I'm see-through,
Totally transparent.

I found it out last week,
when we went shopping,
I'm invisible,
Must be all the pills I'm popping.

I was on the stairs with the kids,
struggling with my crutch,
Clinging to the rail,
It was a bit much.

This man headed towards me,
running to the top stair,
Totally oblivious,
That I was standing there.

He wasn't stopping,
he looked in such a hurry,
I moved across,
Didn't want him to worry.

Then I slipped,
I cried 'cos I jarred my spine,
He didn't even turn,
To see if I was fine.

So I realised I was invisible,
unable to be seen,
No other reason,
Someone could be so mean."

My Own Invisibility Cloak.
By Jackie Portman – HMSA Member

Often the first question that a patient is asked when seeking medical attention for pain is 'what did you do?' In general, for patients with Joint Hypermobility Syndrome (JHS), pain may occur without any obvious cause. Asked how an injury occurred or what triggered the pain, many patients will be unable to trace a specific event. The central nervous system has been bombarded with alarm signals and 'sensitization' may have already begun; ligaments and muscles under stress all the time just keeping a good posture or keeping from falling can cause pain. Activities of daily life such as carrying groceries, babies, working at a computer, or in the garden can send alarm bells. Sitting for long periods, or unaccustomed exercise can bring stiffness and aches that make those things seem impossible. What might otherwise seem 'normal' behaviours may trigger injury; not a readily recognized phenomenon to many health care professionals and hypermobile individuals alike. Moreover, hypermobile patients often complain of 'stiffness' and a sense of being 'clumsy'. What they feel has no relation to the common definition of stiffness that may be experienced by anyone with arthritis or a healthy person who overexerts themselves. Upon examination, unlike a patient with arthritis, they will often appear to be mobile with a range of movement equal to or greater than average and therefore have no apparent functional deficit; likewise no neurological abnormality. When the patient is faced with mounting scepticism from doctors, physiotherapists, friends and family, it is not surprising that the patient will at times doubt their own certitude.

The 'self-concept', the idea of the self constructed from the beliefs one holds about oneself and the responses of others, particularly in relation to the physical self, is in danger when one's body does not behave, indeed is causing pain and even destroying one's life. 'The body is simultaneously a receiver with which the self collects all sensate and cognate information about what lies exterior to it and a projector with which the body declares the self who lives in it' (Charon 2006). If the body is ill and the individual cannot trust it, then the tool by which it communicates with the world is broken; the ability to both gather information from the world, to feel about the world, to communicate back to the world is all filtered through a lens of pain and poor self-concept.

'Fear cannot be without hope nor hope without fear.' Spinoza, Ethics, 1677

The fear of pain can be more crippling than pain itself. The world becomes smaller as social contacts and networks fall away, career goals become shut doors as fitness spirals down, the pain becomes the central character in one's own life. The fear of pain may also prevent compliance with self-management. It requires a great deal of self-efficacy and mindfulness for an individual to pursue, for example, exercise that will result in pain in the near term. Studies have shown success of a mindful, values-based approach to pain and experience, that is, to make a decision to act knowing that there may be pain as consequences, but recognizing the value in the long term (Vowles et al 2009). Studies show that those who accept pain, who are more willing to risk pain, function at a higher level and have more success in the management of their chronic pain (McCracken & Eccleston 2005). When they struggle *against* pain, the patient retains hope of regaining their past identity after vanquishing the enemy of illness. They continue to loathe themselves as well as the illness. On the contrary, when they struggle *with* pain, there is a shift to accepting the body's limitations while exploring what it can still do. In this process, the patient learns to protect the body and gain control over pain. Greater belief in the ability to control the pain leads to greater self-efficacy and thus a better compliance

with self-managed exercise programs and pacing of activities.

Although suffering can be immense, and interventions to control pain not as effective as might be hoped, individual patients can find a pathway to differentiate between pain and suffering.

"Pain is inevitable.
A part of my life.
So I have accepted it.
Avoiding the suffering of bitterness and hate.

Do not confuse this pain
With great suffering profound.
My Life is a pleasure, a privilege.
I live and love all the more for what I have learnt.

Pity those who surround me.
Who see my pain,
And feel its cut.
And see no path but suffering.

They try in vain to ease it,
Not realising that
They fight a reflection
Of their own hurt.

I accepted my pain,
And chose the path without suffering.

May they too find this truth,
So my heart is not wrung
By the unshed tears in their eyes."

Pain is inevitable, suffering is optional.
By Hannah Turner – HMSA Member

A recent study of chronic pain patients found that those who accepted pain as a part of life, set goals and kept them and established rules by which a life could be lived in which pain had a part, appeared to be more successful at management. They were more able to set goals to motivate and to move forward. On the contrary, those patients still seeking a cure were more fatalistic and felt that their life was not controlled by them. They were more subject to mood fluctuations, were more distressed and felt more guilt toward family (Clarke & Iphofen 2007). This is supported by work done by McCracken and Eccleston which found that a group of chronic pain patients who were more accepting of their pain did better over a 3–4 month period of therapy. Those patients who reported greater acceptance initially reported better emotional, social, and physical functioning, less medication consumption, and better work status later. These data suggest that willingness to accept pain, and to engage in activity regardless of pain, can lead to healthy functioning for patients with chronic pain (McCracken & Eccleston 2005). To accept pain one has to understand and to listen to what the body is trying to communicate through pain. From an early age, hypermobile patients experience a variety of sensations from minor stiffness through to severe pain. To have a limited understanding and even a limited vocabulary about these sensations will be problematic for successful self-management. This is a critical issue especially for families affected with this heritable disorder.

A study of over 100 adolescents with chronic pain through self-reporting found that there were many aspects of social development where they lagged behind other children (Eccleston et al 2008). These included independence, emotional adjustment and identity formation. Disability and anxiety had a negative effect on independence, family dysfunction had a negative effect on emotional adjustment, depressive mood on identity formation, and pain intensity on all three factors. Peer relations had a protective effect on psychosocial development, but it was at risk because adolescents in chronic pain had reduced normative school and social exposure. The only aspect where these children felt they were more developed than their peers was at problem solving.

"It's now my secret I try not to tell,
I don't tell them it's hurting,
Or I'm not feeling well.
You see I love to play football,
In goal for the school,
I can't wait for the call.

Last time I told them I sometimes get a sprain,
They called me a risk,
So for the tournament, couldn't train.
I sat in the classroom feeling stupid and sad,
Everyone looked at me,
They asked "Have you been bad?"

I tried to tell them I was fine that day
But I was still stuck there
They wouldn't take me away.

I came home and cried to my Mom, Cass and Dad
They put their arms round me
I got really mad.

Later that night Cass came to my room,
She showed me her wrists
They were like pink balloons.
She still played netball, every single week,
My sister kept it secret,
It never got leaked.

She told me a trick, it was not to tell,
The teachers at school,
When I feel really unwell.
She hugged me some more,
I cried to my sister,
She had been there before.
So now I am silent when it hurts in the class,
I grin and bear it,
I've learned it from Cass."

A Year On And With Cassie's Help.
By Dominic Portman (aged 11) – HMSA Member

Most JHS patients have lived years without diagnosis, some even generations. It is not uncommon for a child's diagnosis to lead to a parent or even a grandparent being diagnosed after many years of pain and humiliation, never knowing what was wrong with them and no doubt experiencing persistent doubt by the medical community.

In the last decades there has been a great deal of good work done to define, diagnose and manage JHS. This is a great benefit for individuals who have languished in pain, without support and often scornfully dismissed as hypochondriacs. With the formation of support groups as well, those affected with the disorder have gained a sense of belonging and solidarity. To know that there is in fact something wrong, and to name it, and even to have a community is important and a vindication. To know the subtleties of treatment may be beyond a generalist though one hopes this book takes them to a new place. However, to be able to listen, realize the impact of pain on quality of life and well-being of a patient and their family, and ultimately to recognize the presence of JHS is not an unreasonable expectation.

References

Broderick JE, Junghaenel DU, Schwartz JE: Written emotional expression produces health benefits in fibromyalgia patients, *Psychosom Med* 67:326–334, 2005.

Charon R: *Narrative Medicine: honoring the stories of illness*, Oxford, 2006, Oxford University Press, p 89.

Clarke KA, Iphofen R: Accepting pain management or seeking pain cure: an exploration of patient's attitudes to chronic pain, *Pain Manag Nurs* 8(2):1087, 2007.

Couser TG: *Recovering Bodies*, Madison, 1997, The University of Winconsin Press, p 22.

Eccleston C, Wastell S, Crombez G, et al: Adolescent social development and chronic pain, *Eur J Pain* 12:765–774, 2008.

Kleinman A: *The Illness Narratives: Suffering, Healing and the Human Condition*, New York, 1988, Basic Books, p 73.

McCracken LM, Eccleston C: A prospective study of acceptance of pain and patient functioning with chronic pain, *Pain* 118:164–169, 2005.

Silver JK: *Chronic pain in the family: a new guide*, Cambridge, 2004, Harvard University Press, pp 10–12.

Smyth JM, Stone AA, Hurewitz A, et al: Effects of writing about stressful experiences on symptom reduction in patients with asthma or rheumatoid arthritis, *JAMA* 281:1304–1309, 1999.

Todd ML, Higginson TW: *Poems by Emily Dickinson*, Boston, 1890, Roberts Brothers, p 3.

Vowles KE, Wetherell JL, Sorrell JT: Targeting acceptance, mindfulness, and values-based action in chronic pain: Findings of two preliminary trials of an outpatient group-based intervention, *Cognitive and Behavioral Practice* 16:49–58, 2009.

Acknowledgements

We gratefully acknowledge the help of Veronika Watkins and her team at Elsevier for their help in the production of this book. Our especial thanks go to Heidi Harrison of Elsevier for the initial inspiration, encouragement and enthusiasm.

We also wish to thank our international team of 36 contributing authors who have given so generously of their time and effort in order to help us create this unique and timely volume.

Finally, we offer a 'thank you' to all our patients who, over the years, have given us such invaluable insight.

Section 1

Clinical science

Chapter 1

The heritable disorders of connective tissue: epidemiology, nosology and clinical features

Alan J Hakim
Fransiska Malfait
Anne De Paepe
With contribution from Anshoo Sahota

INTRODUCTION

Joint hypermobility (JHM) is common and in itself should not be thought of as either a disease or disorder. JHM may be associated with focal, regional or widespread mechanical injury. Equally it may confer advantage to dancers, musicians, sports persons and gymnasts, though perversely these very groups may suffer recurrent injuries if not trained or treated appropriately by taking account of the hypermobility.

Important, however, is the realization that JHM may provide the first insight as to the presence of one of the heritable disorders of connective tissue (HDCT). Further enquiry may reveal an association with skin abnormalities, ligament and tendon pathologies, joint dislocation or subluxation, chronic arthralgia/myalgia, fatigue, early onset osteoarthritis and fragility fractures, abnormal stature, cardiovascular, ocular, autonomic, neuromuscular, visceral, auditory and dental pathologies; a constellation of signs and symptoms constituting the HDCT.

The most common of the HDCT is joint hypermobility syndrome (JHS). It shares some of the signs and symptoms of the Ehlers-Danlos syndrome (EDS) and Marfan syndrome (MFS). Other HDCT include osteogenesis imperfecta (OI) and Stickler syndrome (SS).

This chapter will explore the breadth of clinical manifestations of the HDCT placing JHS in context against the more rare disorders, and setting the scene for the basic science and clinical chapters to follow that will weave together our current understanding of the assessment and management of JHS, fibromyalgia and chronic widespread pain.

DOI: 10.1016/B978-0-7020-3005-5.00001-X

CLASSIFICATION OF THE HDCT

Essential to the correct management and well-being of the hypermobile patient is early identification of the many clinical and often complex symptoms, and second, making a diagnosis. This may seem obvious but it is not necessarily easy. Overlap occurs between JHS (Figure 1.1) (Hakim and Grahame 2003) and the other HDCT. It is a matter of degree with regard to signs and symptoms that lead one to a diagnosis of JHS (Table 1.1) (Grahame et al 2000) rather than EDS (Table 1.2) (Beighton et al 1998) or MFS (Table 1.3) (De Paepe et al 1996). This in itself is a matter of clinical experience. A detailed review by the reader of the table contents is advised as these tables provide a concise source of information upon which to build a clinical history and physical assessment when managing the hypermobile patient.

Specific ultrastructural, biochemical and/or molecular tests of collagen pathology are usually unhelpful in separating JHS from the hypermobility variant of EDS, though may be of value if rarer forms of EDS or OI (Table 1.4) (Byers 1993) are suspected. JHS and EDS hypermobility type are considered to be the same condition (Grahame 1999). A marfanoid body habitus was considered pathognomonic for MFS but is recognized in EDS and SS (Table 1.5) (Stickler et al 1965, 2001, Rose et al 2005) and may be found in up to one third of JHS cases. In the presence of a marfanoid habitus, assessment of cardiac, ocular and dural involvement and eventually genetic study of the *FBN1* gene may be warranted to exclude MFS.

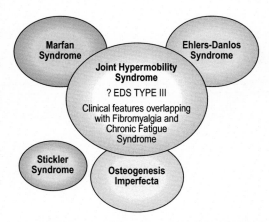

Fig. 1.1 Venn diagram demonstrating the overlap between the HDCT

Table 1.1	The Revised diagnostic criteria for the joint hypermobility syndrome

Major criteria*

1. A Beighton score of 4/9 or greater (either currently or historically)
2. Arthralgia for longer than 3 months in four or more joints

Minor criteria

1. A Beighton score of 1, 2 or 3/9 (0, 1, 2 or 3 if aged 50+)
2. Arthralgia in one to three joints or back pain or spondylosis, spondylolysis/spondylolisthesis
3. Dislocation in more than one joint, or in one joint on more than one occasion
4. Three or more soft tissue lesions (e.g. epicondylitis, tenosynovitis, bursitis)
5. Marfanoid habitus (tall, slim, span > height, upper segment: lower segment ratio less than 0.89, arachnodactily)
6. Skin striae, hyperextensibility, thin skin or abnormal scarring
7. Eye signs: drooping eyelids or myopia or antimongoloid slant
8. Varicose veins or hernia or uterine/rectal prolapse

The JHS is diagnosed in the presence of **two** major criteria or **one** major and **two** minor criteria or **four** minor criteria. **Two** minor criteria will suffice where there is an unequivocally affected first-degree relative. JHS is excluded by presence of Ehlers-Danlos syndromes (other than the EDS hypermobility type formerly EDS III) or Marfan syndrome as defined by the Villefranche 1998 (Beighton et al 1998) and Ghent 1996 (De Paepe et al 1996) criteria respectively.

*The clinical features of JHS are so similar to those seen in the hypermobility subtype of EDS that some experts in the field consider them to be the same condition.

Similarly the brittle bone and blue sclera of OI is seen, to a lesser extent, in EDS and JHS as well. There are, however, well-established classification criteria for each of the HDCT, defined by clinical patterns of disease, identifiable inheritance patterns, and genetic abnormalities of collagen, collagen-modifying enzymes and fibrillin, and histological abnormalities of the dermis. These are shown in each of the classifications in Tables 1.1 to 1.5 and the 'decision tree' (Figure 1.2) (Malfait et al 2006).

THE CLINICAL SPECTRUM

This section will give a broad overview of the nature of symptoms and signs in the HDCT, highlighting their overlap. More detail on the specific clinical picture in JHS can be found in Chapter 2.

PAIN

Pain may occur in any of the HDCT, though perhaps most often in JHS/EDS. It may be localized and acute, secondary to tendon or soft tissue inflammation, joint degeneration, fragility fracture, or chronic widespread and neuropathic in nature. Often there is an association with fatigue and disturbances of mood and psychosocial dysfunction. The complexities of this pattern of pain and fatigue are akin to that seen in fibromyalgia (FM) and chronic fatigue syndrome (CFS). Both conditions are commonly found in EDS (especially in the hypermobility type) and JHS and will be discussed in detail in following chapters. Indeed, given the similarity between EDS hypermobility type and JHS, many experts in the field would now consider these to be the same condition.

In the majority of HDCT cases there is usually no evidence of significant damage to joints, muscles or surrounding structures to account for the widespread pain. There may, however, be evidence of imbalance, poor proprioception, and poor recruitment within muscle groups, as well as features of neural tension potentially related to the presence of hypermobility; again, all these pathologies and the focus for therapeutic interventions will be addressed.

Non-steroidal, opiate-based and tricyclic analgesics may all be of benefit, though for many patients these are ineffective in chronic widespread pain. In this situation physical interventions and cognitive behavioural therapies similar to those employed in the management of FM are of value.

As well as experiencing chronic widespread pain, JHS/EDS hypermobility type patients appear to be resistant to local application of lidocaine (Arendt-Nielsen et al 1990, Hakim et al 2005).

Table 1.2   Classification of Ehlers–Danlos syndromes (Villefranche Nosology 1997)

TYPE	CLINICAL MANIFESTATIONS		IP	PROTEIN	GENE
	Major criteria	*Minor criteria*			
Classic (type I/II)	Skin hyperextensibility Widened atrophic scarring Joint hypermobility	Easy bruising Smooth and velvety skin Molluscoid pseudotumours Subcutaneous spheroids Muscular hypotonia Complications of joint hypermobility Surgical complications Positive family history	AD	Type V procollagen (~50%)	COL5A1 COL5A2
Hypermobility (type III)	Generalized joint hypermobility Mild skin involvement	Recurring joint dislocations Chronic joint pain Positive family history	AD	Tenascin X (~5%)	TNX-B
Vascular (type IV)	Excessive bruising Thin, translucent skin Arterial/intestinal/uterine fragility or rupture Characteristic facial appearance	Acrogeria Early onset varicose veins Hypermobility of small joints Tendon and muscle rupture Arteriovenous or carotid-cavernous sinus fistula Pneumo(hemo)thorax Positive family history, sudden death in close relative(s)	AD	Type III procollagen	COL3A1
Kyphoscoliotic (type VI)	Severe muscular hypotonia at birth Generalized joint laxity Kyphoscoliosis at birth Scleral fragility and rupture of the globe	Tissue fragility, including atrophic scars Easy bruising Arterial rupture Marfanoid habitus Microcornea Osteopenia	AR	Type VIA: Lysyl hydroxylase 1 Type VIB: not known	LH-1 (PLOD1)
Arthrochalasis (type VIIA&B)	Severe generalized joint hypermobility with recurrent subluxations Congenital bilateral hip dislocation	Skin hyperextensibility Tissue fragility, including atrophic scars Easy bruising Muscular hypotonia Kyphoscoliois Mild osteopenia	AD	Type I procollagen	COL1A1 COL1A2
Dermatosparaxis (type VIIC)	Severe skin fragility Sagging, redundant skin Excessive bruising	Soft, doughy skin texture Premature rupture of membranes Large herniae	AR	Procollagen-N-proteinase	ADAMTS-2

AD = autosomal dominant; AR = autosomal recessive.

HYPERMOBILITY

There is wide variation in the prevalence of JHM in the literature dependent on the populations explored. It is three times more common in females than males, of higher prevalence in Asian and African races than Caucasians, and diminishes with age. Generalized or polyarticular hypermobility may be present in 10–30% of males and 20–40% of females in adolescence and young adulthood (Hakim and Grahame 2003a). One survey of Caucasian female twins from the United Kingdom Twin Registry demonstrated that hypermobility is a highly heritable trait (Hakim et al 2004). Polyarticular hypermobility is most often described clinically and in the research literature by applying the Beighton 9-point scoring system (Figure 1.3) (Beighton et al 1973).

Table 1.3	The Ghent 1996 criteria* for Marfan syndrome (*at the time of writing the criteria are being revised)	
Major criteria		
1. Skeletal	Four or more of:	
	Pectus carinatum	
	Pectus excavatum (requiring surgery)	
	Marfanoid habitus arm and height dimensions (see text)	
	Scoliosis > 20 degrees	
	Positive wrist and thumb sign (see text)	
	Reduced extension at the elbow (to < 170 degrees)	
	Pes planus	
	Protrusio Acetabulae	
2. Cardiovascular	Dilatation of the ascending aorta involving at least the sinuses of Valsalva	
	OR	
	Dissection of the ascending aorta	
3. Occular	Ectopia lentis	
4. Dura	Lumbosacral dural ectasia on CT or MRI	
5. Genetic	Parent, child or sibling meeting the criteria	
	OR	
	Presence of a mutation in Fibrillin known to cause MFS	
Minor criteria		
1. Skeletal	Mild-moderate pectus excavatum	
	Joint hypermobility	
	High-arched palate	
	Facies: dolichocephaly, malar hypoplasia, enopthalmos, retrognathia	
2. Cardiovascular	Mitral valve prolapse	
	Dilatation of pulmonary artery below age 40 yrs Dilatation or dissection of the descending thoracic or abdominal aorta below age 50 yrs	
	Calcification of the mitral annulus below age 40 yrs	
3. Occular	Flat cornea, myopia	
4. Skin	Striae, recurrent incisional hernia	
5. Pulmonary	Spontaneous pneumothorax	
	Apical blebs	

In the absence of genetic confirmation, two major criteria and one other system involvement are required for the diagnosis. In a case where genetic mutations are known in the family, one other major criterion is required with involvement of one other organ system.

One point is given for each side of the body for the first four manoeuvres and one for spinal flexion. A value of 4 or more is considered suggestive of generalized hypermobility in males and 5 or more in females, though these figures are arbitrary cut-off points. A study by Van der Giessen et al (2001) of hypermobility in Dutch schoolchildren gave first insight in to the good repeatability of the score (a kappa score of 0.81). Further work by Boyle et al (2003) and Juul-Kristensen et al (2007) showed similar repeatability and reliability between observers. It is recognized however that this classification ignores several other body sites that are often also found to be hypermobile, including the cervical and thoracic spine, shoulders, hips, ankles, and mid-foot, and first metatarsophalangeal joint. It also does not account for the degree of hypermobility at any one site.

A score that occasionally appears in the modern literature is that devised by Rotes-Querol (1957). This incorporates the manoeuvres in the Beighton criteria plus shoulder and neck rotation > 90 degrees, excessive neck and lumbar spine lateral flexion and hip abduction (range not stated), and first MTP dorsiflexion > 90 degrees.

A third tool sometimes used is the Contompasis Score (Table 1.6) (after Contompasis 1974 and described by McNerney and Johnston 1979).

Table 1.4   The classification of osteogenesis imperfecta

TYPE	CLINICAL CHARACTERISTICS	INHERITANCE	GENE
I Mild	Blue sclerae, easy bruising, mild to moderate bone fragility, normal to near-normal stature, no deformities, hearing loss in adolescent to adult life (50%) Dentinogenesis imperfecta: absent – type A; present – type B	AD	COL1A1
II Lethal	Short, deformed extremities, soft thoracic cage and skull with severe bone fragility, absent calvarial mineralization, bony compression, platyspondyly, beaded ribs. Dark sclerae. Death in prenatal period	AD (new mutations) AR (rare)	COL1A1 and COL1A2
III Severe	Bone fragility and progressive deformity, marked short stature, light sclerae, dentinogenesis imperfecta common, hearing loss in early adult life and shortened survival	AD AR	COL1A1 and COL1A2
IV Moderate	Bone fragility, mild to moderate short stature, mild bone deformity, lightly coloured sclerae, hearing loss in early adulthood Dentinogenesis imperfecta: absent – type A; present – type B	AD	COL1A1 and COL1A2
V Moderate to severe	Bone fragility, mild to moderate short stature, no DI, radio-ulnar synostosis, hyperplastic callus formation	AD	Not known
VI Moderate to severe	Moderate to severe skeletal deformity, no blue sclerae, no DI, scale-like appearance of bone lamella, accumulation of osteoid	AD	Not known
VII Severe to lethal	Fractures at birth, bluish sclerae, early deformity of the lower extremities, coxa vara, osteopenia, rhizomelia	AR	CRTAP
VIII Severe to lethal	White sclerae, severe growth deficiency, extreme skeletal undermineralization, bulbous metaphyses	AR	P3H1

Table 1.5   Criteria for the diagnosis of Stickler syndrome

The disorder should be considered in individuals with clinical findings in two or more of the following categories:

Ophthalmologic

Congenital or early-onset cataract
Congenital vitreous anomaly, rhegmatogenous retinal detachment
Myopia greater than –3 diopters
Newborns are typically hyperopic (+1 diopter or greater); thus the finding of any degree of myopia in an at-risk newborn (e.g., a newborn who has Pierre-Robin sequence or an affected parent) is suggestive of the diagnosis of Stickler syndrome

Craniofacial

Midface hypoplasia, depressed nasal bridge, anteverted nares (characteristic facies are typically more pronounced in childhood)
Bifid uvula, cleft hard palate
Micrognathia
Robin sequence (micrognathia, cleft palate, glossoptosis)

Audiologic

Sensorineural or conductive hearing loss
Hypermobile middle ear systems, representing an additional diagnostic feature

Joint

Hypermobility
Mild spondyloepiphyseal dysplasia
Precocious osteoarthritis

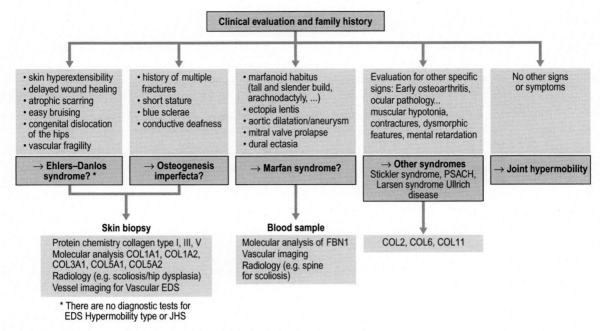

Fig. 1.2 **Differentiating the HDCTs.** *Published (adapted) with permission of the authors*

In this score there is a maximum of 72 points. A normal range of movement scores up to 22 points and an arbitrary cut-off of > 40 was set by McNerny and Johnston as being indicative of JHM. However, as with the Rotes-Querol score it has never been validated and is rarely used in epidemiological studies.

The Beighton score remains the major tool in epidemiology research in this field. It should be noted that a Beighton score of 5 or more was used in the Villefranche criteria for EDS hypermobility type (Table 1.2). Nevertheless the other scores remind us to look beyond the Beighton score in the clinical setting.

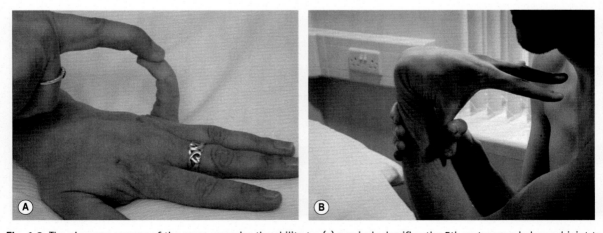

Fig. 1.3 The nine manoeuvres of the score comprise the ability to: (a) passively dorsiflex the 5th metacarpophalangeal joint to ≥ 90°; (b) oppose the thumb to the volar aspect of the ipsilateral forearm;

Continued

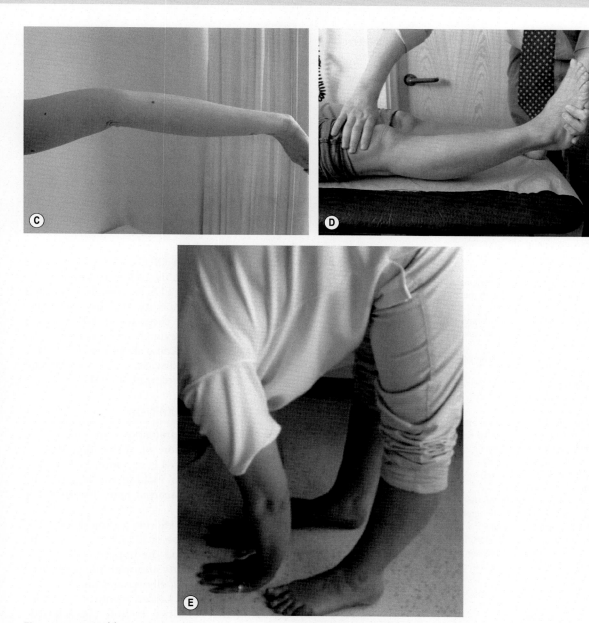

Fig. 1.3—cont'd (c) hyperextend the elbow to ≥ 10°; (d) hyperextend the knee to ≥ 10°; (e) place hands flat on the floor without bending the knees

There has been no study specifically addressing the prevalence of JHS. One study of JHM in a New Zealand Maori and Caucasian population also included an assessment of the JHS phenotype; from this a prevalence of 0.75% could be calculated (Klemp et al 2002). Surveys conducted in the UK and in Chile suggest that 'symptomatic' JHS may be identifiable in over 40% of patients attending routine community hospital clinics (Grahame & Hakim 2004, Bravo & Wolff 2006).

An alternative tool in screening for the presence of JHM is a simple five-part self-report questionnaire (Table 1.7) (Hakim and Grahame 2003b). It does not rely entirely on classifying a group of joints as being hypermobile and for the

Table 1.6	The Contompasis Semi-Quantitative Scoring System for Hypermobility

1. Passive opposition of the thumb to the flexor aspects of the forearm ('thumb to wrist test'). Points are allocated according to the extent to which the thumb meets or passes the forearm as follows:

Thumb and forearm not touching and separated by between 30° and 75°	2
Thumb touches the forearm	4
Thumb digs into the forearm easily	5
Thumb can be pushed beyond the axis of the forearm	6

2. Passive dorsiflexion of the fifth metacarpophalangeal joint. The angle measured is the long axis of the forearm with the long axis of the fifth digit:

Hyperextension between 30° and 85°	2
Hyperextension of 90°–100°	4
Hyperextension of 100°–120°	5
Hyperextension > 120°	6

3. Passive hyperextension of the elbow. The angle measured is the long axis of the forearm with the long axis of the upper arm:

Hyperextension between 0° and 5°	2
Hyperextension between 10° and 15°	4
Hyperextension between 16° and 20°	5
Hyperextension >20°	6

4. Passive hyperextension of the knee:

Hyperextension of 0°–5°	2
Hyperextension of 10°–15°	4
Hyperextension of 16°–20°	5
Hyperextension > 20°	6

5. Forward flexion of the spine, attempting to place the hands flat on the floor in front of the feet (which are together) without bending the knees:

No contact with the ground	2
Fingertips touch the ground	4
Fingers touch the ground	5
Palms can be placed flat on the ground	6
Wrists can be placed on the ground	7
Forearm reaches the ground	8

6. Foot flexibility test (ankle dorsiflexion and calcaneal stance position). The degree of eversion of the calcaneus is recorded:

0°–2° of eversion	2
3°–5° of eversion	4
6°–10° of eversion	5
11°–15° of eversion	6
> 15° of eversion	7

Table 1.7	A five-part questionnaire for identifying hypermobility

Can you now (or could you ever) place your hands flat on the floor without bending your knees?

Can you now (or could you ever) bend your thumb to touch your forearm?

As a child did you amuse your friends by contorting your body into strange shapes OR could you do the splits?

As a child or teenager did your shoulder or kneecap dislocate on more than one occasion?

Do you consider yourself double-jointed?

Answer in the affirmative to two or more questions suggests hypermobility with sensitivity 80–85% and specificity 80–90%.

present in patients with OI (Table 1.4), is usually less obvious in MFS (Table 1.3) and is mild in SS (Table 1.5). The vascular EDS is typically associated with small joint hypermobility affecting the digits, whereas the finding of excessive distal laxity, in combination with proximal contractures and generalized muscle weakness should lead the clinician to consider Ullrich disease, a severe congenital muscular dystrophy (Mercuri et al 2004).

DISLOCATION/SUBLUXATION

Ligament laxity can predispose to soft tissue injuries, joint subluxation or dislocation. Recurrence of these pathologies is common in EDS and JHS. The common sites include the base of the thumb at the carpometacarpal joint, the shoulder and the patella.

Congenital hip dislocation is a clinical hallmark of the arthrochalasia type of EDS, but may also be present in the classic and the hypermobility type. Severe joint hypermobility and multiple congenital joint dislocations of hips, elbows and knees are the main features of the Larsen syndrome. Other symptoms of this condition include characteristic facial appearance of flat face, prominent forehead, widely spaced eyes and a depressed nasal bridge, cleft palate or uvula, dental abnormalities, short metacarpals and cylindrical fingers, equinovarus deformity of the foot and cardiovascular lesions.

THE SKIN

It is fundamentally important to enquire of and assess the skin, identifying skin hyperlaxity, easy bruising, abnormal scarring (such as atrophic or

non-specialist clinician it is a quick screen whilst taking the clinical history that may support the need for physical examination.

The presence of hypermobility can vary considerably between the HDCT and between individuals with the same disorder. It should always therefore be considered as part of a wider clinical picture. It is most pronounced in the variants of EDS (Table 1.2) and JHS (Table 1.1), can sometimes be

---

BOX 1.1	Typical skin features of the HDCTs

- Skin elasticity
- Papyraceous scarring
- Striae
- Easy bruising

---

keloid scarring), and early onset striae at typical and atypical sites. Like the presence of JHM, skin signs are a valuable clue as to the presence of a HDCT (Box 1.1).

HDCTs result from defective protein synthesis within the extracellular matrix (ECM). The ECM includes both structural proteins, such as collagen, fibrillin and fibronectin, and ground substance such as proteoglycans. Together they form a network that provides resistance to mechanical forces while allowing diffusion of small molecules. Four types of macromolecules constitute the ECM: collagens, elastin, proteoglycans and glycoproteins, each of which are produced and maintained by cells specific to the tissue type, such as fibroblasts, chondrocytes, osteocytes and epidermal cells.

Collagens are produced by fibroblasts and are responsible for the strength of skeletal and soft tissues including skin, bone, tendon, ligament and muscle. There are more than 20 types of collagen, however types I and III are the most abundant in the dermis. Types VII and XVII are also important in providing adhesion between the dermis and the superficial layer of the skin, the epidermis. Type V is a minor collagen but it forms heterogeneous collagen fibres with type I, and is also found in the skin. The ubiquitous nature of collagens means that disorders of synthesis or function have diverse clinical effects (see Genetics section below).

Elastin gives skin its elasticity. Elastic fibres are composed of two distinguishable components: an amorphous component, 'elastin', which contributes to the elasticity of the fibre, and a surrounding sheet of microfibrils. An example of a microfibrillar protein is fibrillin-1, which is the protein mutated in patients with MFS. Elastin and other structural proteins are woven onto the microfibrillar array to provide the basic meshwork for the connective tissue matrix. Abnormalities of elastin have been associated with other connective tissue disorders, such as cutis laxa. Proteoglycans are core proteins that are bound to glycosaminoglycans. Essentially, proteoglycans are the glue of the connective tissue protein that seal and cement the underlying

connective tissue matrix. Glycoproteins are macromolecular proteins such as fibronectin, tenascin and fibulins.

SKIN HYPEREXTENSIBILITY

Skin hyperextensibility is characteristic for all EDS-subtypes, except for the vascular type. It is most prominent in the classic type of EDS, but may be present to a lesser extent in the hypermobility type and also in the JHS. In the vascular type of EDS, the skin is not hyperextensible, but thin and transparent, showing the venous pattern over the chest, abdomen and extremities. Skin hyperextensibility should be tested at a neutral site, meaning a site not subjected to mechanical forces or scarring. It is measured by stretching a fold of skin overlying the dorsum of the hand by pinching the skin between one's thumb and second finger and pulling the skin fold (Figure 2.4, p. 26) until resistance is felt. The skin is hyperelastic, which means that it extends easily and snaps back after release. Testing skin hyperextensibility is subjective and requires experience in feeling and stretching normal as well as abnormal skin. In JHS and MFS skin laxity may be subtle; in OI and SS it is usually normal.

From the clinical point of view, the 'hyperextensible' skin in EDS must be distinguished from that of 'cutis laxa' syndromes, which result from the loss or fragmentation of the elastic fibre network, and which are caused by mutations in the elastin gene or other genes that encode proteins related to elastic fibre development of homeostasis (e.g. the fibulins). In the cutis laxa syndromes, the skin is redundant: it hangs in loose folds and returns very slowly to its former position. The skin in cutis laxa is not fragile, and wound healing is normal. Joint hypermobility can, to a variable degree, be present in patients with cutis laxa syndrome.

STRIAE

Stretch marks are most commonly a result of pregnancy, obesity or corticosteroid excess. Typical sites include the abdomen and lower back. In the setting of an HDCT a patient may give a history of onset from an early age and at body sites not usually affected by the other causes. Striae may occur on extensor surfaces such as the elbows or knees, inner thigh, and across the chest. The striae of collagen disorders may also be wide and atrophic. It is a common sign in JHS and EDS, and to a lesser extent in MFS.

EASY BRUISING AND TENDENCY TOWARDS BLEEDING

Easy bruising is a common finding in HDCT, especially in the EDS. In small children it may even be the presenting symptom to the paediatrician. It manifests as spontaneous ecchymoses, frequently recurring in the same areas and causing a characteristic brownish discoloration of the skin, especially in exposed areas such as shins and knees. There is a tendency toward prolonged bleeding, e.g. following brushing of the teeth, in spite of a normal coagulation status. If pronounced, it can raise the suspicion of a haematological disorder, a malignancy, or non-accidental injury (NAI), especially in children. Careful evaluation of the medical and family history, rigorous clinical examination with special attention to skin features that are characteristic for EDS and exclusion of platelet and clotting disorders are mandatory to distinguish between a HDCT and other causes of bruising.

SLOW/POOR WOUND HEALING

The most common causes for poor healing are natural ageing and corticosteroid excess. However these skin features are a typical finding in several HDCT at an early age. Other less common causes of skin fragility and scarring to always consider are the porphyrias (porphyria cutanea tarda), the mechanobullous diseases (epidermolysis bullosa simplex) and vitamin C deficiency.

Delayed wound healing and atrophic scarring is most prominent in EDS classic type, as well as in the rarer subtypes such as the kyphoscoliotic and arthrochalasia type. In JHS the pathology is less obvious and something the patient may not have recognized as 'abnormal', or only comes to light post surgery when the scar becomes atrophic.

THE MARFANOID HABITUS

Marfanoid features include:
- High arched palate
- Arachnodactily:
  'Wrist sign' (Walker): positive if able to wrap the thumb and 5th finger of one hand around the opposite wrist such that the nail bed of the digits overlap with each other (Chapter 2, Figure 2.7b)

'Thumb sign' (Steinberg): positive if the adducted thumb across the palm projects beyond the ulnar border in the clenched hand (Chapter 2, Figure 2.7a)
- Pectus excavatum or carinatum (Chapter 2, Figure 2.7c)
- Scoliosis: Scoliosis >20 degrees is a major criteria in MFS. It is also a sign of EDS kyphoscoliotic type, and can be present in patients with OI. In other EDS variants, and in JHS it may be present, albeit to a milder degree
- Arm span : Height ratio > 1.03 (1.05 in Ghent Nosology for MFS)
- Tall stature with lower limb length (floor to pubis) : upper body (pubis to crown) ratio > 0.89 (0.85 in Ghent Nosology for MFS)
- Foot length (heel to 1st toe) : Height ratio > 0.15
- Hand length (wrist crease to 3rd finger) : Height ratio > 0.11.

The Marfanoid habitus is characteristically encountered in the MFS (Table 1.3). Many of the skeletal features of Marfan syndrome however are common in the general population. When found in combination, such findings usually indicate a disorder of connective tissue.

A marfanoid habitus may also be encountered in patients with the MASS phenotype (**m**itral valve prolapse, myopia, borderline and non-progressive **a**ortic enlargement, and nonspecific **s**kin and **s**keletal findings that overlap with those seen in MFS), and the mitral valve prolapse syndrome (MVPS). Both conditions are autosomal dominant and can be caused by mutations in *FBN1* (see genetic section below).

Other HDCTs that show overlap with the skeletal features of MFS include homocystinuria, congenital contractural arachnodactily and Stickler syndrome.

The marfanoid habitus can, to a somewhat milder degree, be present in patients with JHS, but in this condition it is not associated with the severe ocular and cardiac complications of MFS.

FRACTURES AND POOR DENTITION

Low bone mineral density is seen in EDS (Dolan et al 1998), MFS (Carter et al 2000), and OI (Byers 1993); it is especially common and associated with fragility fractures in OI. Osteopenia is a recognized feature of JHS (Nijs et al 2000, Gulbahar et al 2005).

Risk factors for osteoporosis, particularly personal or family history of low-trauma spinal or peripheral fractures in childhood, and amongst males and pre-menopausal women should be sought alongside other established risks such as corticosteroid treatment and maternal hip fracture. There are no specific guidelines for managing osteoporosis associated with the HDCT.

Poor dentition (dentinogenesis imperfecta) is often present in OI. With the exception of gum pathology in EDS periodontitis type, it is not a common feature of JHS, EDS or MFS, though temporomandibular jaw pain and dislocation can be a significant problem (see Chapter 12.7b).

CARDIOVASCULAR STRUCTURAL AND AUTONOMIC DISORDERS

Potentially life-threatening complications of MFS (Table 1.3) include dilatation and dissection of the aortic root and ascending aorta. In EDS vascular type there is a risk of rupture and/or dilatation/dissection of especially medium-sized arterial vessels, such as the renal or the splenic arteries.

Vascular investigations of MFS should include echocardiography (or CT/MRI angiography when visibility of the aortic root and ascending aorta is limited), which should initially be repeated annually. More frequent imaging should be performed if the aortic diameter is approaching a surgical threshold ($\geq$ 4.5 cm in adults; less well defined in children) or shows rapid change ($\geq$ 0.5 cm/year) or with concerns regarding heart or valve function. Adults with repeatedly normal aortic root dimensions can be seen at intervals of 2–3 years.

Beta-blockade is the accepted therapeutic intervention in trying to delay aortic disease. Angiotensin receptor blockers have shown the ability to prevent aortic enlargement in a mouse model with MFS and several multicentre trials with losartan versus or on top of beta-blockade are underway. Ultimately, however, valve replacement and vascular grafts may be needed.

Mitral valve prolapse (MVP) may also be found in some of these conditions. It is most common in MFS, being present in 60% of cases and audible as a midsystolic click followed by a high-pitched murmur over the mitral area. Contrary to earlier studies it is now thought that MVP is rarely seen in EDS classic or hypermobility type, or in JHS (Dolan et al 1997). There is otherwise no significant

arterial disease in these conditions. Cardiac pathology is not specifically associated with OI and from a recent study of 78 cases of SS in a UK cohort, routine monitoring for MVP in SS is unnecessary (Ahmad et al 2003).

Varicose veins are also associated with JHS (Table 1.1).

AUTONOMIC DISTURBANCE

Patients with JHS often report a number of non-musculoskeletal symptoms that include fainting or feeling faint, palpitations, chest tightness or shortness of breath in the absence of asthma or cardiac disease (Rowe et al 1999, Gazit et al 2003, Hakim and Grahame 2003c). Many of these symptoms may be due to identifiable autonomic disturbances which are discussed in detail in the following chapters.

VISCERAL DISEASE

Intrinsic weakness of supporting structures may lead to complications of the abdominal and pelvic viscera. This is particularly the case in EDS and JHS and more so in relation to uterine and rectal prolapse. Hiatus hernia, abdominal wall herniation and achalasia of the large bowel are other disorders considered to occur in EDS more often than in the general population.

During pregnancy there is the potential for several complications. These might range from the life-threatening such as vascular collapse in MFS and EDS vascular type or premature rupture of the fetal membranes and antepartum haemorrhage in the classic or vascular type of EDS, to the more benign, albeit problematic, worsening of symptoms from abdominal herniation, pelvic floor insufficiency (Chapter 12.6), joint pain, trauma to the vaginal vault and surrounding soft tissues during labour with poor wound healing, and failure of anaesthetic nerve blocks that can be present in JHS and EDS.

PULMONARY DISEASE

MFS is associated with an increased risk of spontaneous pneumothorax. This is said to occur in approximately 5% of cases. Pneumothorax and asthma are also considered to be associated with EDS (Brear et al 1984, Morgan et al 2007) but are not typical features of JHS.

Shortness of breath may be a consequence of a number of pathologies including reduced volume from kypho-scoliosis, articular or neuropathic pain, rib fracture, intercostal or diaphragmatic muscle weakness, intrinsic lung tissue weakness (tracheal to alveolar collapse), or cardiac disease.

OCULAR PATHOLOGY

Ocular pathologies are common in the HDCT. They range from the relatively benign feature of blue sclera seen in OI and sometimes to a milder degree in JHS, to retinal detachments, scarring and visual loss in MFS, SS and EDS kyphoscoliotic type, and the related brittle cornea syndrome.

MFS is also associated with ectopia lentis (lens dislocation), early onset cataract, glaucoma, myopia and hypoplastic iris and ciliary muscles. Myopia is also a feature of JHS.

The Stickler syndrome is subclassified by both ocular and genetic findings. There is an increased risk of retinal detachment and haemorrhage (types I and II); type III SS is a condition in which the systemic features are manifest in the absence of ocular pathology (Table 1.5).

OSTEOARTHRITIS

In EDS and JHS studies suggest an increased risk of articular dysfunction and premature osteoarthritis (OA) (Bridges et al 1992), of the temporomandibular joint (Chapter 12.7), and OA of the knee and hand. An association with chondromalacia patellae is also reported (Chapter 12.4). Other population studies, however, have not shown an association between local or generalized osteoarthritis (Dolan et al 2003, Kraus et al 2004).

Early onset degenerative disease, particularly of the weight-bearing joints is also a feature of SS (Table 1.5) and pseudoachondroplasia (PSACH). PSACH is an autosomal dominant disorder, characterized by short stature, short extremities, and ligamentous laxity usually most prominent in hands and fingers. Premature osteoarthritis, especially in hips and knees, is seen in these conditions.

SUMMARY OF MULTIPLE PATHOLOGIES

Any combination of the above signs and symptoms may occur in the patient with JHS. The reader is encouraged to turn to Chapter 2 for a more

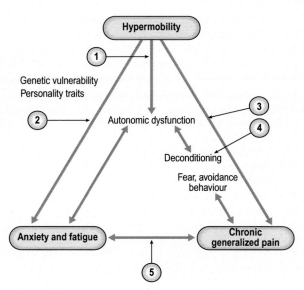

Fig. 1.4 The association between hypermobility, autonomic disorders, anxiety syndromes, pain, physical pathologies and deconditioning, and the interplay of therapies: 1. manage primary autonomic disturbance – beta-blockade, fluid balance etc.; 2. treat primary and secondary anxiety/phobic syndromes; 3. analgesics; 4. physical rehabilitation; 5. behavioural therapies/clinical psychology/antidepressants

detailed discussion of JHS in childhood and adulthood. Figure 1.4 demonstrates the interactions/interdependencies between these varied pathologies and highlights the need for an integrated, multidisciplinary approach to management of complex cases; anxiety and phobic disorders are covered in more detail in Chapter 4.

GENETIC ABNORMALITIES IN THE HDCT

The Villefranche nosology for EDS recognizes six subtypes based on the severity of the clinical features, the underlying biochemical and genetic defect, and the pattern of inheritance (Table 1.2). Mutations in genes encoding collagens I, III and V, and collagen-modifying enzymes have been identified in most forms of EDS (Pope and Burrows 1997).

Procollagen type I contains two proα-1 and an proα-2 polypeptide chain, encoded by single genes *COL1A1* and *COL1A2* on chromosomes 17 and 7 respectively. Type V collagen occurs as two forms of heterotrimers ($[\alpha1(V)]_2\alpha2(V)$ and $\alpha1(V)\alpha2(V)\alpha3$

(V)) or as $\alpha1(V)_3$ homotrimers. In most vertebrate tissues, such as skin, tendon and bone it is present mainly as $[\alpha1(V)]_2\alpha2(V)$ heterotrimers encoded by the genes COL5A1 and COL5A2 being found on chromosomes 9 and 2 respectively. Type III collagen is a homotrimer consisting of three identical proα1-chains, encoded by the COL3A1 gene on chromosome 2.

Mutations in COL1A1 and COL1A2 are usually associated with OI (Sykes et al 1986), while a specific class of mutations, resulting in skipping of exon 6 of either COL1A1 or COL1A2 and hence loss of the procollagen amino-proteinase cleavage site results in EDS arthrochalasia type (Eyre et al 1985, Byers et al 1997). EDS classic type is an autosomal dominant disorder caused by mutations in COL5A1 or COL5A2 (Lichtenstein et al 1973, Wenstrup et al 1996, Loughlin et al 1995, Burrows et al 1996, De Paepe et al 1997, Michalickova et al 1998), whereas EDS vascular type is caused by mutations in the COL3A1 gene. The kyphoscoliotic and dermatosparaxis subtypes of EDS are recessive conditions caused by deficient activity of proteins involved in post-translational modification of the fibrillar collagens. There are in addition many rare unclassified variants of EDS, the molecular basis of which is unknown.

SS is caused by mutation in the genes encoding collagens type II and XI. These collagen types are components of vitreous, cartilage and other connective tissues. (Francomano et al 1988, Ahmad et al 1991, Brunner et al 1994, Sirko-Osadsa et al 1998.)

MFS is associated with mutations in fibrillin-1, encoded by the FBN1 gene on chromosome 15q21 (Lee et al 1991, Kainulainen et al 1994, Dietz and Pyeritz 1995).

The defect underlying the most common EDS hypermobility subtype is unknown. The genetics of JHS also remains ill understood with only a few family case reports in the literature (Malfait et al 2006). In a small subset of patients (5–10%) with EDS hypermobility type/JHS, diminished levels of tenascin-X, due to heterozygous mutations in the TNX-B gene, have been identified (TNX-B haplo-insufficiency) (Zweers et al 2004). Tenascin-X is a large extracellular matrix glycoprotein that plays a role in the maturation and/or the maintenance of the dermal collagen and elastin network. In the vast majority of patients however, no molecular defects have been identified either in this gene or in any of the fibrillar collagen-encoding genes.

The heritability of JHS has not been determined; however anecdotal observations from large family pedigrees would suggest a dominant inheritance as per HM with variable penetrance.

If an HDCT is suspected additional morphological, biochemical and/or molecular analyses are available to confirm the diagnosis. A skin biopsy is required in order to perform biochemical analysis of collagen subtypes, and additional DNA analysis can be performed from the cultured fibroblasts. Molecular analysis of the fibrillin-1 gene can be performed on DNA extracted from leucocytes (Figure 1.2).

References

Ahmad NN, Ala-kokko L, Knowlton RG, et al: Stop codon in the procollagen gene II in a family with the Stickler Syndrome, Proc Natl Acad Sci USA 88:6624–6627, 1991.

Ahmad N, Richards AJ, Murfett HC, et al: Prevalence of mitral valve prolapse in Stickler Syndrome, Am J Med Genet 116A:234–237, 2003.

Arendt-Nielsen L, Kaalund S, Bjerring P, et al: Insufficient effect of local analgesics in Ehlers-Danlos type III patients, Acta Anaesthesiol Scand 34:358–361, 1990.

Beighton PH, Solomon L, Soskolne CL: Articular mobility in an African population, Ann Rheum Dis 32:413–417, 1973.

Beighton P, De Paepe A, Steinmann B, et al: Ehlers-Danlos syndromes: revised nosology, Villefranche 1997. Ehlers-Danlos National Foundation (USA) and Ehlers-Danlos Support Group (UK), Am J Med Genet 77:31–37, 1998.

Boyle KL, Witt P, Riegger-Krugh C: Intrarater and Interrater reliability of the Beighton Mobility Index, J Athl Train 38 (4):281–285, 2003.

Bravo JF, Wolff C: Clinical study of hereditary disorders of connective tissues in a Chilean population: joint hypermobility syndrome and vascular Ehlers-Danlos syndrome, Arthritis Rheum 54(2):515–523, 2006.

Brear SG, Beton D, Slaven Y, et al: Spontaneous pneumothoraces are associated with mitral valve prolapse, Arthritis Rheum 39:219, 1984.

Bridges AJ, Smith E, Reid J: Joint hypermobility in adults referred to rheumatology clinics, Ann Rheum Dis 51(6):793–796, 1992.

Brunner HG, van Beersum SEC, Warman ML, et al: A Stickler Syndrome gene is linked to chromosome 6 near COL11A2 gene, *Hum Mol Genet* 3:1561–1564, 1994.

Burrows NP, Nicholls AC, Yates JR, et al: The gene encoding collagen alpha-1 (V)(COL5A1) is linked to mixed Ehlers-Danlos syndrome type I/II, *J Invest Dermatol* 106:1273–1276, 1996.

Byers PH: Osteogenesis imperfect. In Royce PLSB, editor: *Connective Tissue and its Inheritable Disorders*, New York, 1993, Wiley-Liss, pp 317–350.

Byers PH, Duvic M, Atkinson M, et al: Ehlers-Danlos syndrome type VIIA and VIIB result from splice-junction mutations or genomic deletions that involve exon 6 in the COL1A1 and COL1A2 genes of type 1 collagen, *Am J Med Genet* 72:94–105, 1997.

Carter N, Duncan E, Wordsworth P: Bone mineral density in adults with Marfan syndrome, *Rheumatology (Oxford)* 39:307–309, 2000.

De Paepe A, Devereux RB, Dietz HC, et al: Revised diagnostic criteria for the Marfan syndrome, *Am J Med Genet* 62:417–426, 1996.

De Paepe A, Nuytinck L, Hausser I, et al: Mutations in the COL5A1 gene are causal in the Ehlers-Danlos syndromes I and II, *Am J Hum Genet* 60:547–554, 1997.

Dietz HC, Pyeritz RE: Mutations in the human gene for fibrillin-1 in the Marfan syndrome and related disorders, *Hum Mol Genet* 4:1799–1809, 1995.

Dolan AL, Mishra MB, Chambers JB, et al: Clinical and echocardiographic survey of the Ehlers-Danlos syndrome, *Br J Rheumatol* 36:459–462, 1997.

Dolan AL, Arden NK, Grahame R, et al: Assessment of bone density in Ehlers-Danlos syndrome by ultrasound and densitometry, *Ann Rheum Dis* 57:630–633, 1998.

Dolan AL, Hart DJ, Doyle DV, et al: The relationship of joint hypermobility, bone mineral density, and osteoarthritis in the general population: the Chingford Study, *J Rheumatol* 30:799–803, 2003.

Eyre DR, Shapiro FD, Aldridge JF: A heterogeneous collagen defect in a variant of the Ehlers-Danlos syndrome type VII, *J Biol Chem* 260:11322–11329, 1985.

Francomano CA, Liberfarb RM, Hirose T, et al: The Stickler Syndrome is closely linked to COL2A1, the structural gene for type II collagen, *Pathol Immunopathol* 7:104–106, 1988.

Gazit Y, Nahir AM, Grahame R, et al: Dysautonomia in the joint hypermobility syndrome, *Am J Med* 115:33–40, 2003.

Grahame R: Joint hypermobility and genetic collagen disorders. Are they related, *Arch Dis Child* 80:188–191, 1999.

Grahame R, Bird HA, Dolan AL, et al: The revised (Brighton 1998) criteria for the diagnosis of benign joint hypermobility syndrome, *J Rheumatol* 27:1777–1779, 2000.

Grahame R, Hakim AJ: High prevalence of joint hypermobility syndrome in clinic referrals to a North London community hospital, *Rheumatology* 43 (3 Suppl 1):198, 2004 [Abstract].

Gulbahar S, Sahin E, Baydar M, et al: Hypermobility syndrome increases the risk for low bone mass, *Clin Rheumatol* 26:1–4, 2005.

Hakim AJ, Grahame R: Joint Hypermobility, *Best Pract Res Clin Rheumatol* 17:989–1004, 2003a.

Hakim AJ, Grahame R: A simple questionnaire to detect hypermobility: an adjunct to the assessment of patients with diffuse musculoskeletal pain, *Int J Clin Pract* 57:163–166, 2003b.

Hakim A, Grahame R: Symptoms of autonomic nervous system dysfunction in the Benign Joint Hypermobility Syndrome, *Rheumatology (Oxford)* 42 (Suppl 1):47, 2003c [Abstract].

Hakim AJ, Cherkas LF, Grahame R, et al: The genetic epidemiology of joint hypermobility: a female twin population study, *Arthritis Rheum* 50(8):2640–2646, 2004.

Hakim AJ, Norris P, Hopper C, et al: Local Anaesthetic Failure; Does Joint Hypermobility Provide The Answer? *J R Soc Med* 98(2):84–85, 2005.

Juul-Kristensen B, Rogind H, Jensen DV, et al: Inter-examiner reproducibility of tests and criteria for generalized joint hypermobility and benign joint hypermobility syndrome, *Rheumatology (Oxford)* 46(12): 1835–1841, 2007.

Kainulainen K, Karttunen L, Puhakka L, et al: Mutations in the fibrillin gene responsible for dominant ectpopia lentis and neonatal marfan syndrome, *Nat Genet* 6:64–69, 1994.

Klemp P, Williams SM, Stansfield SA: Articular mobility in Maori and European New Zealanders, *Rheumatology* 41(5):554–557, 2002.

Kraus VB, Li YJ, Martin ER, et al: Articular hypermobility is a protective factor for hand osteoarthritis, *Arthritis Rheum* 50:2178–2183, 2004.

Lee B, Godfrey M, Vitale E, et al: Linkage of Marfan syndrome and a phenotypically related disorder to two different fibrillin genes, *Nature* 352:330–334, 1991.

Lichtenstein JR, Martin GR, Kohn LD, et al: Defect of conversion of procollagen to collagen in a form of Ehlers-Danlos syndrome, *Science* 182:298–299, 1973.

Loughlin J, Irvin C, Hardwick LJ, et al: Linkage of the gene that encodes the alpha-1 chain of type V collagen to type II Ehlers Danlos syndrome, *Hum Mol Genet* 4:1649–1651, 1995.

McNerney JE, Johnston WB: Generalised ligamentous laxity, hallux abducto-valgus and the first metatarsocuneiform joint, *J Am Podiatr Assoc* 69:69–82, 1979.

Malfait F, Hakim AJ, De Paepe A, et al: The genetics of Joint Hypermobility Syndrome, *Rheumatology* 45(5):502–507, 2006.

Mercuri E, Lampe A, Straub V, et al: Congenital muscular dystrophy with short stature, proximal contractures and distal laxity, *Neuropediatrics* 35:224–229, 2004.

Michalickova K, Susic M, Willing MC, et al: Mutations of the alpha-2 (V) chain of type V collagen impair matrix assembly and produce Ehlers-Danlos syndrome type I, *Hum Mol Genet* 7:249–255, 1998.

Morgan AW, Pearson SB, Davies S, et al: Asthma and airways collapse in two heritable disorders of connective tissue, *Ann Rheum Dis* 66:1369–1373, 2007.

Nijs J, Van Essche E, De Munck M, et al: Ultrasound, axial, and peripheral measurements in female patients with benign hypermobility syndrome, *Calcif Tissue Int* 67:37–40, 2000.

Pope FM Burrows NP: Ehlers-Danlos syndrome has varied molecular mechanisms, *J Med Genet* 34:400–410, 1997.

Rose PS, Levy HP, Liberfarb RM, et al: Stickler Syndrome: Clinical Characteristics and Diagnostic Criteria, *Am J Med Genet* 138:199–207, 2005.

Rotes-Querol J: Articular laxity considered as factor of changes of the locomotor apparatus, *Rev Rhum Mal Osteoartic* 24(7–8):5359, 1957.

Rowe PC, Barron DF, Calkins H, et al: Orthostatic intolerance and chronic fatigue syndrome associated with Ehlers-Danlos syndrome, *J Pediatr* 135:494–499, 1999.

Sirko-Osadsa DA, Murray MA, Scott JA, et al: Stickler syndrome without eye involvement is caused by mutations in COL11A2, the gene encoding the alpha2(XI) chain of type XI collagen, *J Pediatr* 132:368–371, 1998.

Stickler GB, Belau PG, Farrell FJ, et al: Hereditary progressive arthroopthalmopathy, *Mayo Clin Proc* 40:433–455, 1965.

Stickler GB, Hughes W, Houchin P: Clinical features of hereditary arthroophthalmopathy (Stickler Syndrome): A survey, *Genet Med* 3:192–196, 2001.

Sykes B, Ogilvie D, Wordsworth P, et al: Osteogenesis imperfecta is linked to both type I collagen structural genes, *Lancet* 12:69–72, 1986.

Van der Giessen LJ, Liekens D, Rutgers KJ, et al: Validation of the beighton score and prevalence of connective tissue signs in 773 Dutch children, *J Rheumatol* 28(12):2726–2730, 2001.

Wenstrup RJ, Langland GT, Willing MC, et al: A splice-junction mutation in the region of COL5A1 that encodes for the carboxyl propeptide of pro alpha-1 (V) chains result in the gravis form of the Ehlers-Danlos syndrome (type I), *Hum Mol Genet* 5:1733–1736, 1996.

Zweers M, Hakim AJ, Grahame R, et al: Tenascin-X deficiency and haploinsufficiency as a cause of generalized joint hypermobility, *Arthritis Rheum* 50:2742–2749, 2004.

Chapter 2

What is the joint hypermobility syndrome?

JHS from the cradle to the grave

Rodney Grahame

With contributions from: Jaime F Bravo, Nathan Hasson, Rosemary Keer, Susan M Maillard and Gonzalo Sanhueza

INTRODUCTION

WHAT IS JOINT HYPERMOBILITY?

There is widespread misunderstanding over the use of the terms joint hypermobility (JHM) and joint hypermobility syndrome (JHS). Hypermobility implies a range of joint movement that exceeds what is considered to be normal for that joint taking into consideration the individual's age, gender and ethnic background. It does not necessarily lead to symptoms; it is not a disease state; it is not a diagnosis. Many, if not most, hypermobile people may not even be aware that they are hypermobile. They generally assume that their range of movement represents the norm (which, of course, is not the case!). For many performing artists it acts as a positive selection factor in their successful recruitment (McCormack et al 2004).

JHM is measured by the ability to perform a number of manoeuvres. The two scales that have received greatest popularity are the Beighton 9-point scale (Beighton et al 1973) (Chapter 1, Figure 1.3), and the Rotes-Querol Scale (Bulbena et al 1992), the latter being favoured in Spanish-speaking countries. The reproducibility of the Beighton scale has recently been tested (Juul-Kristensen et al 2007) showing a higher kappa value in the Beighton tests (generally above 0.80) than in the Rotes-Querol tests (generally > 0.57). Despite the survival of these scoring systems for over three decades, and their good reproducibility, they have been subjected to criticism from clinicians for several reasons: they are 'all or none' tests and give

no indication of the severity of JHM; the count diminishes over time and may fall to zero with ageing; injury may reduce apparent range of movement; they favour the upper as opposed to the lower limbs; and they only sample few body sites, so that JHM at other sites may be overlooked. Perhaps, the most serious accusation is that rheumatologists and others see the score as the be all and the end all of JHM and fail to seek (and hence to find) the other features of JHS (Grahame 2008).

WHAT IS THE JOINT HYPERMOBILITY SYNDROME?

Joint hypermobility only becomes JHS when it is deemed to be responsible for emerging symptoms, of which pain and instability are the most important. The term hypermobility syndrome (HMS) was first coined in 1976 and defined as the occurrence of musculoskeletal symptoms in the presence of joint hypermobility in healthy individuals (Kirk et al 1967). In this context, 'healthy individuals' should be interpreted as meaning an absence of other (inflammatory) rheumatic diseases. At the time it represented an important historical landmark, but over the last four decades burgeoning evidence has revealed overlapping features with other heritable disorders of connective tissue (HDCTs) (Chapter 1) suggesting that JHS is, itself, a *forme fruste* of an HDCT (Grahame et al 1981, Grahame 1999).

Over the past four decades the perception of JHS has changed from being a mild or even trivial

DOI: 10.1016/B978-0-7020-3005-5.00002-1

condition of lax joints, pain on exercise, joint dislocation with possible osteoarthritis in later life to a genetically determined multisystemic disorder of connective tissues rendering them more vulnerable to injury and mechanical failure.

THE BRIGHTON CRITERIA FOR JHS

The Revised 1998 Brighton Criteria for the benign joint hypermobility syndrome, promulgated by the British Society for Rheumatology Special Interest Group on the Heritable Disorders of Connective Tissue represents a validated set of Classification Criteria for the BJHS (now generally termed JHS) (Grahame et al 2000). Like its sister sets of criteria for Marfan (De Paepe et al 1996) and Ehlers-Danlos (Beighton et al 1998) syndromes, the Brighton Criteria comprise sets of major and minor criteria (Chapter 1, Table 1.1). The criteria are met when either two major, or one major and two minor, or four minor are satisfied. Two minor criteria alone suffice in the presence of an unequivocally affected first-degree relative. Although designed primarily as a tool to identify JHS in the research setting, anecdotally they are also useful as a diagnostic aid in the clinical setting. Reproducibility of the Brighton Criteria has been found to be excellent with a kappa value above 0.73 (with the exception of the skin stretch (0.63)) (Juul-Kristensen et al 2007). It should be noted that the Brighton Criteria were conceived in the 1990s, since when there has been a veritable explosion of new information and knowledge regarding JHS. There is general consensus that the Criteria need to be regularly reviewed and updated in the light of this new knowledge (Juul-Kristensen et al 2007).

Successive studies using the Brighton Criteria have demonstrated that JHS is a multifaceted disorder that frequently affects body systems remote from the confines of the locomotor system and bearing little obvious direct relationship to it. These intriguing nuances will be revealed in the coming chapters. The stark reality is that clinicians appear by and large to be unaware of them (Grahame 2008).

Bravo in Santiago, Chile, has undertaken a detailed clinical evaluation of his patients and finds an exceptionally high prevalence of previously undiagnosed HDCTs (overwhelmingly patients with JHS) in his clinic. He advocates the use of the 1998 Brighton Criteria in preference to the 9-point Beighton score for the recognition of

JHS, the latter in his series gave a 35% false-negative diagnosis rate. He draws attention to important clinical signs of JHS which have not yet received widespread recognition including blue sclera, osteopenia/osteoporosis, typical facies and the recognition of hypermobile hand postures as in the 'hand holding the head' sign (Bravo & Wolff 2006).

IS JHS THE SAME AS THE HYPERMOBILITY TYPE OF EHLERS–DANLOS SYNDROME?

There has been a lively debate as to whether JHS and the hypermobility type of the Ehlers-Danlos syndrome (HT-EDS) (Chapter 1, Table 1.2) are one and the same or represent two phenotypically related conditions. The recently published Position Statement from the Professional Advisory Network of the Ehlers-Danlos National Foundation (of the USA) has clearly and unequivocally expressed the present consensus trend (Tinkle et al 2009). It states that 'it is our collective opinion that BJHS/HMS and EDS hypermobility type represent the same phenotypic group of patients that can be differentiated from other HCTD but not distinguished from each other'.

HYPERMOBILITY IN CHILDREN

JHS is the one rheumatological disorder, par excellence, that transcends the child–adult divide. It casts its shadow across the whole age range, literally, from the cradle to the grave, as this chapter will attempt to illustrate. One's genetic profile is established at the moment of conception. By the time of birth, one of the earliest known associations with hypermobility, namely congenital hip dysplasia, manifesting either as a 'clicky hip' or as a frank congenital dislocation (CDH) may already be apparent (Wynne-Davies 1971) and should always be sought in the neonatal period by careful clinical examination and, where appropriate, by ultrasound examination (Poul et al 1998). Maternal pre- and perinatal issues are covered in Chapter 12.6.

The Brighton Criteria have, strictly speaking, not yet been fully validated in children. However, their potential use in children has been explored in 36 patients clinically diagnosed as JHS aged 4–18 (median 11) years seen in the Hypermobility Clinic at Great Ormond Street Hospital for Children in

London between October 2004 and March 2006; 31/36 (86%) satisfied the Brighton Criteria for JHS giving a specificity of 86%. Sensitivity was not studied. A comparison of the performances of the individual Brighton Criteria in these children with that seen in an adult JHS cohort of 558 shows that they performed reasonably well. This is seen in Figure 2.1 (authors correspondence, unpublished data).

In the photographs a young patient is seen demonstrating her ability to perform the Beighton Score as well as the increased extensibility of her skin (Figure 2.2a–f).

A novel suggestion has been put forward recently by a paediatric group in Australia suggesting that the term JHS should be extended to include all hypermobile children with musculoskeletal symptoms irrespective of genetic cause so that potentially they may all benefit from a programme of multidisciplinary rehabilitation, as well as identifying the genetic cause of joint hypermobility (where possible). They propose the use of both diagnostic labels, i.e. JHS, *and* the individual's HDCT diagnosis (Tofts et al 2009).

THE CLINICAL SPECTRUM IN CHILDREN

JHM in children is common but often missed by clinicians. It is one of those conditions which 'you see if you look for it, but not if you don't'. Yet as

has been suggested in a paper from Turkey, 'evaluating (child) patients for hypermobility in routine rheumatologic examination will obviate the need for unnecessary diagnostic studies and treatments' (Toker et al 2009).

MOTOR DELAY AND ABNORMAL GAIT

One of the most common features of JHS in early life is motor delay. It was observed in approximately one third of children with generalized JHM in one series (Engelbert et al 2005). Delay in onset of walking independently, omitting to crawl and the use of bottom-shuffling or sometimes commando crawl is seen as an alternative means of locomotion. There is often also a clumsiness of movement (that may persist into adult life), as well as an irrepressible fidgetiness in affected children. When they do start to walk, hypermobile toddlers find walking on tiptoes, or with an inward or outward toeing gait, splints the ankle. This gives them a sense of better support and so they employ an abnormal gait. However the toeing gait often leads to frequent falls as the feet trip over one another. This is often the time when parents notice easy bruising especially on the shins. Many hypermobile children have been investigated for bruising which is a common feature in this condition. Test of bleeding diatheses are almost invariably normal, and the bruising can be explained on the basis of lack of the normal capillary support

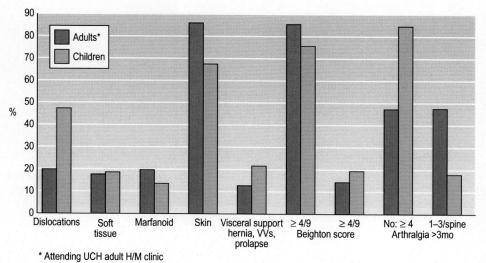

Fig. 2.1 A comparison of the performances of individual Brighton criteria in children with those seen in an adult JHS cohort of 558

* Attending UCH adult H/M clinic

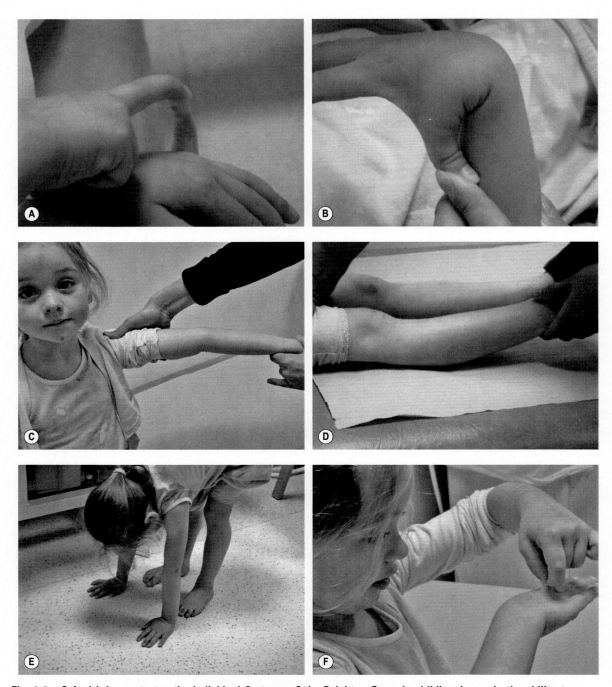

Fig. 2.2a–f A girl demonstrates the individual features of the Beighton Score in childhood namely the ability to:
a, dorsiflex the fifth metacarpophalangeal joint passive to beyond 90°; b, oppose the thumb to the volar aspect of the ipsilateral forearm; c, hyperextend the elbow to beyond 10°; d, hyperextend the knee to beyond 10°; e, place the hands flat on the floor without bending the knees; f, shows her also testing her own skin stretchiness

afforded by the inherently weak collagen infrastructure. Once walking, parents often notice that their child has very flat, pronated feet (see later). Reassurance along the lines that all infants are like this is misleading. Flat pronated feet lead to abnormal gaits (Chapter 12.5) with features such as:

● squinting of the patella
● tibial torsion
● femoral anteversion
● hyperlordosis.

Fortunately, the motor delay diminishes as the infant develops (Davidovitch et al 1994). A recent study of 29 infants from the same group reveals that this catch-up can be helped by a programme of monthly physical therapy combined with a home treatment protocol administered by caregivers. Weekly physical therapy offered no advantage over a monthly regimen (Mintz-Itkin et al 2009).

Children with JHS often have poor ball-catching skills and difficulty with using scissors due to an associated developmental coordination disorder (dyspraxia) (Kirby & Davies 2007).

Proprioception is often poor in hypermobility persisting into adulthood (Chapter 6.4). This leads to frequent falls, and also clumsiness with walking into door frames and furniture, tripping over, and knocking objects over being common complaints. Once the infant has mastered walking other milestones such as climbing and running are difficult due to suppleness and weakness of muscles. The gait is further disrupted as in pronation the first metatarsophalangeal joint is locked and thus toeing off may be difficult if not impossible.

Much of the locomotor difficulty encountered by children with JHS derives from impairment of muscle power and proprioceptive acuity which can be detected both clinically and experimentally. In one study of 37 healthy children (mean age ± s.d. = 11.5± 2.6 years) and 29 children with JHS (mean age ± s.d. = 11.9 ± 1.8 years) the children with JHS had significantly poorer joint kinaesthaesia, joint position sense and muscle torque than that found in control subjects (both $P < 0.001$). Knee extensor and flexor muscle torque was also significantly reduced (both $P < 0.001$) in children with JHS compared with healthy counterparts. The authors concluded that these findings provided a rationale for the use of proprioceptive training and muscle strengthening in treatment (Fatoye et al 2009) as has been advocated clinically (Maillard et al 2004) (Chapter 11). A recent Dutch study demonstrated in 41 hypermobile children (mean age 9 years) that only muscle strength correlated with motor performance (Hanewinkel-van Kleef et al 2009) adding yet further weight to the primacy of muscle strength and stamina in children with JHS.

SCOLIOSIS AND JHS IN CHILDREN

Scoliosis is a frequently encountered finding in children and adults with JHS. A recent study of joint laxity during scoliosis screening of 1273 children (males 598; females 675; mean age 10.4 years) using the Bunnell scoliometer (Bunnell 1993) showed a correlation between the Beighton score and trunk rotation of $\geq 7°$ (Erkula et al 2005).

JOINT PAIN AND HYPERMOBILITY IN CHILDREN

Paediatric rheumatologists now acknowledge that many if not most children and adolescents attending paediatric rheumatology clinics will have a non-inflammatory origin for their complaints or disorder. Mechanical causes are frequently identified, and hypermobility or ligamentous laxity of joints is increasingly recognized as an aetiological factor in the presentation (Murray 2006).

In spite of this several authorities are sceptical about the link between hypermobility and pain and doubt the existence of a causative link between JHM and musculoskeletal pain (MSKP) thereby challenging the very existence of JHS. One typical example was a recently published Italian study of 1046 schoolchildren (mean age 10.8; range 7–15 years). MSKP was found in 18%. The study group was composed of children experiencing pain once per week; 22% of children with MSKP had a Beighton Score of $\geq 5/9$ compared with 23% of controls who had pain only rarely or never. Because they have only looked at the Beighton Score (rather than for JHS using the Brighton criteria), the authors have failed to distinguish between subjects with JHM and those with JHS (Leone et al 2009).

Restricting evaluation to the Beighton Score (rather than taking a broader view using the Brighton Criteria) may have led to an erroneous conclusion of no influence of JHM on the outcome of neck pain in 1756 Finnish 9–12-year-olds followed for 1–4 years. Other factors (now known to be strongly associated with JHS) such as concurrence of frequent other musculoskeletal pains, headache, abdominal pain, day tiredness, depressive mood and sleep difficulties were found to be risk factors for both the occurrence and persistence of weekly neck pain during the subsequent 4-year period (Stahl et al 2008).

By contrast, in a study of 829 Mumbai children aged 3–19 years from an urban lower socio-economic population with a high prevalence of JHM, 59% showing a Beighton score of > 4/9, 26% of the JHM children had MSKP symptoms compared with only 17.7% in the non-JHM children ($P < 0.05$). A striking novel finding was the higher prevalence of JHM in those with malnutrition (61.5%) compared with those with normal nutrition or mild grades of malnutrition (36.8%) (Hasija et al 2008).

FLAT FEET (PES PLANUS) IN CHILDREN

Examining the feet barefoot (see Chapter 12.5) is an essential part of the examination of the child, and it is an obvious and easy way to spot hypermobility. It might provide the instant clue to a diagnosis of JHS. In a recent study a significant statistical correlation was found between JHM and the occurrence of both pes planus and arthralgia in pre-pubertal children (Yazgan et al 2008). An example of pes planus in JHS is seen in Figure 2.3a, b.

GROWING PAINS

The nature of so-called growing pains (GP) has mystified paediatricians and family practitioners since the term was introduced in 1823 by the French physician Marcel Duchamp (Duchamp 1823). Peterson viewed the term as a nebulous entity that can be diagnosed only by exclusion. He wisely warned that 'the greatest diagnostic error is to make a diagnosis of growing pains while overlooking some serious underlying condition'. He defined growing pains as bilateral, intermittent non-articular pains involving the lower limbs; typically occurring during late afternoons or evenings with a normal physical examination and normal laboratory parameters whenever performed (Peterson 1986). There is a growing impression amongst clinicians that JHS provides the key to GP. This assertion is now beginning to acquire an evidence base. In a study of 433 (219 boys and 214 girls – age range 3–9 years) 177 (41%) had JHM (Beighton ≥ 5/9) and 122 (28%) satisfied Peterson's criteria for GP. Of the 177 with JHM, 75 (42%) had GP. Of the 122 with GP, 75 (62%) had JHM. Using chi square statistical analysis, the authors found that JHM and GP were strongly

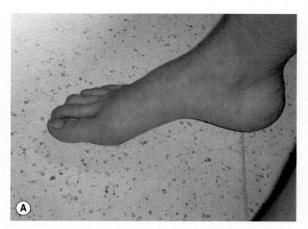

Fig. 2.3a A hypermobile child's foot – non–weight–bearing. Note the normal appearance of the longitudinal arch and of the foot when not subjected to the weight of the body

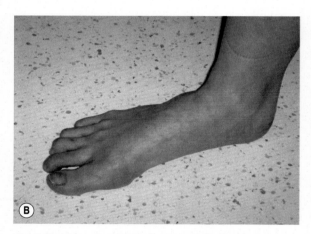

Fig. 2.3b The same child's foot – weight–bearing. Note the complete collapse of the longitudinal arch with pronation of the foot under the weight of the body

associated. They also showed a particularly strong association between knee hypermobility and GP (Viswanathan & Khubchandani 2008).

There is now increasing evidence that much of the pain experienced by patients, in particular, children with JHM, is associated with the increased muscle fatigue due to deconditioning and the increased demands falling on to muscles attempting to control joints in the hypermobile range. Ergometric testing on 32 children (mean age 12 years) revealed a significantly reduced absolute peak oxygen consumption and relative peak oxygen consumption in patients with JHS compared to control subjects (Engelbert et al 2006).

PROGNOSIS OF JHS IN CHILDHOOD

For many if not most patients the symptoms of JHS in childhood are relatively mild and unobtrusive. Others with more persistent pains in over-stressed muscles will continue to have difficulties until their musculature is strengthened by appropriate exercises or as a result of the adolescent growth spurt and puberty (Chapters 10 and 11). There is, however, a severely debilitated and disabled group whose lives and education are disrupted due to the development of a secondary chronic pain syndrome. An association between hypermobility and chronic pain in children is not new. A link with fibromyalgia has been known and acknowledged for nearly two decades (Gedalia et al 1993) (Chapter 5). In a retrospective study of 125 children referred to a tertiary hypermobility clinic in London (highly selected sample) the scope and array of adverse clinical features are described. The striking findings (Table 2.1) included the delay in diagnosis resulting

Table 2.1	Most frequently encountered symptoms and other features occurring in 25% or more of patients attending Great Ormond Street Hospital for Children, London with a diagnosis of JHS between 1999 and 2002 (Adib et al 2005)
CLINICAL FEATURE	**PROPORTION (%)**
Pes planus	88/99 (89)
Pain exacerbated by exercise	80/99 (81)
Anterior knee pain	85/116 (73)
Sport hobbies difficulties	35/52 (67)
Joint laxity in first-degree relative	57/90 (63)
Clumsy	44/92 (48)
Physical education missed	49/103 (48)
Easy bruising	39/91 (43)
Back pain	46/116 (40)
School missed	42/102 (41)
Handwriting problems	42/106 (40)
Pain exacerbated by infection	30/83 (39)
Weakness	41/106 (39)
Sleep disturbance	41/111 (37)
Poor coordination	30/86 (36)
Foot pain	37/110 (34)
Walked after 15 months	19/57 (33)
'Growing pains' diagnosed	32/98 (33)
Clicky joints	25/84 (30)
Joint stiffness	31/103 (30)
Skin extensibility increased	27/87 (31)
Wheelchair/crutches used	27/107 (25)

in poor pain control, and the disruption of normal home life, schooling and physical activities (Adib et al 2005). There is also some evidence to suggest that JHS acts as a predisposing factor in the pathogenesis of complex regional pain syndrome in children (Stoler & Oaklander 2006).

RELATED EXTRA-ARTICULAR SYMPTOMS IN JHS

GASTROINTESTINAL SYMPTOMS

A recent Australian study has demonstrated an association between constipation and JHM in 39 children (aged 7–17 years) with slow transit constipation (STC), a form of chronic constipation, with delayed colonic passage of stool when compared with 41 controls without constipation. JHM was defined as a Beighton score of $\geq 4/9$. The relationship was only statistically significant in boys (Reilly et al 2008). This study nicely matches similar studies in adults which point towards panintestinal dysmotility being a common, though hitherto unrecognized, feature of JHS (Zarate et al 2009) (Chapter 6.2, 6.3).

FATIGUE

Joint hypermobility undoubtedly makes extra physical demands on the muscles of affected patients. Muscular fatigue after exercise is, therefore, not surprisingly, frequently reported in JHS. More severe and enduring chronic fatigue occurs when JHS is complicated by chronic pain. It is, of course, the cardinal symptom of chronic fatigue syndrome (CFS) so that there may be some difficulty in distinguishing between CFS and JHS. The question is further complicated by the finding that JHM occurs more frequently among children with CFS than in controls (Barron et al 2002).

For further information about JHS in children the reader is encouraged to turn to Chapter 11.

JHS IN ADOLESCENCE

The presence of musculoskeletal pain was evaluated in adolescents. Pain was reported by 40% of respondents, benign joint hypermobility syndrome by 10%, myofascial syndrome by 5%, tendonitis by

2%, and fibromyalgia by 1%. Logistic regression analysis indicated that sex and age were predictive of pain (Zapata et al 2006a). Surprisingly, pain in this cohort was not related to computer and video games (Zapata et al 2006b).

Hypermobility in adolescents is dealt with comprehensively in Chapter 10.

THE CLINICAL SPECTRUM OF JHS IN ADULTS

KEY FEATURES OF JHS

There are four principal components of JHS. Each can contribute to the clinical diagnosis and should be sought in all cases. They comprise joint hypermobility, skin involvement, marfanoid habitus and the supporting structures. The skill is not only to identify them but also to understand how one might distinguish the distribution and severity of signs and symptoms from that of the rarer HDCT (Chapter 1).

Joint hypermobility

The Beighton Score has not been abandoned in favour of the Brighton Criteria. On the contrary, it forms their central pillar. But, relying on hypermobility alone for the recognition for JHS is a recipe for diagnostic disaster. Yet, that is what most rheumatologists do (Grahame 2008). The 9-point Beighton scoring system was introduced as an epidemiological tool and for this it worked well. As a diagnostic tool it may fail to register hypermobility in joints that are not included in the test. It is fruitful for the examiner to look further afield, e.g. to the shoulders, cervical and thoracic spine and to the toes and feet to glean additional evidence of hypermobility. There is much discussion as to what should be the cut-off point; whether it should be 3/9, 4/9 or 5/9. This becomes a rather sterile argument when one considers that the Beighton score is not per se a measure of the degree of joint hypermobility, but merely of the number of joints (out of a rather small arbitrarily chosen selection) affected. So that it is more of a qualitative rather than a quantitative measure. There is a semi-quantitative adaptation called the Contompasis score (Chapter 1, Table 1.6), which has more credibility as a measuring instrument for hypermobility.

Skin involvement

Skin is very rich in collagen, which represents 70% of its dry weight. It also happens to be the most widely distributed of all human proteins. Skin represents a readily accessible means of observing collagen's physical properties by observing, feeling and stretching it. The skin in JHS is often semi-transparent, silky soft to the touch and it stretches like an elastic glove. This is best appreciated by observing the lines of force stretching some distance away from the point of application of the traction (Figure 2.4). This is quite a subtle technique which requires practice and experience to perfect. It is several orders of magnitude less stretchy than what is seen in the classical forms of Ehlers-Danlos syndrome (Figure 2.5), which is what most clinicians are expecting to find. It is four decades since the discovery that the difference between EDS and normal skin stretch lies in the first phase of the stress/strain curve, which represents the taking up of slack, during which the bundles of collagen are lined up in the direction of force (Grahame & Beighton 1969).

Scar tissue is also composed of collagen. The appearance of the scar can give information of diagnostic importance. In JHS the scar is often paper-thin, shiny and easily wrinkles when compressed from side to side between the examiner's index finger and thumb. It is often visibly and

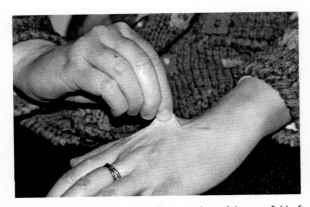

Fig. 2.4 Skin stretch in JHS. The examiner picks up a fold of skin on the dorsum of the hand tugging gently and observes how the early phase of stretching requires little force whereas the phase thereafter is very resistant to stretch. The first phase represents the taking up of slack followed by the much more resistant linear second phase which represents the actual stretching of the collagen fibrils. It is better recognized by tactile sense rather than visually

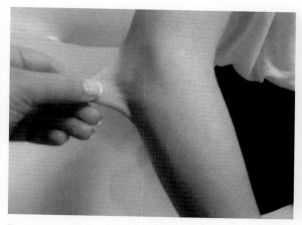

Fig. 2.5 The greater degree of stretch seen in an example of the EDS classical type. By comparison, the more subtle degree of skin stretch seen in JHS patients (Fig. 2.4) may be overlooked or discounted

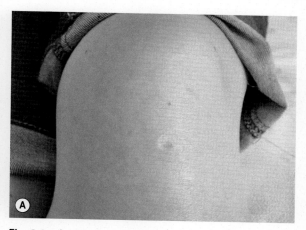

Fig. 2.6a A typical paper-thin scar seen in a JHS patient

palpably sunken below the surface of the surrounding skin as shown in Figure 2.6a. A typical papyraceous scar from a patient with the classical form of EDS is shown in Figure 2.6b for the purposes of comparison. Another reliably constant skin feature is the appearance of stretch marks (striae atrophicae) during the phase of maximal adolescent growth, which is usually between the ages of 11 and 13 years. It is always worth looking for skin involvement as its identification adds a minor criterion towards the Brighton Criteria for JHS and helps to make the diagnosis.

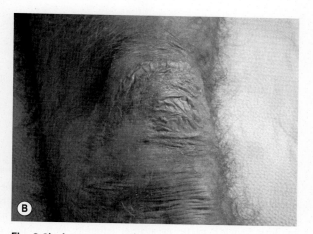

Fig. 2.6b A papyraceous (parchment-like) scar of the distinct type seen in the classical type of EDS

Marfanoid habitus

The features of the marfanoid habitus (MH) are listed in Chapter 1. The recognition that features of MH are seen in JHS dates back nearly three decades (Grahame et al 1981). It is always worthwhile looking for MH in any musculoskeletal examination as in JHS the features are not always obvious and incomplete forms abound. Nevertheless, the identification of MH adds a minor criterion towards the Brighton Criteria for JHS and thereby assists in diagnosis. Because JHS is so much more common than Marfan syndrome (MFS), in clinical practice MH is statistically much more likely to indicate JHS than MFS. Some of the features of MH are shown in Figure 2.7a–c.

Weakness of supporting structures and other signs

The presence or history of inguinal, abdominal or hiatus hernia, varicose veins, pelvic floor problems such as uterine or rectal prolapse, cystocele, rectocele with or without stress incontinence, all constitute diagnostic support for JHS and any one satisfies a minor criterion towards the Brighton Criteria. Other diagnostic signs, not forming part of the Criteria include Gorlin sign, the ability to touch the nose with the tip of the tongue, and the absence of the lingual frenulum (De Felice et al 2001). An example of the latter is shown in Figure 2.8.

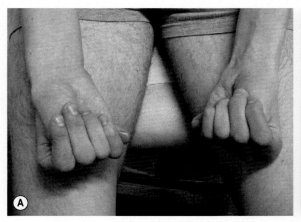
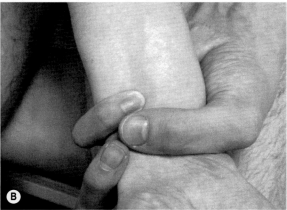
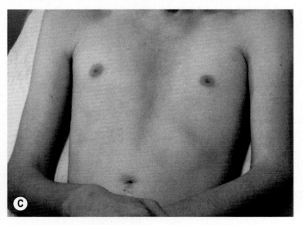

Fig. 2.7a–c Diagnostic features of the marfanoid habitus: **a**, the Steinberg test for arachnodactyly. In a positive test the subject is able to extend the thumb beyond the hypothenar edge of the hand; **b**, the Walker (wrist) sign for arachnodactyly. In a positive test the subject is able to overlap finger/thumb nails while encircling the contralateral wrist with the thumb and little finger; **c**, pectus excavatum deformity. Note sunken ribs below left nipple

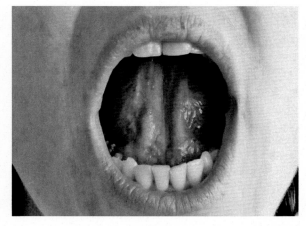

Fig. 2.8 Absence of the lingual frenulum (together with the superior and inferior labral frenula) has been described by De Felice (2001)

OTHER CLINICAL FEATURES OF JHS IN ADULTS

Vulnerability to injury

As with children and adolescents the connective tissues of adults with JHS are both lax and fragile. This renders them more vulnerable to injuries of various kinds. These may result in damaged ligaments, ligamentous attachments, fractures, dislocations and subluxations. Overuse injuries sustained include tendonitis, tenosynovitis, epicondylitis, plantar fasciitis, carpal and tarsal tunnel syndromes, chondromalacia patellae and work-related and performance-related upper limb disorders. A diagrammatic representation of the pathogenesis of the JHS is shown in Figure 2.9.

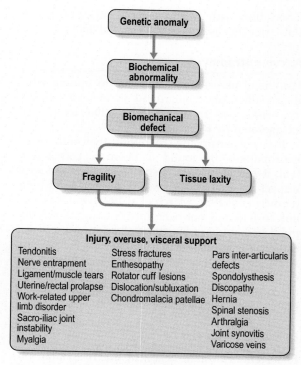

Fig. 2.9 A representation of the pathogenesis of JHS.
A genetic anomaly (yet to be determined in the case of JHS) gives rise to biochemical abnormality in the structural protein, which, in turn results in a biomechanical defect. This has two opposing results; on the one hand there is tissue laxity which is responsible for (amongst other effects) joint hypermobility and flexibility; the other is tissue fragility resulting in tissue injury and mechanical breakdown and fracture or rupture depending on the site or organ involved. In clinical terms this, potentially, may manifest in a host of traumatic or overuse lesions listed in the box which are regarded as manifestations of JHS, since their pathogenesis can be traced back to mechanical failure of one kind or another in all cases

Anxiety, pain perception and autonomic disturbance

Over the past two decades it has become increasingly clear that the clinical manifestations of JHS are by no means limited to the musculoskeletal system. Extra-articular features comprise:

- Increased pain perception (Chapters 3 and 5)
- Joint proprioception impairment (Chapter 6.4)
- Lack of efficacy of local anaesthetics (Hakim et al 2005)
- Autonomic dysfunction (Gazit et al 2003) (Chapter 6.1)

- Anxiety and phobias (Chapter 4)
- Gastrointestinal dysmotility (Chapter 6.2).

In the majority of patients with JHS the syndrome will have already become established by the time adulthood is reached (40 out of 45 adults in one series (Sacheti et al 1997)). The evolution of the symptom complex associated with JHS untreated can be seen as a slowly developing crescendo of painful short-lived soft tissue traumatic incidents, occurring sequentially and building up a momentum of severity, frequency and duration over time. Slow and often incomplete healing of individual lesions results in a blurring of their margins, so that pain transforms from discontinuous to continuous, from recurrent acute to sub-acute and ultimately, to chronic. Two other factors reinforce the downward trend. Firstly, the apparent lack of efficacy of potent analgesic drugs starts progressively to intensify (Chapter 7). Secondly, since movement in general becomes painful, patients adopt a strategy of pain-avoidance through movement-avoidance (a process known as kinesiophobia), which rapidly leads to progressive muscle deconditioning. The result is destabilization of a locomotor system already compromised by inherent ligament laxity and resultant/potential joint instability. This sequence of events is illustrated in Figure 2.10.

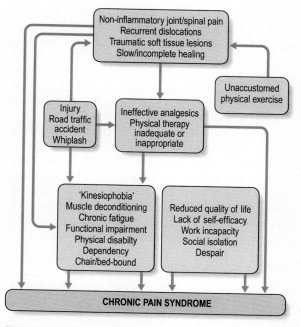

Fig. 2.10 A schematic representation of the pathogenesis of chronic pain in JHS

Pathogenetic mechanisms surrounding pain amplification are the subject of discussion in Chapter 3 and are frequently operating in patients with JHS by the time of their first presentation in the Hypermobility Clinic. A high proportion (24% in the author's series of 700 JHS patients) already has an established chronic pain syndrome in advance of their obtaining specialist advice.

Fatigue

Chronic fatigue (CF) is a frequent and disturbing symptom that may significantly adversely affect the quality of life of patients and is a feature of many conditions including depressive disorders, chronic fatigue syndrome (CFS) and fibromyalgia (FM). CF is also frequently seen in joint hypermobility syndrome (JHS), usually in young adults and especially in adolescent girls.

The CF in JHS is usually but not exclusively associated with autonomic nervous system (ANS) dysfunction (Chapter 6.1). A number of other factors may conspire to accentuate CF in JHS patients including chronic pain, years of suffering and poor physical fitness (with muscle deconditioning) (Figure 2.10).

JHS/JHM and CF frequently concur both in adults and in children. In one study of patients with CFS aged 18–65 years, 40/68 (58.5%) fulfilled the Brighton Criteria for the JHS compared to 0/69 of the controls (Fisher exact test, $P < 0.004$) (Nijs et al 2006). A similar result emerged when 58 children with CFS were found to have higher median Beighton scores (4/9 compared with 1/9) compared with healthy controls. The odds ratio for hypermobility in all patients with CFS versus healthy controls was 3.5 ($P < 0.001$; 95% CI, 1.6–7.5) (Barron et al 2002).

It is not surprising, therefore, that patients with fatigue in JHS may be misdiagnosed as suffering from CFS or FM, especially as JHS is the least widely appreciated or understood of the three conditions (Grahame 2008). There is clearly overlap between JHS, CFS and FM, which confuses all clinicians and which only future research can disentangle in the course of time.

Osteopenia and osteoporosis

Evidence has been growing for some time for an association between JHS and osteopenia (Mishra et al 1996), but this did not apparently extend to osteoporosis. Now there is better evidence for an

association with osteopenia but, alas, only with JHM, not JHS as yet (Gulbahar et al 2006).

Nerve entrapment

Peripheral nerves are vulnerable to trauma when their path takes them round wide-angled bends. The risks are increased when the angles are exaggerated by hypermobility.

It is not surprising, therefore, that entrapment neuropathies are found to be more common in JHS. It has long been suspected that this is so in respect of carpal and tarsal tunnel syndromes (Francis et al 1987, March et al 1998), but a proven link to JHS had not been forthcoming. A recently published study of 55 patients has shown a highly significant correlation ($r = 0.59$, $P = 0.0001$) between the presence of electrophysiologically proven carpal tunnel syndrome and the occurrence of JHS diagnosed on the basis of the Brighton 1998 criteria (Aktas et al 2008).

Orthostatic headache

Recurrent orthostatic headache due to spontaneous intracranial hypotension is becoming increasingly recognized, the mechanism being leakage of cerebrospinal fluid from the sub-arachnoid space. Of 18 patients thus presenting in one series, no less than seven (38%) showed evidence of a connective tissue disorder including types of EDS. The authors postulate that leakage from the dural membranes may have resulted from their inherent fragility (Schievink et al 2004).

Pelvic floor problems

Weakness of the pelvic floor is a common occurrence in post-partum women. Because of its musculotendinous nature and its high collagen content, pelvic floor problems occur in women with JHS with increased frequency and severity (Al-Rawi & Al-Rawi 1982) (see Chapter 12.6).

In a recent Turkish study 65 women recommended for surgery with pelvic organ prolapse (POP) were compared with 52 age-matched healthy controls. Patients with POP had a significantly higher prevalence of JHM (53.8%) when compared with controls (9.6%). No significant correlation was demonstrated between Beighton scores and incontinence, exercise pattern and hormone replacement therapy (Aydeniz et al 2009). Unfortunately, JHS was not recorded.

Anecdotally, pelvic floor problems also encountered occasionally in nulliparous women as well. In one study 100 pairs of nulliparous and parous postmenopausal sisters were recruited for assessment of pelvic organ prolapse. High concordance of pelvic organ prolapse in nulliparous and parous sister pairs suggests a familial predisposition toward developing this condition. Interestingly, vaginal delivery did not confer a risk for more advanced pelvic organ prolapse (Buchsbaum et al 2006).

Jha et al (2007) compared 30 JHS patients with 30 controls using The International Consultation on Incontinence Questionnaire-Short Form (ICIQ-SF) and the Manchester Health Questionnaire. Incontinence in the study group was present in 18/30 and in the control group was 9/30 (60 vs 30%; $P = 0.037$); 23% (7/30) of the women with JHS had a problem with anal incontinence compared to none of the controls (23 vs 0%; $P = 0.01$). Therefore, the prevalence of both urinary and anal incontinence appears to be significantly higher in women with JHS when compared to women without this condition. The same group also conducted a survey among 148 members of the Hypermobility Syndrome Association, a patients' self-help group in the UK (40% response rate). The survey revealed a prevalence of urinary and faecal incontinence of 68.9% and 14.9% respectively, compared to 30% and 2.2% respectively in the general population (Arunkalaivanan et al 2009). Data of this kind clearly need to be interpreted with caution, but in spite of this the figures are striking and further studies are needed.

HYPERMOBILITY AND THE ELDERLY

Anecdotally, patients with JHM and JHS retain their generous range of joint motion well into old age so that they remain fitter, more agile and more active than their non-hypermobile counterparts. This enhances their ability to maintain socially integrated lifestyles and mentally stimulating activities, which would be expected to reduce the risk or postpone the clinical onset of dementia, including Alzheimer's disease (Qiu et al 2009).

There is some epidemiological support for this optimistic outlook. As an offshoot of the 15-year-long Chingford follow-up study of 1000 healthy women in East London hypermobility was included in 2003. It was found that JHM in the community was not associated with the development of osteoarthritis (OA) or osteoporosis. Contrary to popular belief and to the investigators' expectations, the study showed JHM may even be a marker for fitness in old age, with reduced knee OA and increased hip bone mineral density (Dolan et al 2003). Clearly, more epidemiology is needed to explore this further.

CONCLUDING CONUNDRUM

Could there, therefore, exist two hypermobile populations: one in the community who appear to thrive and derive benefit from their hypermobility, and another, who attend hospital clinics for treatment of their wide array of musculoskeletal and systemic complications? Could this explain an often expressed conundrum, 'Why do some hypermobile subjects have so much pain, while others have none?'

A clearer understanding would come from large-scale prospective general population and family studies where the presence and degree of hypermobility, skin and other connective tissue pathologies is recorded at base-line, and the prevalence and then incidence of injuries, pain, anxiety, and autonomic syndromes tracked against risk factors over time.

References

Adib N, Davies K, Grahame R, et al: Joint hypermobility syndrome in childhood. A not so benign multisystem disorder, *Rheumatology (Oxford)* 44(6): 744–750, 2005.

Aktas I, Ofluoglu D, Albay T: The relationship between benign joint hypermobility syndrome and carpal tunnel syndrome, *Clin Rheumatol* 27(10):1283–1287, 2008.

Al-Rawi ZS, Al-Rawi ZT: Joint hypermobility in women with genital prolapse, *Lancet* 1(8287):1439–1441, 1982.

Arunkalaivanan AS, Morrison A, Jha S, et al: Prevalence of urinary and faecal incontinence among female members of the Hypermobility Syndrome Association (HMSA), *J Obstet Gynaecol* 29(2):126–128, 2009.

Aydeniz A, Dikensoy E, Cebesoy B, et al: The relation between genitourinary prolapse and joint hypermobility in Turkish women, *Arch Gynecol Obstet* 281(2):301–304, 2009.

Barron DF, Cohen BA, Geraghty MT, et al: Joint hypermobility is more common in children with chronic fatigue syndrome than in healthy controls, *J Pediatr* 141(3):421–425, 2002.

Beighton PH, Solomon L, Soskolne CL: Articular mobility in an African population, *Ann Rheum Dis* 32(5):413–418, 1973.

Beighton P, De PA, Steinmann B, et al: Ehlers-Danlos syndromes: revised nosology, Villefranche, 1997. Ehlers-Danlos National Foundation (USA) and Ehlers-Danlos Support Group (UK), *Am J Med Genet* 77(1):31–37, 1998.

Bravo JF, Wolff C: Clinical study of hereditary disorders of connective tissues in a Chilean population: joint hypermobility syndrome and vascular Ehlers-Danlos syndrome, *Arthritis Rheum* 54(2):515–523, 2006.

Buchsbaum GM, Duecy EE, Kerr LA, et al: Pelvic organ prolapse in nulliparous women and their parous sisters, *Obstet Gynecol* 108 (6):1388–1393, 2006.

Bulbena A, Duro JC, Porta M, et al: Clinical assessment of hypermobility of joints: assembling criteria, *J Rheumatol* 19(1):115–122, 1992.

Bunnell WP: Outcome of spinal screening, *Spine* 18:1572–1580, 1993.

Davidovitch M, Tirosh E, Tal Y: The relationship between joint hypermobility and neurodevelopmental attributes in elementary school children, *J Child Neurol* 9(4):417–419, 1994.

De Felice C, Toti P, Di MG, et al: Absence of the inferior labial and lingual frenula in Ehlers-Danlos syndrome, *Lancet* 357 (9267):1500–1502, 2001.

De Paepe A, Devereux RB, Dietz HC, et al: Revised diagnostic criteria for the Marfan syndrome, *Am J Med Genet* 62(4):417–426, 1996.

Dolan AL, Hart DJ, Doyle DV, et al: The relationship of joint hypermobility, bone mineral density, and osteoarthritis in the general population: the Chingford Study, *J Rheumatol* 30(4):799–803, 2003.

Duchamp M: Maladies de la croissance. In Levrault FG, editor: *Memoires de Médecine Practique*, Paris, 1823, Jean-Frederic Lobstein.

Engelbert RH, Kooijmans FT, van Riet AM, et al: The relationship between generalized joint hypermobility and motor development, *Pediatr Phys Ther* 17(4):258–263, 2005.

Engelbert RH, van Bergen M, Henneken T, et al: Exercise tolerance in children and adolescents with musculoskeletal pain in joint hypermobility and joint hypomobility syndrome, *Pediatrics* 118(3):e690–e696, 2006.

Erkula G, Kiter AE, Kilic BA, et al: The relation of joint laxity and trunk rotation, *J Pediatr Orthop B* 14(1):38–41, 2005.

Fatoye F, Palmer S, Macmillan F, et al: Proprioception and muscle torque deficits in children with hypermobility syndrome, *Rheumatology (Oxford)* 48(2): 152–157, 2009.

Francis H, March L, Terenty T, et al: Benign joint hypermobility with neuropathy: documentation and mechanism of tarsal tunnel syndrome, *J Rheumatol* 14(3): 577–581, 1987.

Gazit Y, Nahir AM, Grahame R, et al: Dysautonomia in the joint hypermobility syndrome, *Am J Med* 115(1):33–40, 2003.

Gedalia A, Press J, Klein M, et al: Joint hypermobility and fibromyalgia in schoolchildren, *Ann Rheum Dis* 52(7):494–496, 1993.

Grahame R, Beighton P: Physical properties of the skin in the Ehlers-Danlos syndrome, *Ann Rheum Dis* 28(3):246–251, 1969.

Grahame R, Edwards JC, Pitcher D, et al: A clinical and echocardiographic study of patients with the hypermobility syndrome, *Ann Rheum Dis* 40(6):541–546, 1981.

Grahame R: Joint hypermobility and genetic collagen disorders: are they related? [Review] [29 refs], *Arch Dis Child* 80(2):188–191, 1999.

Grahame R, Bird HA, Child A, et al: The revised (Brighton 1998) criteria for the diagnosis of benign joint hypermobility syndrome (BJHS) [see comment], *J Rheumatol* 27(7):1777–1779, 2000.

Grahame R: Hypermobility: an important but often neglected area within rheumatology, *Nat Clin Pract Rheumatol* 4(10):522–524, 2008.

Gulbahar S, Sahin E, Baydar M, et al: Hypermobility syndrome increases the risk for low bone mass, *Clin Rheumatol* 25(4): 511–514, 2006.

Hakim AJ, Grahame R, Norris P, et al: Local anaesthetic failure in joint hypermobility syndrome, *J R Soc Med* 98(2):84–85, 2005.

Hanewinkel-van Kleef YB, Helders PJ, Takken T, et al: Motor performance in children with generalized hypermobility: the influence of muscle strength and exercise capacity, *Pediatr Phys Ther* 21(2):194–200, 2009.

Hasija RP, Khubchandani RP, Shenoi S: Joint hypermobility in Indian children, *Clin Exp Rheumatol* 26(1):146–150, 2008.

Jha S, Arunkalaivanan AS, Situnayake RD: Prevalence of incontinence in women with benign joint hypermobility syndrome, *Int Urogynecol J Pelvic Floor Dysfunct* 18(1):61–64, 2007.

Juul-Kristensen B, Rogind H, Jensen DV, et al: Inter-examiner reproducibility of tests and criteria for generalized joint hypermobility and benign joint hypermobility syndrome, *Rheumatology (Oxford)* 46(12): 1835–1841, 2007.

Kirby A, Davies R: Developmental Coordination Disorder and Joint Hypermobility Syndrome–overlapping disorders? Implications for research and clinical practice, *Child Care Health Dev* 33(5):513–519, 2007.

Kirk JA, Ansell BM, Bywaters EG: The hypermobility syndrome. Musculoskeletal complaints associated with generalized joint hypermobility, *Ann Rheum Dis* 26(5):419–425, 1967.

Leone V, Tornese G, Zerial M, et al: Joint hypermobility and its relationship to musculoskeletal pain in schoolchildren: a cross-sectional study, *Arch Dis Child* PM:19465584, 2009.

Maillard SM, et al: Physiotherapy management of benign joint hypermobility syndrome, *Arthritis Rheum* 50(Suppl):S78, 2004.

March LM, Francis H, Webb J: Benign joint hypermobility with neuropathies: documentation and mechanism of median, sciatic, and common peroneal nerve compression, *Clin Rheumatol* 7(1):35–40, 1988.

McCormack M, Briggs J, Hakim A, et al: Joint laxity and the benign joint hypermobility syndrome in student and professional ballet dancers.[see comment], *J Rheumatol* 31(1):173–178, 2004.

Mintz-Itkin R, Lerman-Sagie T, Zuk L, et al: Does physical therapy improve outcome in infants with joint hypermobility and benign hypotonia? *J Child Neurol* 24(6):714–719, 2009.

Mishra MB, Ryan P, Atkinson P, et al: Extra-articular features of benign joint hypermobility syndrome, *Br J Rheumatol* 35(9):861–866, 1996.

Murray KJ: Hypermobility disorders in children and adolescents, *Best Pract Res Clin Rheumatol* 20(2): 329–351, 2006.

Nijs J, Aerts A, De Meirleir K: Generalized joint hypermobility is more common in chronic fatigue syndrome than in healthy control subjects, *J Manipulative Physiol Ther* 29(1):32–39, 2006.

Peterson H: Growing pains, *Pediatr Clin North Am* 33(6):1365–1372, 1986.

Poul J, Garvie D, Grahame R, et al: Ultrasound examination of neonate's hip joints, *J Pediatr Orthop B* 7(1):59–61, 1998.

Qiu C, Kivipelto M, von Strauss E: Epidemiology of Alzheimer's disease: occurrence, determinants, and strategies toward intervention, *Dialogues Clin Neurosci* 11(2):111–128, 2009.

Reilly DJ, Chase JW, Hutson JM, et al: Connective tissue disorder–a new subgroup of boys with slow transit constipation? *J Pediatr Surg* 43(6):1111–1114, 2008.

Sacheti A, Szemere J, Bernstein B, et al: Chronic pain is a manifestation of the Ehlers-Danlos syndrome, *J Pain Symptom Manage* 14(2):88–93, 1997.

Schievink WI, Gordon OK, Tourje J: Connective tissue disorders with spontaneous spinal cerebrospinal fluid leaks and intracranial hypotension: a prospective study, *Neurosurgery* 54(1):65–70, 2004.

Stahl M, Kautiainen H, El-Metwally A, et al: Non-specific neck pain in schoolchildren: prognosis and risk factors for occurrence and persistence. A 4-year follow-up study, *Pain* 137(2):316–322, 2008.

Stoler JM, Oaklander AL: Patients with Ehlers Danlos syndrome and CRPS: a possible association? *Pain* 123(1–2):204–209, 2006.

Tinkle BT, Lavallee M, Levy H, et al: Position Statement from the Professional Advisory Network of the Ehlers-Danlos National Foundation, 2009.

Tofts LJ, Elliott EJ, Munns C, et al: The differential diagnosis of children with joint hypermobility: a review of the literature, *Pediatr Rheumatol Online J* 7:1, 2009.

Toker S, Soyucen E, Gulcan E, et al: Presentation of two cases with hypermobility syndrome and review of the related literature, *Eur J Phys Rehabil Med* May 21, 2009 (Epub ahead of print).

Viswanathan V, Khubchandani RP: Joint hypermobility and growing pains in school children, *Clin Exp Rheumatol* 26(5):962–966, 2008.

Wynne-Davies R: Familial Joint Laxity, *Proc R Soc Med* 64:689–690, 1971.

Yazgan P, Geyikli I, Zeyrek D, et al: Is joint hypermobility important in prepubertal children? *Rheumatol Int* 28(5):445–451, 2008.

Zapata AL, Moraes AJ, Leone C, et al: Pain and musculoskeletal pain syndromes in adolescents, *J Adolesc Health* 38(6):769–771, 2006a.

Zapata AL, Moraes AJ, Leone C, et al: Pain and musculoskeletal pain syndromes related to computer and video game use in adolescents, *Eur J Pediatr* 165 (6):408–414, 2006b.

Zarate N, Farmer AD, Grahame R, et al: Unexplained gastrointestinal symptoms and joint hypermobility: is connective tissue the missing link? *Neurogastroenterol Motil* 22(3): 252–278, 2010 Mar; Epub 2009 Oct 15.

Chapter 3

The physiology of pain

Maliha Shaikh

Alan J Hakim

Nicholas Shenker

INTRODUCTION

The International Association for the Study of Pain defines pain as 'an unpleasant sensory or emotional experience associated with actual or potential tissue damage or described in terms of such damage' (Merskey 1979). It is an experience influenced by sensory, affective, motivational and sociocultural elements, with many factors apart from the intensity of the noxious stimulus determining the way in which it is perceived (Shipton 1999). Pain is always subjective (Prologue). Although it is an unpleasant experience, the absence of pain is far from blissful. Individuals with congenital absence of pain either due to failure of nociceptor survival in the embryo or channelopathies have congenital pain hyposensitivity leading to damaged limbs and joints and early death which highlights the importance of nociception as a protective mechanism.

The pain perception threshold is the threshold at which a subject perceives pain. Interestingly this shows little interindividual variability. For a thermal stimulus, this is around 44–45°C. However, the pain tolerance threshold, the maximum amount of pain that a person is able to tolerate, differs widely (Baldry 2001). Pain is greatly affected by the context in which the pain is experienced. For example, soldiers sustaining severe battlefield injuries often feel little pain at the time, while the pain of fibromyalgia, with little evidence of tissue damage can lead to an individual functioning at a very low level (Chapter 5). Pain caused by tissue damage cannot be differentiated from that without tissue damage (Merskey 1979).

The nervous system is highly adaptive. The variable and non-linear nature of these properties means adaptation of the nervous system at an individual level is inherently unpredictable and, like any complex adaptive system, can only be observed after the fact, rather than predicted (Plsek & Greenhalgh 2001).

A deeper understanding of pain has paralleled the understanding of the nervous system. In 1664, the philosopher and scientist Rene Descartes described in his 'Treatise of Man' the transmission of pain through a single hardwired channel from the skin to the brain. Its stimulation led to involuntary withdrawal of a foot on application of a noxious stimulus. Signals transmitted along the pain pathway are in fact subject to modulation at different levels. Rather than being hardwired as proposed by Descartes, neurological pathways are in fact plastic, reorganizing and learning from previous experience. This plasticity remains possible even in adult life (Pearce & Merletti 2006). The brain and spinal cord learn to facilitate activity in commonly utilized pathways. Such changes occur in relation to useful information such as practical tasks, innocuous details as well as unpleasant information such as pain (Deleo 2006, Holdcroft 2005).

CLASSIFICATION OF PAIN

Several parallel classification systems exist for categorizing pain. These have been based on characteristics such as the area involved (somatic/visceral; regional/widespread), duration (acute/

DOI: 10.1016/B978-0-7020-3005-5.00003-3

chronic), causative agent (cancer, inflammatory, neuropathic) and mechanism (nociceptive/peripheral/central). It is often necessary to use more than one classification system to describe a pain experience.

TERMINOLOGY

Hyperalgesia and allodynia

Common signs are hyperalgesia and allodynia. Hyperalgesia is an exaggerated pain response to a noxious stimulus, while allodynia is a pain response produced by a non-noxious stimulus. Sensitization of the peripheral and central nervous system are the underlying mechanisms for these signs (Table 3.1).

Nociceptive and neuropathic pain

Nociceptive pain occurs upon stimulation of nociceptors by mechanical, thermal or chemical stimuli (Woolf 1991). Neuropathic pain occurs as a result of damage to the peripheral or central nervous system rather than stimulation of nociceptors and can continue even after cessation of the original stimulus (Woolf 1991).

Somatic and visceral pain

Somatic pain arises from the skin, bones and joints whereas visceral pain comes from the internal organs.

Acute versus chronic

Acute pain resolves within hours, days or weeks and is caused by trauma or inflammation. Pain over more than three months is artificially defined as chronic. The boundary blurs between when an acute pain becomes chronic, but pain persisting beyond what is 'normal' for a certain injury may also be considered chronic (Breivik et al 2006). Spontaneous pain is a common symptom in chronically painful conditions (Woolf 1995).

Peripheral versus central

Peripheral pain originates in the peripheral tissues and nerves while central pain originates from pathology in the central nervous system (CNS) such as stroke, multiple sclerosis, trauma and Parkinson's disease.

PAIN IN THE EVOLUTIONARY CONTEXT

The primary function of pain can be understood from the evolutionary perspective. Acute pain serves as a warning system and alerts the organism to tissue damage or injury that needs to be addressed. Nociceptive pain has an essentially protective role as it results in a flexion withdrawal response. The CNS allows learning to avoid similar potentially tissue-damaging stimuli in future (Woolf 1989).

Somatic pain is protective, encouraging the person to escape from the noxious stimulus. The natural response of immobility prevents further tissue damage. Hypersensitivity in the injured area prevents contact with other external stimuli, while hypervigilance causes a range of protective behaviours to prevent further damage (e.g. licking, rubbing, looking and holding) (Woolf 1995).

When pain becomes a chronic phenomenon, it changes the physical, emotional and psychological state. The changes that occur in the nervous system become the pathology. The pain becomes maladaptive and offers no survival advantage to the individual.

Table 3.1 A mechanism–based classification system for pain (Woolf 1998)		
PAIN CATEGORY	POSSIBLE PRIMARY AFFERENT MECHANISM	POSSIBLE CENTRAL MECHANISM
Transient pain (response to noxious stimulus with no long-term effect e.g. pin prick)	Nociceptor specialization	–
Tissue injury pain	Sensitization, recruitment of silent nociceptors, alteration in phenotype, hyperinnervation	Central sensitization and recruitment, summation, amplification
Nervous system injury pain	Acquisition of spontaneous and stimulus evoked activity by nociceptor axons at loci other than peripheral terminals, phenotype change	Central sensitization, deafferentation of second-order neurons, disinhibition and structural reorganization

NEUROANATOMY: THE PAIN NETWORK

THE PERIPHERAL NERVOUS SYSTEM

Primary sensory neurons have cell bodies outside of the spinal cord within the dorsal root ganglion. A receptor at the end of each neuron lies in the peripheral tissue and transduces environmental signals into an action potential (see later). This is transmitted along an axon which terminates in the dorsal horn of the spinal grey matter (Table 3.2). Sensory neurons can be classified according to cell body size, axon diameter, conduction velocity, degree of myelination and response to various neurotrophic factors.

A-fibres have large cell body diameters and are divided into three subgroups: A-alpha, A-beta and A-delta fibres. A-alpha fibres innervate muscle spindles and golgi tendon organs and their main function is proprioception (Chapter 6.4). A-beta fibres are low-threshold, cutaneous mechanoreceptors.

Nociceptive neurons are divided into A-delta fibres (20%) and C-fibres (80%). A-delta fibres tend to be associated with mechanical and thermal nociceptors (Holdcroft 2005) and respond to one stimulus only (unimodal). Stimulation of A-delta fibres results in sharp, well-localized pain felt almost immediately (Davies & Blakeley 2001). C-fibres have small diameter, unmyelinated axons with free nerve endings (Rang et al 1991, Woolf 1991) associated with polymodal nociceptors which can be stimulated by thermal, mechanical or chemical stimuli. C-fibres cause slower, poorly localized pain. Both C and A-delta fibres may be associated with 'silent nociceptors'. These have very high thresholds for mechanical stimulation and do not fire under normal circumstances (Meyer et al 2006). Nociceptive neurons are found in somatic tissues such as skin, joints, muscle, fascia, tendons, cornea and tooth pulp (Cimino 1992). The concentration of nociceptive neurons within a tissue is positively correlated to that tissue's sensitivity to pain. Nociceptive neurons are also found in viscera, but there are relatively fewer A-delta fibres.

Nociceptive neurons are further divided into two major subgroups: those expressing peptides (peptidergic) and those that do not (non-peptidergic). The majority of peptidergic neurons co-localize substance P (SP) and calcitonin gene-related peptide (CGRP) whilst others contain vaso-active intestinal peptide (VIP) and somatostatin (SS) (Woolf & Ma 2007). Peptidergic nociceptive neurons also contain excitatory neurotransmitters (glutamate). Peptidergic C-fibres project mainly to lamina I and lamina II outer layers of the dorsal horn. Non-peptidergic neurons project to areas within lamina II and contain only neurotransmitters.

Peptidergic and non-peptidergic fibres have different processes of signal transduction and demonstrate different sensitivities to the same stimulus (McMahon et al 2006). Nociceptors are dynamic and shift their properties according to their environment (Schmidt et al 1994). This plasticity allows mediation of homeostatic functions under physiological conditions and sensitization following injury or inflammation.

Table 3.2	The classification of nerve fibres				
FIBRE TYPE (Erlanger and Gasser, 1937)	FUNCTION	GROUP (Lloyd 1943)	FUNCTION	AVERAGE FIBRE DIAMETER (mm)	AVERAGE CONDUCTION VELOCITY (m/s)
A-alpha	Primary muscle spindle afferents, motor fibres to motor neurons	I	Primary muscle spindle afferents for proprioception	15	95
A-beta	Cutaneous touch and pressure afferents	II	Afferents from tendon organs and cutaneous mechanoreceptors	8	50
A-gamma	Motor fibres to muscle spindles	—	—	6	20
A-delta	Thinly myelinated, cutaneous temperature and pain afferents	III	Afferents from deep pressure receptors in muscle	3	15
B	Sympathetic preganglionic C-fibres	—	—	3	7
C	Unmyelinated cutaneous pain afferents, sympathetic postganglionic C-fibres	IV	Unmyelinated nerve fibres	0.5	1

Nociceptive neurons develop from neural crest stem cells that migrate from the dorsal part of the neural tube and are formed late in neurogenesis under the neurotrophic influence of nerve growth factor (NGF) interacting with the tyrosine kinase A (trkA) receptor in the periphery. During perinatal and postnatal development approximately half the nociceptive population switch off the genes necessary for (TrkA) expression. Most of these fibres switch to expressing Ret, the transmembrane signalling component of the receptor for glial cell-derived neurotrophic factor (GDNF) as well as other neurotrophic factors (McMahon et al 2006). These neurons become the non-peptidergic C-fibres and express surface glucoconjugates that bind the lectin IB4 (Molliver et al 1997). Tyrosine kinase activity continues in the remaining half of C-fibres. A-delta fibres express the high-affinity receptor for neurotrophin 3 and tyrosine kinase C. Sensory neurons remain responsive to neurotrophic factors into adulthood and they have effects on the pain experience.

Primary afferent neurons can switch their phenotype as the result of changes in gene expression leading to an up-regulation of various transmitters, receptors, ion channels and growth factors (Table 3.3). After inflammation or injury A-beta fibres can produce and release SP which they do not contain under normal circumstances. This is important for the development of mechanical allodynia which is mediated by A-beta fibres (Coderre et al 2003). Neurotrophins are thought to play an important part in this.

Table 3.3	Molecules up-regulated in phenotypic changes of primary sensory afferents
MOLECULE	EXAMPLE
Transmitter	SP
	CGRP
	Glutamate
	Nitric oxide
Receptors	NK1
	Galanin1
Ion channels	TRPV-1
	Sensory neuron specific sodium channels
Growth factors	NGF
	BDNF

THE SPINAL CORD

The cells in the spinal cord are arranged in laminae. The dorsal horn of the grey matter of the spinal cord is conventionally divided into six layers or laminae (I–VI) on the basis of Rexed's descriptions of their appearance under light microscopy; the ventral horn is divided into three further laminae (laminae VII–IX); and another column of cells arranged around the central canal is lamina X (Cramer & Darby 2005). A-delta and C-fibres carrying nociceptive information terminate in laminae I and II (also known as the substantia gelatinosa because of its translucent appearance on light microscopy).

Primary afferent input to the dorsal horn is mostly ipsilateral (same side), however, there is some contralateral (opposite side) input. Many dorsal horn neurons, especially in lamina II are interneurons which project locally within the spinal cord. Excitatory interneurons contain glutamate, whereas inhibitory interneurons contain GABA, enkephalins and dynorphin. The deep laminae of the dorsal horn contain many pre-motor interneurons and have many projections to ventral horn neurons, the cerebellum and reticular formation where they influence sensorimotor coordination and behaviour (Dostrovsky & Craig 2006).

Microglia and astrocytes are glial cells in the CNS. They are important in modulating neuronal excitability and synaptic transmission and are involved in the initiation and maintenance of neuropathic pain (Hains & Waxman 2006, Hashizume et al 2000).

Projection neurons in the spinal cord transmit information supraspinally and have indirect polysynaptic input from excitatory and inhibitory interneurons allowing processing of information (Coderre et al 2003). Transmission of different types of nociceptive information occurs through two separate pathways, each with its own conduction velocity and termination in the brain (Kerr et al 1955). Phylogenetically, the younger tract is the neospinothalamic tract (STT) while the spinoreticular tract (paleo-spino-reticulo-diencephalic pathway) is older.

The STT is the most prominent ascending nociceptive pathway and arises mainly from laminae I and V of the dorsal horn where most A-delta nociceptive fibres terminate. It passes contralaterally over several spinal cord levels via Lissauer's tract to ascend to the thalamus. This pathway is arranged topographically and placed laterally (predominantly from lamina I) and anteriorly (predominantly from laminae V and VII) within the spinal cord (Dostrovsky & Craig 2006). It is responsible for the identification and localization of a noxious stimulus and determining when this crosses the pain threshold (Melzack & Casey 1968).

STT fibres terminate in either the medial laminae (lateral spinal tracts) or the lateral laminae of the thalamus (anterior spinal tracts). STT terminations from lamina V neurons tend to occur in the ventroposterior nucleus and in the ventral lateral nucleus (VPL). These lateral tracts project from here to the primary somatosensory cortex (Dostrovsky & Craig 2006) and are responsible for the 'sensory-affective' aspects of the pain experience. The posterior part of the ventral medial nucleus of the thalamus (VMpo) serves as a thalamocortical relay nucleus for lamina I STT cells to the insula. Other medial tracts project to the insula and anterior cingulated cortex.

The spinoreticular tract carries noxious information from sensory afferents which terminate in laminae I and II. The tract ascends contralaterally alongside the STT. It separates in the brain and takes a medial route to the brainstem. The tract terminates in four main areas: catecholamine cell groups (ventrolateral medulla, nucleus of the solitary tract, and locus coeruleus) involved in sympathetic outflow; the parabrachial nucleus; the periaqueductal grey matter; and the reticular formation (Dostrovsky & Craig 2006). There are also projections to the anterior cingulate, limbic and frontal cortices. This tract is responsible for the slow, aching, emotional aspects of the pain experience and important for overall cognitive effects (Dostrovsky & Craig 2006).

Some ascending nociceptive information is also transmitted along the spinomesencephalic tract, cervicothalamic tract and spinohypothalamic tract (Basbaum & Jessell 2000). The spinomesencephalic tract arises from laminae I and V neurons and projects to the mesencephalic limbic system and via the parabrachial nuclei to the amygdala and is also involved in the affective component of pain. The cervicothalamic tract arises from the lateral cervical nucleus of the upper two cervical segments of the spinal cord which receives input from nociceptive neurons in laminae III and IV. Most of these axons ascend contralaterally to nuclei in the midbrain and the ventroposterolateral and posteromedial nuclei of the thalamus (Basbaum & Jessell 2000). The spinohypothalamic tract arises from laminae I, V and VIII and projects directly to supraspinal

autonomic control centres and activates neuroendocrine responses (Basbaum & Jessell 2000).

Descending pathways

A descending inhibitory system was first discovered by stimulation of the periaqueductal grey area which produced a profound analgesia allowing surgery without any apparent distress in conscious animals (Reynolds 1969). There are three endogenous descending pathways from the brain for inhibiting pain which are mediated by either serotonin (5-hydroxytryptamine), noradrenaline (norepinephrine) or opioids. Associated brain areas influencing these pathways include the frontal lobe, anterior cingulate cortex, insula, amygdala, hypothalamus, nucleus cuneiformis. The descending pathways involve the medulla, especially the rostroventral medulla (RVM) and the nucleus raphe magnus (NRM) (Gebhart 2004).

Descending noradrenergic input to the spinal cord originates from the dorsolateral pons, locus coeruleus and to some extent the parabrachial nuclei and adrenergic neurons of the ventrolateral medulla (Scholz 2005). Axons then descend to the spinal cord.

The projections of the raphe spinal pathway from the nucleus raphe magnus in the medulla use serotonin (5-hydroxytryptamine) as the neurotransmitter (Dubner & Ren 1999). Axons descend in the dorsolateral funiculus of the spinal cord and synapse with stalked enkephalinergic inhibitory interneurons in the dorsal horn (Basbaum & Jessell 1977). There are also SP and inhibitory enkephalinergic connections between the nucleus raphe magnus and the noradrenergic neurons of the dorsolateral pons (Westlund 2005).

Finally, the diffuse noxious inhibitory control system (DNIC) describes the reduction in pain perception in one part of the body by the application of a noxious stimulus to another area and is mediated by opioids. Endogenous opiate-like substances comprise three groups: the enkephalins, endorphins and dynorphins. These occur throughout the body and act upon mu, kappa and delta opioid receptors within and outside the pain pathways. Mu opioid receptors occur extensively in certain parts of the brain including the medial thalamic nuclei, the reticular formation and the limbic system, as well as within the substantia gelatinosa of the dorsal horn. Only a few occur in the ventrobasal thalamus and post central gyrus associated with the neospinothalamic tract. DNIC is possibly mediated by collaterals linking the neospinothalamic pathway to the subnucleus reticularis dorsalis in the medulla (Villaneuva et al 1988). Axons from here descend in the dorsolateral funiculus and exert an inhibitory effect via the opioid system on neurons responsible for transmitting noxious information to the brain (Bernard 1990).

THE BRAIN

Nociceptive information is transmitted to and processed by a number of brain areas forming a distributed network known as the pain 'neuromatrix' (Tracey & Mantyh 2007). On a simplistic level this can be divided into lateral and medial neuroanatomical components with the former having mainly sensory-discriminatory function and the latter having affective and cognitive functions (Tracey & Mantyh 2007) (Fig. 3.1).

The thalamus

All the sensory pathways synapse with thalamic neurons before reaching the cortex. This allows the thalamus to act as the gateway to the cerebral cortex (Tracey & Mantyh 2007).

The cerebral cortex

The outermost neocortex has a characteristic cytoarchitecture with the cell bodies of cortical neurons arranged in six layers parallel to the surface of the brain. Neurons of layer IV receive synaptic input from outside the cortex, mainly from the thalamus, and make short-distance connections with other layers of cortex (Fatterpekar et al 2002). Neurons in the outer layers II and III tend to project to other neurons of the neocortex while those of layers V and VI transmit information out of the cortex to the thalamus, brainstem and spinal cord. The insula cortex is phylogenetically older than neocortex and the anterior and mid-parts are active in human pain experiences. These neurons are dysgranular in microscopic appearance.

The neospinothalamic pathway projects to the primary somatosensory cortex (S1) which receives a large nociceptive input from the ventroposterolateral nucleus of the thalamus (Fatterpekar et al 2002). Like the spinal cord, S1 is arranged somatotopically so

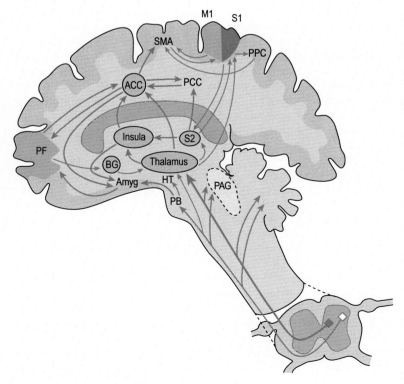

Fig. 3.1 Neuroanatomy of brain areas involved in pain processing. HT, hypothalamus; Amyg, amygdala; PAG, periaqueductal grey; PF, prefrontal cortex; BG, basal ganglia; ACC, anterior cingulate cortex; PCC, posterior cingulate cortex; PPC, posterior parietal cortex; M, motor; S, sensory; SMA, supplementary motor area; PB, pineal body.

that the body homunculus is mapped onto the surface of the cortex with the legs arranged medially and the face laterally. Information is further processed in the secondary somatosensory cortex (S2) and there are close connections with the primary motor cortex as well as parietal inputs.

Limbic system

The limbic system is a set of specialized cortical and subcortical structures bordering the corpus callosum involved in emotions. Areas include the cingulate cortex, hippocampus and amygdala.

The main nociceptive inputs to the anterior cingulate cortex (ACC) are from the thalamus (six medial nuclei: midline, intralaminar, central, parafascicular, reuniens and mediodorsal nuclei) and the amygdala. It also links closely to the prefrontal cortex and is involved in cognitive functions. There are many reciprocal connections with the hypothalamus which allows it to play a part in the regulation of autonomic activity (Luu & Posner 2003). Lesions most consistently result in affective changes: patients are apathetic and unconcerned when significant events occur, such as making mistakes (Luu & Posner 2003).

The hippocampus lies medial to the lateral ventricle and is distinguishable by the pattern in which it is folded upon itself. It is involved in the consolidation of memory. The amygdala is situated in the medial part of the pole of the temporal lobe, just below the cortex. It consists of three groups of nuclei: the basolateral, corticomedial and central nucleus. Input to the amygdala comes from the neocortex of all the lobes of the brain, the hippocampus and the cingulate cortex. Information from the different sensory systems is received by the amygdala and integrated across sensory modalities (Fatterpekar et al 2002).

Frontal lobe

The frontal lobe is involved in personality and behavioural traits. It also contains the motor cortex which is involved in carrying out movement. The prefrontal cortex is involved in sensorimotor incongruence sensing to ensure motor outputs are congruent with intentions (Fink et al 1999). The right ventral area of the lateral prefrontal cortex monitors proprioceptive and visual feedback and is activated by discrepancies between these different sensory signals. A dorsolateral prefrontal area is activated when actions need to be actively maintained in the presence of such conflict between intention and sensory outcome (Fink et al 1999).

NEUROPHYSIOLOGY: THE PAIN NETWORK

PERIPHERAL NERVES AND ION CHANNELS

A neuron or nerve cell is the basic unit of the nervous system and is adapted to transmit information.

Nerves transmit information through action potentials (electrical impulses). A voltage difference exists across the cell membrane with respect to the outside (membrane potential). This is approximately −65 millivolts when the cell is at rest. It is dependent upon the concentration and charges of intra- and extracellular ions which are maintained by ion pumps. Potassium is concentrated inside the cell and sodium and calcium outside (Bear et al 2006).

An action potential is a rapid change in the electrical state of the cell such that for a brief period of time the normally negative interior becomes positively charged with respect to the outside. The initial depolarization needs to reach a threshold in order to generate an action potential. It is important to note that the closer the resting potential is to the threshold, the more excitable the cell will be. The whole action potential lasts approximately two milliseconds at any given part of the neuron.

Sodium and potassium

Depolarization is caused by the influx of sodium ions through voltage-gated sodium channels. This protein forms a pore in the neuronal membrane that is highly selective to sodium ions. It is opened and closed by changes in the electrical potential of the membrane. A conformational change opens the pore and allows the passage of sodium into the cell (Bear et al 2006). Voltage-gated sodium channels open quickly, stay open for approximately 1 millisecond and then close. Once closed, they cannot be opened again until the membrane potential reaches a value near to the resting potential.

There are at least nine different genes encoding different voltage-gated sodium channels with similar structures. These are expressed selectively in different types of neuron (Waxman 2000). Properties such as the threshold, refractory period and pattern of the action potential are determined by the type of sodium channel expressed by a neuron. Changes in transcription can have significant effects on neuronal function (Waxman 2000). A single neuron can switch gene expression to change its phenotype of sodium channels in response to stimuli.

Channelopathies are genetic or acquired diseases caused by alterations in the structure and function of ion channels. They have been described as part of pain syndromes such as erythromelalgia. Mutations in the *SCN9A* gene leading to a loss of function in the Nav1.7 voltage-gated sodium channel result in a congenital indifference to pain without loss of nociceptors or their associated neurons (Cox et al 2006, Goldberg et al 2007). Acquired channelopathies are usually part of an autoimmune process but may be due to dysregulated transcription of a normal gene which results in altered function (Waxman 2001).

Axonal injury can cause such transcriptional channelopathies with abnormal expression of the various subtypes of voltage-gated sodium channel proteins in dorsal root ganglion neurons. This can account for the hyperexcitability of such cells after injury and the propagation of neuropathic pain. These changes may be due to the interruption of access to peripheral pools of neurotrophic factors (Waxman 2001).

Neurons also express voltage-gated potassium channels which open approximately 1 millisecond after the opening of the sodium channel. They allow potassium to leave the cell, prevent any further depolarization and reset the membrane potential.

Potassium channelopathies also cause pathology although they tend to be mediated by autoimmune diseases.

Ligand–gated ion channels and chemical synapses

The action potential is transmitted from the pre-synaptic neuron to the post-synaptic neuron across a synapse. Most synapses in the mature nervous system are chemical, consisting of two nerve endings separated by a synaptic cleft 20–50 nm wide. The pre-synaptic terminal contains many small vesicles containing neurotransmitters (Sudhof 2004).

The release of neurotransmitter is triggered by an action potential at the axon terminal. Depolarization opens voltage-gated calcium channels and the calcium influx causes exocytosis and release of neurotransmitter (Sudhof 2004). This diffuses across the synaptic cleft and binds to specific receptor proteins on the post-synaptic membrane (Sudhof 2004).

The receptors on the postsynaptic membrane responsible for the fast transmission of information are ligand-gated ion channels (Bear et al 2006). If the channel is permeable to sodium, it depolarizes the postsynaptic cell and brings it closer to the threshold. As this effect is excitatory the transient depolarization is termed an excitatory post-synaptic potential (EPSP). The most important excitatory neurotransmitter in the central nervous system is glutamate. Activation of glutamate-gated channels results in EPSPs. If the channel is permeable to chloride, it hyperpolarizes the membrane and takes it further from the threshold, making it more difficult to generate an action potential. This is inhibitory and the transient hyperpolarization is an inhibitory post-synaptic potential (IPSP). The transmitters of inhibitory synapses are glycine or GABA (acting on $GABA_A$ receptors) and result in the movement of chloride ions to cause hyperpolarizing IPSPs (Giuliodori & Zuccolilli 2004).

Neurons integrate the total input into the pre-synaptic terminal into a single output through the process of synaptic integration. The simplest form of this is spatial or temporal summation of EPSPs. Spatial summation is the addition of EPSPs generated simultaneously at many different synapses of the neuron. Temporal summation is the addition of EPSPs generated at the same synapse within close succession of each other (Giuliodori & Zuccolilli 2004). The net activity between IPSPs and EPSPs determines the likelihood of a neuron generating an action potential (Giuliodori & Zuccolilli 2004).

The likelihood of transmission is complicated by activation of G-protein-coupled receptors which generate secondary messengers rather than opening ion channels. These messengers produce changes in gene expression and thus protein synthesis producing slower, longer-lasting changes. Secondary messengers also phosphorylate ligand-gated or voltage-gated ion channels. Phosphorylation causes changes in the properties of these channels and their ionic flow. SP, bradykinin, prostaglandins (EP_3 receptors) and histamine (H_1 receptors) act on receptors positively coupled to phospholipase C (PLC). This enzyme triggers the release of intracellular calcium and protein kinase C (PKC) which phosphorylates the neuronal membrane and increases sodium and calcium flow through the channel. Adenosine, CGRP ($CGRP_1$, $CGRP_2$ receptors), histamine, prostaglandins (EP_2, EP_4 receptors), serotonin ($5HT_4$, $5HT_7$ receptors) act on receptors positively coupled to adenylate cyclase to increase cyclic AMP (cAMP) which causes membrane phosphorylation (Coderre 2003). $GABA_B$ receptors are negatively coupled to adenylate cyclase and reduce calcium influx, increase potassium influx and cause hyperpolarization and reduced release of neurotransmitter (Coderre et al 2003).

SP and CGRP are co-localized with aspartate and glutamate in a subset of primary afferents. Neuropeptide receptors are coupled to PLC by G-proteins and cause slow, long-lasting depolarization of dorsal horn neurons. They act as neuromodulators and enhance the response of dorsal horn neurons to excitation. They may also relieve the magnesium block of NMDA receptors and facilitate glutamate and aspartate release from primary afferents (Coderre et al 2003).

Complex interactions between neurotransmitters and neuropeptides determine the transmission activity. For example, glutamate is an important excitatory transmitter in the nervous system and in the dorsal horn activates both NMDA and AMPA receptors (Carpenter & Dickenson 2005). AMPA receptors are ligand-gated sodium ion channels and experimental excitation produces short-lived depolarization. It is a fast method of relaying nociceptive information. Blocking AMPA receptors in rats reduces thermal hyperalgesia and mechanical allodynia (Bardoni et al 2004).

Activation of NMDA receptors results in membrane depolarizations which are slower to rise and longer-lasting. The receptor is tightly controlled by magnesium ions which block the channel and is only released during sustained membrane depolarization. Activation of large numbers of NMDA receptors change the likelihood of nociceptive transmission and allow 'sensitization' to occur (Carpenter & Dickenson 2005).

THE SPINAL CORD

At this level the pain pathway may be modulated by either sensory afferents at the same spinal level, by neural pathways descending from higher centres in the brain or by interneurons. Furthermore, the previous state of the system (for example sensitization) influences the likelihood of transmission.

Three types of transmission neuron within the spinal cord transmit sensory information to the brain. Nociceptive neurons are present mainly in lamina I and transmit A-delta and C-fibre nociceptive inputs from the skin to the brain (Christensen & Perl 1970). Wide dynamic-range neurons are present in all the laminae but are concentrated in laminae V, VII and VIII and respond to a wide range of stimuli both noxious and innocuous. Non-nociceptive neurons are located mainly in laminae III and IV and transmit proprioceptive information.

Descending pathways

Noradrenergic, serotonergic and opioid systems all have inhibitory effects on pain transmission at the spinal cord. Descending axons have direct contacts with pain-relay neurons in the dorsal horn. Electrical stimulation of the brainstem has been shown to produce inhibitory post-synaptic potentials in nociceptive neurons of the spinal dorsal horn (Westlund et al 1990, Giesler et al 1981). There are very few direct synapses between central neurons and primary afferents however, and most effects are thought to be mediated by interneurons or neurotransmitter diffusion (Stone et al 1988, Rudomin & Schmidt 1999).

Stimulation of noradrenergic neurons produces an inhibitory effect on dorsal horn cells by acting pre-synaptically at the spinal level to inhibit the release of SP. This has an important role in regulating morphine-induced analgesia in response to mechanical nociceptive stimuli (Dubner & Ren 1999).

There are two different types of serotonergic neurons in the RVM and the NRM. 'On' cells mediate descending facilitation of pain, whereas 'off' cells mediate descending inhibition (Dubner & Ren 1999). Descending facilitation of pain may be due in part to reduced activity of 'off' cells.

The observation that 'pain inhibits pain' underpins DNIC. Dorsal horn neuronal responses are reduced when a second noxious stimulus is applied outside their receptive field. DNIC occurs in a widespread non-somatotopic fashion and its effect increases in proportion to the strength of the noxious counter-stimulus. Opioids cause spinal pre-synaptic inhibition and post-synaptic hyperpolarization of excitatory interneurons (Trafton et al 2000).

THE BRAIN

Certain brain areas are consistently activated in experimentally induced pain using imaging modalities such as positron emission tomography (PET), functional magnetic resonance imaging (fMRI), electroencephalography (EEG) and magnetoencephalography (MEG). These include the thalamus, S1, S2/parietal cortex, insula, anterior cingulate and pre-frontal cortices (Fig. 3.1) (Apkarian et al 2005).

Pain perception is altered by context, attention, stimulus-type, learning and emotional state. Most of the neuromatrix is activated by anticipation of a painful stimulus (Jones et al 2003). A painful stimulus decreases auditory perception, language processing and visuospatial brain activations. Pain demands attention over other brain functions, it 'fills the space of consciousness' (Hsieh et al 1995).

The thalamus

The thalamus is an important integration centre. Thalamic neurons have small receptive fields, allowing precise location of injury (Basbaum & Jessell 2000). Lateral inhibition emphasizes somatopic information.

Primary somatosensory cortex

Neuronal activity in S1 is correlated with the duration and intensity of nociceptive stimuli. Receptive fields are restrictive and there is somatotopic organization of activation. Inhibition as well as excitation occurs.

Secondary somatosensory cortex and posterior parietal cortex

Neurons exhibit bilateral receptive fields to nociceptive stimuli with polymodal activation, especially from visual cues. There are mainly excitatory effects and very little inhibition. The posterior parietal cortex holds intra- and extra-personal spatial representations, including a body scheme allowing individuals a sense of 'self' (Hsieh et al 1995). Lesions in and around this region, especially in the white matter underlying the posterior parietal cortex can give rise to pain perception abnormalities in humans (Berthier et al 1988, Greenspan & Winfield 1992) as well as pain asymbolia (neglect), hypoalgesia, analgesia and spontaneous pain. This implies that the region may be uniquely involved in the conscious subjective experience of pain (Schmahmann & Liefer 1992, Apkarian et al 1999). There are direct outputs to the insula and temporal lobe structures involved in memory and learning.

Insula

The insula acts as a relay of sensory information into the limbic system and is important in memory, motivational and affective components including the 'unpleasantness' of the pain experience and autonomic activation (Hsieh et al 1995). This is the only area consistently activated by noxious and innocuous thermal stimuli, suggesting an important role in thermal monitoring (Craig et al 1996).

Anterior cingulate cortex

These neurons have non-somatotopic, large receptive fields sometimes of the entire organism. Many neurons are nociceptive unimodally whereas others behave polymodally, responding to noxious heat and noxious pressure. The only non-noxious stimulus to activate these neurons is 'tapping'. The anterior cingulate cortex is most reliably activated by applying differing noxious stimuli (Apkarian et al 2005). Simultaneously applying non-noxious, non-activating warm and cold stimuli is found to cause both activity in the ACC and the perception of pain (Thunberg's illusion). The ACC also forms connections with the motor system and is important in avoidance learning and in processing the affective component of pain (Vogt et al 1993). It is extremely important in attributing emotional overtones and attention to pain and cingulotomy has been shown to reduce the affective impact, attention and cognitive appraisal of intractable pain while maintaining pain perception (Ploner et al 2002).

Prefrontal cortex

Prefrontal cortex activity is closely related to ACC activity after noxious stimuli. The medial and dorsolateral prefrontal areas are most active. Damage here results in reduced planning, behavioural control, affective attachment and directed or prolonged attention (Fink et al 1999, Hsieh et al 1995).

Primary motor cortex

There is a large confluent activation of the primary somatosensory cortex and motor cortex. Activity of these two areas can be correlated to the intensity of the painful stimulus. This activation may be due to the function of these two areas in integrating the sensorimotor response (Hsieh et al 1995).

Amygdala

The amygdala is involved in fear, as reported by conscious patients upon direct electrical stimulation. It is involved in emotional learning and the memory formation of emotional events (McGaugh 2004). It is activated when emotional significance is assigned to events through the learning of associations between cues and positive experiences (Gallagher & Holland 1994). The latero-capsular division of the central nucleus is considered the 'nociceptive amygdala' and integrates nociceptive information with polymodal sensory information regarding the internal and external environment. Nerves from the central nucleus project to the peri-aqueductal grey matter and hypothalamus causing changes in the autonomic nervous system (Neugebauer et al 2004).

Hypothalamus

Spinal nociception goes to the hypothalamic centres including the autonomic and neuroendocrine control centres which modulate the stress responses (Kupferman 2000). Stress hormones and the neuroendocrine response are mediated through nociceptive effects via the hypothalamus.

MECHANISMS OF PAIN

GATE–CONTROL THEORY

The gate-control theory (Melzack & Wall 1965) states that in each dorsal horn there exists a 'gate' responsible for inhibiting or facilitating afferent impulses. The control of this 'gate' depends upon the relative activity in large-diameter (A-beta) fibres and small-diameter (A-delta and C-) fibres. Large-diameter fibre activity closes the 'gate', while small-diameter fibre activity opens it. Descending pathways from the brain also close the gate.

Lamina II of the dorsal horn where many inhibitory neurons are situated is the physical location of the gate. Large-diameter myelinated fibres excite inhibitory interneurons and reduce the presynaptic input to the transmission cells, thereby inhibiting pain. Activity in small-diameter unmyelinated A-delta and C-fibres inhibits the inhibitory neurons (disinhibition) and facilitates the transmission of noxious impulses to the transmission cells, resulting in pain.

This theory explains the scientific rationale of the efficacy of transcutaneous electrical nerve stimulation (TENS) in reducing pain and why rubbing an injured area helps to reduce the pain. Both of these stimulate A-beta fibres and block the transmission of nociceptive information.

PERIPHERAL SENSITIZATION

Trauma, inflammation or nerve damage can cause changes to the properties of nociceptive neurons that result in increased sensitivity to pain. This is known as peripheral sensitization. It occurs outside the CNS and results in low-intensity stimulation causing primary hyperalgesia, most commonly associated with damaged tissue (Scholz & Woolf 2007).

The cardinal signs of acute inflammation are *dolor* (pain), *tumor* (swelling), *calor* (heat), *rubor* (redness) coupled with *functio laesa* (loss of function). These are mediated by the release of inflammatory substances from various cells (Table 3.4). Many of these act on both nociceptors and their primary afferents. Furthermore, neuropeptides (e.g. SP, CGRP) contained in nociceptive neurons can also cause neurogenic inflammation when they are released in the periphery. These induce vasodilation, plasma extravasation and activation of inflammatory cells (Scholz & Woolf 2007).

Within the nociceptor, transduction molecules are activated such as transient receptor potential ion channel (TRPV1). This excitatory cation channel is activated by noxious heat, capsaicin and protons. Following inflammation, the proportion of TRPV1 unmyelinated axons in the periphery increases almost two-fold with a corresponding increase in the sensitivity of DRG neurons and primary afferent fibres (Meyer et al 2006).

Prostaglandin PGE_2 and bradykinin via the activation of PKA and PKC cause changes in the expression of the voltage-gated sodium channel Nav1.8. This changes the resting potential and increases the excitability of the terminal membrane leading to increased transmission of pain (Ji et al 2003).

Table 3.4	Algesic substances involved in peripheral sensitization	
SUBSTANCE	**SOURCE**	**ACTION**
Bradykinin	Mast cells	Vasodilation, extravasation
Substance P	Primary afferents	Vasodilation, extravasation, nociceptor sensitization
Calcitonin gene-related peptide	Primary afferents	Vasodilation, extravasation, nociceptor sensitization
Hydrogen ions	Damaged tissue	Direct depolarization of sensory neurons
Prostaglandins and leukotrienes	Membrane phospholipid	Reduced pain threshold, vasodilation and extravasation
Catecholamines (noradrenaline, adrenaline)	Sympathetic nerves	Sensitization of nociceptors
Interleukins (pro-IL1, IL1b, IL6, TNFa)	Fibroblasts, macrophages, keratinocytes, mast cells	Stimulate SP release

Other substances involved in peripheral sensitization include potassium (from damaged tissue) and serotonin.

Nerve damage recruits inflammatory cells which release pro-inflammatory cytokines (Table 3.4) (Scholz & Woolf 2007). Proinflammatory cytokines contribute to further axonal damage, but are also involved in modulating spontaneous nociceptor activity and sensitivity. The recruitment of macrophages and T cells leads to up-regulation of *c-fos* and other genes in the dorsal horn which increase synthesis of cytokines such as interleukins (IL1, IL6) and tumour necrosis factor alpha (TNFα). These can have direct effects on neuronal activity by generating spontaneous action potentials (Costigan 2002). These cytokines also modulate the synthesis of neuropeptide transmitters which has an effect upon the presynaptic input to the spinal cord.

CENTRAL SENSITIZATION

Central sensitization describes the changes in the spinal processing of information from primary afferent neurons leading to continued hyperalgesia and widened areas of hyperalgesia and allodynia (Carpenter & Dickenson 2005). It is an important aspect of neuroplasticity in the nociceptive system in the response to injury. As the resting potential of a dorsal horn neuron increases towards threshold, it becomes more excitable; it responds to weaker stimuli and fires with input that is not normally sufficient to produce an action potential. This expands the peripheral receptive field, creating an area of secondary hyperalgesia in the surrounding undamaged tissue. This central sensitization occurs in classic and neurogenic inflammation. Continuous nociceptive activity shifts the state of the dorsal horn from basal to suppressed and then sensitized modes. There is an abrupt switching from a system that suppresses to one that enhances its response to a stimulus (Woolf & Mannion 1999).

Long-term potentiation occurs in the dorsal horn, especially lamina I, due to a synergistic activation of NMDA and NK1 receptor activation as well as low-threshold T-type calcium channels to increase intracellular calcium levels above a certain threshold (Ji et al 2003). Intense nociceptor activity causes activation of glutamate NMDA receptors, SP neurokinin 1 (NK1) receptors, and brain-derived neurotrophic factor (BDNF) trkB receptors. There is then PKA, PKC and ERK activation. ERK leads to phosphorylation of cAMP-response-element binding protein (CREB). There is also increased expression of early response genes encoding *c-fos* and COX-2 and late-response genes encoding prodynorphin, NK1 and trk B in the dorsal horn. Blocking ERK activation reverses these transcriptional changes (Ji et al 2003).

Glial cells are involved in the development of central sensitization in pathological pain. Activated microglia cause up-regulation of proinflammatory cytokines (e.g. IL-6, -12, and -18). Pain processing is facilitated by presynaptic release of neurotransmitter and increased postsynaptic excitability (McMahon et al 2006). This is then followed by astrocytic activation which is thought to maintain exaggerated pain in both neuropathic and inflammatory pain (Cao & Zhang 2008). Activated microglia in the CNS release brain-derived growth factor (BDNF) causing depolarization of lamina I neurons. This reverses the polarity of currents activated by GABA. Blocking BDNF can reverse these membrane potential changes and reduce allodynia (Coull et al 2005).

Damaged fibres are activated by sympathetic noradrenergic stimulation.

Noradrenaline (norepinephrine) acts on α_1 receptors coupled to PLC to increase inflammatory hyperalgesia (Coderre et al 2003). Noradrenaline α_2 receptors usually present on dorsal root ganglion sensory neurons increase five-fold in number following injury leading to an abnormal sensitivity to noradrenaline. This may contribute to neuropathic pain (Scholz 2005).

WIND UP

The phenomenon known as 'wind-up' describes the abnormal temporal summation that corresponds with increasing neuronal activity caused by repeated subthreshold stimulation of C-fibres with impulses less than 5 Hz. Repetitive low-intensity stimuli which usually act on A-beta fibres elicit pain as there is a summation of these impulses within the secondary neuron. There is a cumulative depolarization that removes the voltage-gated magnesium block on NMDA receptors and increases glutamate sensitivity. This leads to a progressive increase in the action potential elicited by each stimulus (Ji et al 2003). Wind-up pain can be produced by mechanical, thermal and chemical stimuli.

Substance P is a key mediator of wind-up and central sensitization in chronic pain states and knockout mice for the NK1 receptor do not exhibit these phenomena (De Felipe et al 1998).

AUTONOMIC AND ENDOCRINE INFLUENCES ON PAIN

The hypothalamus, amygdala and peri-aqueductal grey matter integrate the responses to aversive stimuli and modulate the endocrine and autonomic responses to pain and aggressive–defensive behaviours.

The autonomic nervous system consists of two parallel, functionally opposing parts: the sympathetic and parasympathetic divisions (Chapter 6.1). The sympathetic nervous system coordinates the behavioural response to tissue trauma and the 'fight-or-flight' response to threatening stimuli. Hypothalamic activation of the hypothalamo–pituitary–adrenal axis results in the release of adrenaline (epinephrine) which prepares the organism for escape or confrontation. Cognitive hypervigilance, pupillary dilatation, increased cardiac output, respiratory rate and blood glucose level result (Donaldson et al 2003). Fear responses and aversive emotional arousal are related.

Growth hormone deficiency parallels many of the symptoms present in patients with fibromyalgia. Replacement of growth hormone leads to normalization of IGF-1 levels and improvement in symptoms (Jones et al 2007).

Melatonin is a hormone synthesized by the pineal gland. In animal models of acute pain, intrathecal or systemic administration produces dose-dependent analgesia. It significantly reduces activity of spinal dorsal horn neurons caused by C-fibre activation by reducing voltage-gated calcium currents and inhibits wind-up (Ambriz-Tututi & Granados-Soto 2007). Activation of the endogenous melatonin system within the spinal cord reduces the development and propagation of central sensitization (Tu et al 2004).

Pain is a stressor and results in cortisol release. Cortisol levels prior to noxious stimulation can predict lower pain rating, especially in men. Reduced adrenocortical activity is associated with various chronic pain syndromes, such as fibromyalgia and chronic fatigue syndrome (Al-Absi & Petersen 2003).

PSYCHOLOGICAL ASPECTS

Psychological influences are important factors contributing to an individual's experience of a noxious stimulus as well as determining those at risk of developing chronic pain after an acute injury. Pain is intimately related to fear and anxiety (Buer & Linton 2002). Both result in a similar activation of the sympathetic nervous system. Persistent pain is more commonly associated with anxiety disorders than with other psychiatric diagnoses (Chapter 5). Acute pain is characterized by a pattern of physiological responses similar to that seen in anxiety disorders while chronic pain follows that seen in depressive disorders (Vlaeyen & Linton 2000).

The transition from acute to chronic pain may be determined by the concept of fear-avoidance (Chapter 8). This model (Fig. 3.2) describes the 'fear of pain' and subsequent avoidance of movement (Vlaeyen 2000). Avoidance describes a learned behaviour that postpones or prevents an aversive event. Patients learn that avoiding situations which provoke or increase pain reduces the likelihood of further painful episodes (Fordyce et al 1982, Lohnberg 2007). A non-noxious pain-associated stimulus leads to avoidance learning so that this neutral stimulus causes a negative

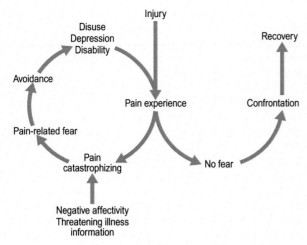

Fig. 3.2 Fear–avoidance model. There are two opposing behavioural responses to pain: confrontation and avoidance. This determines whether the individual falls into a vicious cycle of increasing avoidance, disability and pain

reaction. Avoidance of the threatening situation is reinforced as it leads to a reduction in fear, anxiety and pain, whereas fear returns when the avoidance behaviour cannot be performed. In the long term this causes functional disability as well as depression and disuse, both of which reduce pain tolerance and promote further pain (Vlaeyen & Linton 2000).

PLASTICITY, LEARNING AND PAIN MEMORY

Although the capacity of neurons to regenerate in adult life is limited, they can undergo significant reorganization (Feldman & Brecht 2005). Plasticity describes these anatomical and functional changes that come about as a result of experience. The effects of plasticity can improve recovery after injury to the central nervous system but excessive maladaptive plasticity is implicated in the development of chronic pain (Cheetham & Finnerty 2007).

Cortical reorganization consists of early functional modification followed by long-term structural changes (Cheetham & Finnerty 2007). Functional modifications include alterations in synaptic strength due to long-term potentiation or depression (Cheetham et al 2007). Structural changes can occur in the shape of the dendritic spines (the postsynaptic component of the synapse) as a result of modification in synaptic strength. Strengthening or

weakening of connections between neurons reflect the number of synapses involved (Cheetham & Finnerty 2007). New connections may be formed by axonal growth and dendritic remodelling, although such rewiring only occurs extensively following damage (Chklovskii et al 2004).

Plastic changes can take place in the periphery with changes in neurotransmitter, receptor and ion-channel reorganization. In the spinal cord, sensitization and disinhibition reflect plasticity. In the brain there can be functional changes in representational fields (May 2008). The interaction between these levels and the immune system, autonomic nervous system and higher cognitive functions is also subject to change. The most consistent changes in chronic pain are a decrease in the grey matter of the cingulate cortex, the orbitofrontal cortex, the insula and the dorsal pons. This may be due to a change in cell size, shrinkage or atrophy of neurons or glia as well as loss of synapses through changes in the intracortical axonal architecture (May 2008).

Changes in functional organization can be examined by studying the cortical representation of a body part on the somatosensory cortex. There may be a change in the area of cortex representing the painful body part suggesting that chronic pain leads to an expansion of the cortical representation zone related to nociceptive input. This is also positively correlated with the chronicity of the pain implying that this reorganization develops over time (Flor 2003). Such alterations in the cortex may be considered a somatosensory pain memory, similar to that occurring in phantom limb patients. These memories can be explicit, for example patients' recollection that the phantom pain was similar to their previous pain. They may also be implicit, based on changes in the brain which do not enter conscious awareness but cause changes in behaviour or perception such as hyperalgesia and allodynia. As the patient is unaware of these memories, they cannot be counteracted and may lead to pain perception in the absence of peripheral stimulation (Flor 2003). This pain is centrally represented (Katz & Melzack 1990).

Pain is a conscious experience and the brain actively alters the input of conscious information to create an adaptable model of the body, the world around it and its sense of 'self'. Memories are reconstructions of the past rather than exact replications (Mountcastle 1998, Schachter et al 1998). The brain deals with an internal representation of reality which it builds and revises by integrating sensory information and networks of association. It constructs pain from complex patterns of massive parallel processing within each individual's model of their self, their world and previous value-laden experiences to influence future responses and perceptions (Chapman 2005).

Learning mechanisms such as habituation (repeated stimulus ceases to have an effect), sensitization (repeated stimulus has an enhanced effect), operant (association made between a behaviour and a consequence) and classical conditioning (association made between two stimuli) can affect implicit pain memories. This affects pain behaviours and the subjective experience of pain and importantly, the physiological processing of painful stimulation (Flor 2003). This is evidenced by the increased cortical electrical signal elicited by painful stimuli in patients whose spouses reinforce pain.

SUMMARY

The mechanisms for pain perception are extremely complex, highly developed and plastic. Chronic pain is a significant cause of morbidity. There is altered nervous system function that underlies the development and persistence of chronic pain, even in the absence of tissue damage. Many different brain areas are activated in the perception of pain and various factors determine pain perception and the individual's response.

As our understanding of the basic science improves we can hope for the development of more effective pharmacological and non-pharmacological treatments.

References

Al-Absi M, Petersen KL: Blood pressure but not cortisol mediates stress effects on subsequent pain perception in healthy men and women, *Pain* 106:285–295, 2003.

Ambriz-Tututi M, Granados-Soto V: Oral and spinal melatonin reduces tactile allodynia in rats via activation of MT_2 and opioid receptors, *Pain* 132:273–280, 2007.

Apkarian AV, Darbar A, Krauss BR, et al: Differentiating cortical areas related to pain perception from stimulus identification: temporal analysis of fMRI activity, *J Neurophysiol* 81:2956–2963, 1999.

Apkarian AV, Bushnell MC, Treede RD, et al: Human brain mechanisms of pain perception in health and disease, *Eur J Pain* 9:463–484, 2005.

Baldry PE: *Myofascial pain and fibromyalgia syndromes*, Edinburgh, 2001, Churchill Livingstone, pp 17–39.

Bardoni R, Torsney C, Tong CK, et al: Presynaptic NMDA receptors modulate glutamate release from primary sensory neurons in rat spinal cord dorsal horn, *J Neurosci* 24:2774–2781, 2004.

Basbaum AI, Maley JE, O'Keefe J, et al: Reversal of morphine and stimulus-produced analgesia by subtotal spinal cord lesion, *Pain* 3:43–56, 1977.

Basbaum AI, Jessell TM: The perception of pain. In Kandel ER, Schwartz JH, Jessell TM, editors: *Principles of neural science*, ed 4, New York, 2000, McGraw-Hill, pp 472–483.

Bear MF, Connors BW, Paradiso MA: *Neuroscience: Exploring the brain*, ed 3, 2006, Lippincott Williams and Wilkins.

Bernard JF, Villaneuva L, Carroue J, et al: Efferent projections from the subnucleus reticularis dorsalis (SRD): a phasolus vulgaris leucoagglutinin study in the rat, *Neurosci Lett* 116:257–262, 1990.

Berthier M, Starkstein S, Leigurda R: Asymbolia for pain: a sensory-limbic disconnection syndrome, *Ann Neurol* 24:41–49, 1988.

Breivik H, Collett B, Ventafridda V, et al: Survey of chronic pain in Europe: prevalence, impact on daily life and treatment, *Eur J Pain* 10:287–333, 2006.

Buer N, Linton SJ: Fear-avoidance beliefs and catastrophising: occurrence and risk factor in back pain and ADL in the general population, *Pain* 99:485–491, 2002.

Cao H, Zhang YQ: Spinal glial activation contributes to pathological pain states, *Neurosci Biobehav Rev* 32:972–983, 2008.

Carpenter K, Dickenson A: Peripheral and central sensitization. In Holdcroft A, editor: *Core topics in pain*, Cambridge, 2005, Cambridge University Press, pp 29–32.

Chapman CR: Psychological aspects of pain: a consciousness studies perspective. In Pappagallo M, editor: *The neurological basis of pain*, New York, 2005, McGraw-Hill, pp 157–169.

Cheetham CE, Finnerty G: Plasticity and its role in neurological diseases of the adult nervous system, *Advances in Clinical Neuroscience and Rehabilitation* 7:8–9, 2007.

Cheetham CE, Hammond MS, Edwards CE, et al: Sensory experience alters cortical connectivity and synaptic function site specifically, *J Neurosci* 27:3455–3465, 2007.

Chklovskii DB, Mel BW, Svoboda K: Cortical rewiring and information storage, *Nature* 431:782–788, 2004.

Christensen BN, Perl ER: Spinal neurons specifically excited by noxious or thermal stimuli: marginal zone of the dorsal horn, *J Neurophysiol* 33:293–307, 1970.

Cimino C: Painful neurological syndromes. In Aronoff GM, editor: *Evaluation and treatment of chronic pain*, ed 2, Baltimore, 1992, Williams and Wilkins, pp 56–66.

Coderre TJ, Mogill JS, Bushnell MC: The biological psychology of pain. In Gallagher M, Nelson RJ, Weiner IB, editors: *Handbook of psychology*, vol 3, New Jersey, 2003, John Wiley & Sons, pp 237–257.

Costigan M: Replicate high-density rat genome oligonucleotide microassays reveal hundreds of regulated genes in the dorsal root ganglion after peripheral nerve injury, *BMC Neurosci* 3:16, 2002.

Coull JAM, Beggs S, Boudreau D, et al: BDNF from microglia causes the shift in neuronal anion gradient underlying neuropathic pain, *Nature* 438:923–927, 2005.

Cox JJ, Reimann F, Nicholas AK, et al: An SCN9A channelopathy causes congenital inability to experience pain, *Nature* 44:894–898, 2006.

Craig AD, Reiman EM, Evans A, et al: Functional imaging of an illusion of pain, *Nature* 385:258–260, 1996.

Cramer GD, Darby SA: *Basic and clinical anatomy of the spine, spinal cord and ANS*, 2005, St. Louis, Elsevier Mosby, pp 88–93.

Davies A, Blakeley AGH, Kidd C: *Human Physiology*, Edinburgh, 2001, Churchill Livingstone, pp 265–275.

De Felipe C, Herrero JF, O'Brien JA, et al: Altered nociception, analgesia and aggression in mice lacking the receptor for substance P, *Nature* 392:394–397, 1998.

Deleo JA: Basic science of pain, *J Bone Joint Surg* 88A(S2):58–62, 2006.

Descartes R: *Treatise of man* (Hall TS, translator), Cambridge, MA, 1972, Harvard University Press.

Donaldson GW, Chapman CR, Nakamura Y, et al: Pain and the defense response: structural equation modelling reveals a coordinated psychophysiological response to increasing painful stimulation, *Pain* 102:97–108, 2003.

Dostrovsky JO, Craig AD: Ascending projection systems. In McMahon SB, Koltzenburg M, editors: *Wall and Melzack's Textbook of Pain*, ed 5, London, 2006, Elsevier Churchill Livingstone, pp 187–203.

Dubner R, Ren K: Endogenous mechanisms of sensory modulation, *Pain* Suppl 6:545–553, 1999.

Erlanger J, Gasser HS: *Electrical signs of nervous activity*, USA, 1937, University of Pennsylvania Press, H. Milford, Oxford University Press in Philadelphia, pp 206–216.

Fatterpekar GM, Naidich TP, Delman BN, et al: Cytoarchitecture of the human cerebral cortex: MR microscopy of excised specimens at 9.4 Tesla, *AJNR Am J Neuroradiol* 23:1313–1321, 2002.

Feldman DE, Brecht M: Map plasticity in the somatosensory cortex, *Science* 310:810–815, 2005.

Fink GR, Marshall JC, Halligan PW, et al: The neural consequences of conflict between intention and the senses, *Brain* 122:497–512, 1999.

Flor H: Cortical reorganisation and chronic pain: implications for rehabilitation, *J Rehabil Med* 41 (Suppl):66–72, 2003.

Fordyce WE, Shelton JL, Dundore DE: The modification of avoidance learning in pain behaviours, *J Behav Med* 5:405–414, 1982.

Gallagher M, Holland PC: The amygdala complex: multiple roles in associative learning and attention, *Proc Natl Acad Sci U S A* 91:11771–11776, 1994.

Gebhart GF: Descending modulation of pain, *Neurosci Biobehav Rev* 27:729–737, 2004.

Giesler GJ, Gerhart KD, Yezierski RP, et al: Postsynaptic inhibition of primate spinothalamic neurons by stimulation in nucleus raphe magnus, *Brain Res* 204:184–188, 1981.

Giuliodori MJ, Zuccolilli G: Post-synaptic potential summation and action potential initiation: function following form, *Adv Physiol Educ* 28:79–80, 2004.

Goldberg YP, MacFarlane J, MacDonald ML, et al: Loss of function mutations in the Nav1.7 gene underlie congenital indifference to pain in multiple human populations, *Clin Genet* 71:311–319, 2007.

Greenspan JD, Winfield JA: Reversible Pain and Tactile Deficits in a Patient with a Tumor Compressing the Posterior Insula and Parietal Operculum, *Pain* 50:29–39, 1992.

Hains BC, Waxman SG: Activated microglia contribute to the maintenance of chronic pain after spinal cord injury, *J Neurosci* 26:4308–4317, 2006.

Hashizume H, Deleo JA, Colburn RW, et al: Spinal glial activation and cytokine expression after lumbar root injury in the rat, *Spine* 25:1206–1217, 2000.

Holdcroft A: Peripheral and central sensitization. In Holdcroft A, editor: *Core topics in pain*, Cambridge, 2005, Cambridge University Press, pp 29–32.

Hsieh JC, Stahle-Backdahl M, Hagermark O, et al: Traumatic nociceptive pain activates the hypothalamus and the periaqueductal gray: a positron emission tomography study, *Pain* 64:303–314, 1995.

Ji RR, Kohno T, Moore KA, et al: Central sensitization and LTP: do pain and memory share similar mechanisms? *Trends Neurosci* 26(12):696–703, 2003.

Jones AKP, Kulkarni B, Derbyshire SWG: Pain mechanisms and their disorders, *Br Med Bull* 65:83–93, 2003.

Jones KD, Deodhar P, Lorentzen A, et al: Growth hormone perturbations in fibromyalgia: a review, *Semin Arthritis Rheum* 354–376, 2007.

Katz J, Melzack R: Pain 'memories' in phantom limbs: review and clinical observations, *Pain* 43:319–336, 1990.

Kerr DIB, Haughen FP, Melzack R: Responses evoked in the brainstem by tooth stimulation, *Am J Physiol* 183:252–258, 1955.

Kupferman I: Hypothalamus and limbic system: peptidergic neurons, homeostasis and emotional behaviour. In Kandel ER, Schwartz JH, Jessell TM, editors: *Principles of neural science*, ed 4, New York, 2000, McGraw-Hill, pp 735–749.

Lloyd DPC: Neuron patterns controlling transmission of ipsilateral hind limb reflexes in cat, *J Neurophysiol* 6:293–315, 1943.

Lohnberg JA: A review of outcome studies on cognitive-behavioral therapy for reducing fear-avoidance beliefs among individuals with chronic pain, *J Clin Psychol Med Settings* 14:113–122, 2007.

Luu P, Posner MI: Anterior cingulate cortex regulation of sympathetic activity, *Brain* 126:2119–2120, 2003.

May A: Chronic pain may change the structure of the brain, *Pain* 137:7–15, 2008.

McGaugh JL: The amygdala modulates the consolidation of memories of emotionally arousing experiences, *Annu Rev Neurosci* 27:1–28, 2004.

McMahon SB, Bennett DL, Bevan S: Inflammatory mediators and modulators of pain. In McMahon SB, Koltzenburg M, editors: *Wall and Melzack's Textbook of Pain*, ed 5, London, 2006, Elsevier Churchill Livingstone, pp 49–73.

Melzack R, Wall PD: Pain mechanisms: a new theory, *Science* 150:971–979, 1965.

Melzack R, Casey KL: Sensory, motivational and central control determinants of pain: a new conceptual model. In Kenshalo D, editor: *The skin senses*, Springfield IL, 1968, CC Thomas, pp 423–443.

Merskey H: Pain terms: a list with definitions and notes on usage International Association for the Study of Pain, *Pain* 6:249–252, 1979.

Meyer R, Ringkamp M, Campbell JN, et al: Peripheral mechanisms of cutaneous nociception. In McMahon SB, Koltzenburg M, editors: *Wall and Melzack's Textbook of Pain*, ed 5, London, 2006, Elsevier Churchill Livingstone, pp 3–35.

Molliver DC, Wright DE, Leitner ML, et al: IB4-binding DRG neurons switch from NGF to GDNF dependence in early life, *Neuron* 19:849–861, 1997.

Mountcastle VB: Brain science at the century's ebb, *Daedalus* 127:1–36, 1998.

Neugebauer V, Weidong L, Bird GC, et al: The amygdala and persistent pain, *Neuroscientist* 10:221–234, 2004.

Pearce N, Merletti F: Complexity, simplicity and epidemiology, *Int J Epidemiol* 35(3):515–519, 2006.

Ploner M, Gross J, Timmermann L, et al: Cortical representation of first and second pain sensation in humans, *Proc Natl Acad Sci U S A* 99(19):12444–12448, 2002.

Plsek PE, Greenhalgh T: The challenge of complexity in health care, *BMJ* 323:625–628, 2001.

Rang HP, Bevan S, Dray A: Chemical activation of nociceptive peripheral neurons, *Br Med Bull* 47(3):534–548, 1991.

Reynolds DV: Surgery in the cat during electrical analgesia induced by focal brain stimulation, *Science* 164:444–445, 1969.

Rudomin P, Schmidt RF: Presynaptic inhibition in the vertebrate spinal cord revisited, *Exp Brain Res* 129:1–37, 1999.

Schachter DL, Norman KA, Koutstaal W: The cognitive neuroscience of constructive memory, *Annu Rev Psychol* 49:289–318, 1998.

Schmahmann JD, Leifer D: Parietal pseudothalamic pain syndrome, clinical features and anatomic correlates, *Arch Neurol* 49:1032–1037, 1992.

Schmidt RF, Schaible HG, Meblinger K, et al: Silent and active nociceptors: structure, functions and clinical implications. In Gebhardt GF, Hammond DL, Jensen TS, editors: *Progress in pain research and management-Proceedings of the 7th World Conference on Pain*, vol 2, Seattle, 1994, IASP Press, pp 213–250.

Scholz J: Mechanisms of neuropathic pain. In Pappagallo M, editor: *The neurological basis of pain*, New York, 2005, McGraw-Hill, pp 71–95.

Scholz J, Woolf CJ: The neuropathic pain triad: neurons, immune cells and glia, *Nat Neurosci* 10(11):1361–1368, 2007.

Shipton EA: *Pain acute and chronic*, London, 1999, Arnold Hodder Headline Group, pp 2–11.

Stone LS, Broberger C, Vulchanova L, et al: Differential distribution of alpha 2A and alpha 2C adrenergic receptor immunoreactivity in the rat spinal cord, *J Neurosci* 18:5928–5937, 1988.

Sudhof TC: The synaptic vesicle cycle, *Annu Rev Neurosci* 27:509–547, 2004.

Tracey I, Mantyh PW: The cerebral signature for pain perception and its modulation, *Neuron* 55:377–391, 2007.

Trafton JA, Abbadie C, Marek K, et al: Post-synaptic signalling via the mu-opioid receptor: responses of dorsal horn neurons to exogenous opioids and noxious stimulation, *J Neurosci* 20 (23):8578–8584, 2000.

Tu Y, Sun RQ, Willis WD: Effects of intrathecal injections of melatonin analogues on capsaicin-induced secondary mechanical allodynia and hyperalgesia in rats, *Pain* 109:340–350, 2004.

Villaneuva L, Bouhassira B, Bing Z, et al: Convergence of heterotopic nociceptive information on to subnucleus reticularis dorsalis neurons in the rat medulla, *J Neurophysiol* 23:197–210, 1988.

Vlaeyen JWS, Linton SJ: Fear-avoidance and its consequences in chronic musculoskeletal pain: a state of the art, *Pain* 85:317–332, 2000.

Vogt BA, Sikes RW, Vogt LJ: Anterior cingulate cortex and the medial pain system. In Vogt BA, Gabriel M, editors: *Neurobiology of the cingulate cortex and limbic thalamus*, Boston, MA, 1993, Birkhauser, pp 313–344.

Waxman SG: The neuron as a dynamic electrogenic machine: modulation of sodium channel expression as a basis for functional plasticity in neurons, *Philos Trans R Soc Lond B Biol Sci* 355:199–213, 2000.

Waxman SG: Transcriptional channelopathies: an emerging class of disorders, *Nat Neurosci* 2:652–659, 2001.

Westlund KN, Carlton SM, Zhang D, et al: Direct catecholaminergic innervation of primate spinothalamic tract neurons, *J Comp Neurol* 299:178–186, 1990.

Westlund KN: Neurophysiology of nociception. In Pappagallo M, editor: *The neurological basis of pain*, New York, 2005, McGraw-Hill, pp 3–20.

Woolf CJ: Recent advances in the pathophysiology of acute pain, *Br J Anaesth* 63:139–146, 1989.

Woolf CJ: Generation of acute pain: central mechanisms, *Br Med Bull* 47(3):523–533, 1991.

Woolf CJ: Somatic pain-pathogenesis and prevention, *Br J Anaesth* 75:169–176, 1995.

Woolf CJ, Bennet GJ, Doherty M, et al: Towards a mechanism-based classification of pain? *Pain* 77:227–229, 1998.

Woolf CJ, Mannion R: Neuropathic pain, *Lancet* 353:1959–1964, 1999.

Woolf CJ, Ma Q: Nociceptors-noxious stimulus detectors, *Neuron* 55:353–364, 2007.

Chapter 4

Anxiety disorders, their relationship to hypermobility and their management

Rocío Martín-Santos

Anthony Bulbena

José Alexandre Crippa

INTRODUCTION

Anxiety is a universal human experience, with psychological, physiological, behavioural and cognitive manifestations. Anxiety becomes abnormal when its intensity and duration is disproportionate or when it occurs without recognizable threat.

The most recent mental disorders classifications (DSM-IV and ICD-10) describe different anxiety disorders:

- Panic with and without agoraphobia – characterized by attacks of extreme anxiety accompanied by sympathetic arousal that can be associated with the fear of having another attack, and with avoidance behaviour
- Agoraphobia – an extended avoidance behaviour
- Generalized anxiety disorder – a chronic disturbance characterized by excessive anxiety and worry
- Social phobia disorder – e.g. public-speaking phobia
- Specific phobia – e.g. animal phobia
- Post-traumatic stress disorder
- Anxiety in medically ill – e.g. thyroiditis.

PREVALENCE AND ASSOCIATION OF ANXIETY DISORDERS

The life-time prevalence of anxiety disorders is approximately 28% in the general population (Kessler & Wang 2008). They are more prevalent in women than men, and in some such as phobias and separation anxiety disorder, the greatest frequency of onset is found in early childhood.

Other anxiety disorders such as panic disorder, generalized anxiety, and post-traumatic stress disorder, typically occur in adulthood. The 12-month-prevalence estimates of the DSM-IV disorders showed that the highest of these is specific phobia (8.7%), social phobia (6.8%), and major depression disorder (6.7%). Among school children, anxiety disorders are the most prevalent (18.1%), followed by mood disorders (9.5%), and substance disorders (3.8%) (Kessler & Wang 2008). Moreover, there is a considerable degree of overlap in these disorders. Most of the anxiety disorders run a chronic course.

GENETICS

Genetic epidemiology studies suggest that anxiety disorders are familial and moderately heritable. Linkage studies have implicated several chromosomal regions. However, candidate gene association studies have not established a role for any specific loci to date. It seems that genes underlying these disorders overlap and transcend diagnostic boundaries. Understanding animal models of anxiety, the neuroimaging of phenotypes, and intermediate phenotypes such as anxiety-related personality ('neuroticism', 'harm avoidance', 'behavioural inhibition temperament to the unfamiliar') may provide better clues in future (Smoller et al 2008).

RECOGNIZING ANXIETY DISORDERS

There are many rating scales measuring anxiety or depression. Methods to improve the recognition of anxiety disorder in busy medical settings include

DOI: 10.1016/B978-0-7020-3005-5.00004-5

the integration of simple screening questions into clinical interviews and the application of short screening questionnaires.

One of the most commonly used validated screening questionnaires in medical settings is the Hospital Anxiety and Depression Scale (HADS) (Zigmond & Snaith 1983). The HADS consists of seven items.

Another validated screening instrument frequently used is the PRIME-MD Patient Health Questionnaire (PHQ) (Spitzer et al 1999, Díez-Quevedo et al 2001, Kroenke et al 2001, 2002). It includes a panic disorder module, and a generalized anxiety module as well as a depression module which has been validated in large sample populations against the diagnosis of mental health professionals. The PHQ is self-administered and gives diagnoses approaching the DMS-IV criteria.

Both PHQ and HADS can be recommended as valid and practicable screening instruments for anxiety disorder. In particular the PHQ has the best operating characteristics with overall accuracy and specificity superior to other measures in medical as well as in psychosomatic cases (Löwe et al 2003).

The SF-36 item is a questionnaire of quality of life with good psychometric properties (McHorney et al 1993, Sareen et al 2006). It is often used in studies of musculoskeletal pain.

ANXIETY DISORDERS AND MEDICAL ILLNESS

Emerging evidence suggests that anxiety disorders are related to other medical illnesses. Anxiety disorders are associated with high rates of medically unexplained symptoms, increased utilization of healthcare resources (Katon & Walker 1998, McLaughlin et al 2006), and poor quality of life and disability (Sareen et al 2006). Aside from the association with other conditions, anxiety disorders can manifest in a number of ways (Table 4.1).

They have been associated with several physical conditions such as functional gastrointestinal disease, cardiovascular disease, asthma, neoplasia and chronic pain (Roy-Byrne et al 2008). Results from the National Co-morbidity Survey-Replication (NCS-R) (Kessler et al 2003) showed that various anxiety disorders had equal or greater association than depression with four chronic physical disorders, namely hypertension, arthritis, asthma and gastrointestinal ulcers.

Table 4.1	Physiologic, cognitive and behaviour factors of anxiety	
SOMATIC	COGNITIVE	BEHAVIOUR
Muscular:	Worry	Flushing
Tremor, spasm	Fear	Pallor
Muscle weakness	Anticipation	Strained voice
Discomfort	Fear of being unable	Tense facial
Pain regions	to cope	Restlessness
Autonomic:	Fear of developing	Immobilization
Palpitations	anxiety	Laughing
Flushing	Feelings of	Crying
Feeling of heat	depression	Over
Perspiration	*Hyper–arousal:*	talkativeness
Clammy hands	Alertness	
Dryness of mouth	Excessive vigilance	
Rapid breathing	Feeling excessive	
Tightness in the	stimulation	
chest	Distractibility	
	Insomnia	

Panic disorder and agoraphobia are intensely associated with cardiovascular illness and joint and bone diseases (Sareen et al 2005). Recent data from clinical settings showed that patients with panic disorder with or without agoraphobia had a 4.2-fold increase in the risk of neurological disorders, 3.9-fold increased risk of cardiovascular disease, a 3.8-fold increased risk of musculoskeletal disorders, and 2-fold increase in the risk of digestive diseases (Pascual et al 2008). These results support previous research in co-morbid anxiety disorders and chronic pain (Norton & Asmundson 2004; McWilliams et al 2003, 2004).

The co-morbidity of anxiety disorders and pain has received little attention even though recent studies show that these disorders are as likely to co-occur with chronic pain conditions as depressive disorder. A cross-national population-based study of the association of chronic back or neck pain with a broad spectrum of mental disorders (Demyttenaere et al 2007) found that, after adjusting for age and gender, anxiety, alcohol and mood disorders all occurred with greater frequency among patients with chronic back or neck pain. The World Mental Health Survey, undertaken in 18 countries ($N = 85\ 088$), highlighted the importance of assessing mental disorder status in the community and the need for specific care and management among those with back or neck chronic pain (Chapter 12.8 – Yellow Flags). Data from the same survey showed a higher prevalence of chronic pain conditions among females and older persons. Interestingly, the association between chronic pain and depression-anxiety disorders was similar in developed and developing countries (Tsang et al 2008).

ANXIETY TRAITS AND HYPERMOBILITY

There are some data to show that anxiety is common among subjects with joint hypermobility (JHM).

Hypermobile individuals with high levels of anxiety traits are more prone to have fears, anxiety sensitivity, anxiety expectations, illness fears, and to develop avoidance behaviour. They may respond to anxiety symptomatology with catastrophic misinterpretations of the physical arousal, pain and hypervigilance. These personality characteristics occur in both genders (Bulbena et al 2004a). In one study of 553 workers (61.4% male) attending a routine medical check-up, the presence of JHM and anxiety traits was evaluated using the Spielberg Trait Anxiety Scale (Spielberg et al 1986). Twenty-six percent of women and 17.6% of men demonstrated presence of JHM. Hypermobile women showed significantly higher anxiety traits than non-hypermobile women (P value = 0.0008). A similar pattern was seen among men (P value = 0.03).

The relationship between anxiety and JHM has also been studied in a survey of university students in Brazil ($N = 2300$). Hypermobility was assessed by a screening questionnaire (Chapter 1 – Table 1.7) and anxiety was measured by the self-administered questionnaire the Beck Anxiety Scale (Beck & Steer 1993). This anxiety scale assesses four factors: autonomic symptoms, neuroticism, panic and subjective symptoms. Hypermobile students had higher scores on the autonomic symptoms compared with non-hypermobile subjects (P value <0.005) (Crippa et al, authors' correspondence, unpublished). These results may add support to the growing evidence in the literature of autonomic dysfunction found in JHS (Chapter 6.1), though one must note that the individuals in the study were only identified as having presence of JHM and not necessarily as having JHS by the Brighton Criteria (Chapter 1).

FEAR TRAITS AND HYPERMOBILITY

Hypermobility has been associated with the presence of intense fears. In a sample of 1305 subjects from a rural town in Catalonia the prevalence of JHM was assessed using the Beighton Criteria (Bulbena et al 2006). Fear intensity and frequency was explored using a modified version of the Fear Survey Schedule (FSS-III) (Wolpe & Lang 1964). Intense fears, defined as a score of 3–4, were compared between JHM and non-JHM subjects. Hypermobility was found in 19.9% ($N = 141$) of women and 6.9% ($N = 41$) of men; typical population prevalence values compared to other large studies. The comparison of both groups showed that the mean total scores for fear in both genders were significantly higher in the JHM group. Hypermobile men had more fears related to social phobia ('being rejected by others', 'being ignored', and 'being watched while working') and to simple phobia ('worms', 'insects', and 'flying insects'). Hypermobile women had more fears related to death ('deaths', 'cadavers'), to being rejected ('failure', 'being ignored', 'being rejected'), to agoraphobia ('graveyards', 'open crowded', 'travelling by subways', 'closed places'), and simple phobia ('flying insects', 'insects', 'animal blood'). These associations with intense fears might represent a susceptibility factor or intermediate phenotype for anxiety conditions.

ANXIETY DISORDERS AND JOINT HYPERMOBILITY SYNDROME (JHS)

The clinical association between anxiety disorders and JHS has been observed in clinic populations (Bulbena et al 1993, Martín-Santos 1993, Martín-Santos et al 1998) and in general population studies (Bulbena et al 2004b, Gago 1992).

One case-control study of a rheumatology clinic population found that anxiety disorders were highly associated with JHS, with age- and gender-adjusted risk ratios of >10. The authors studied 114 patients who were initially referred for pain and then diagnosed with JHS. These were compared to 59 control subjects randomly selected from patients seen at the same clinic in the same period of time. Both cases and controls were examined by a psychologist who used the Structured Clinical Interview for DSM-III-R (SCID) to diagnose mental disorders

(Spitzer et al 1985). Panic disorder, agoraphobia, and simple phobia, but not generalized anxiety disorder, dysthymic disorder, or major depression, were found to be highly associated with JHS.

In a study of outpatients within a psychiatric clinic of a general hospital, the prevalence of JHS among cases of panic disorders with or without agoraphobia ($N = 99$) was found to be 67.7%, and significantly higher than that observed in two control groups (10.1% and 12.5%) (Martín-Santos et al 1998). Two gender/age-matched control groups were studied, one psychiatric patients without anxiety disorders ($N = 99$) and the other medical outpatients without mental disorders ($N = 64$). The study showed that women and younger subjects with anxiety disorders were over 29 times more likely to have JHS than controls. All patients were interviewed using the SCID-DSM-III-R by a trained clinician. Moreover, all subjects were examined for presence of JHM using the Beighton Criteria by an expert rheumatologist in hypermobility syndrome blinded to the outcome of any psychiatry assessment. Table 4.2 shows the type of psychiatric disorders identified in this study.

Panic and agoraphobia disorder patients with hypermobility had higher scores in the stress reactivity index and neuroticism as well as level of anxiety and depression. The correlation between the scores of both psychic anxiety and somatic anxiety subscales of the Hamilton anxiety scale items and the total score of the Beighton Scale showed a significant correlation ($P < 0.05$) with cardiovascular, respiratory and autonomic symptomatology.

A smaller clinical study compared 30 JHS patients with two age-matched control groups of 25 healthy individuals and 30 patients with fibromyalgia. Considerable emotional symptoms were identified in the patient groups (Ercolani et al 2008). The hypermobile group scored significantly higher in psychological distress and frequency and intensity on somatic symptoms. When compared to the hypermobile group, the fibromyalgia group showed elevated scores in illness behaviour questionnaire subscales for psychological versus somatic focus, disease affirmation and discriminating factors.

Similar clinical associations have been identified in other large general populations (Gago 1992, Bulbena et al 2004b). In a two-stage epidemiological study inhabitants of one village were assessed. Subjects with dementia, severe physical disease, and known heritable diseases of connective tissue were excluded. In the first phase of the study all

Table 4.2	Correlations between Hamilton anxiety scale items and the total score of the presence of JHM		
HAMILTON ANXIETY SCALE ITEMS	CASES $N=99$	PSYCHIATRIC CONTROLS $N=99$	MEDICAL CONTROLS $N=64$
Psychic anxiety			
1. Anxious mood	0.16	−0.08	−0.17
2. Tension	0.24	0.03	−0.18
3. Fear	0.12	0.04	−0.01
4. Insomnia	0.21	−0.27	−0.13
5. Intellectual problems	0.20	−0.05	−0.29
6. Depressed mood	0.05	−0.08	−0.27
7. Nervous behaviour	0.23	−0.07	−0.06
Somatic anxiety			
8. Muscular symptoms	0.10	−0.02	−0.04
9. Sensorial symptoms	0.16	0.14	−0.12
10. Cardiovascular symptoms	0.28*	−0.08	−0.15
11. Respiratory symptoms	0.29*	0.14	−0.17
12. Gastrointestinal symptoms	0.20	−0.02	−0.06
13. Genitourinary symptoms	0.23	−0.04	−0.33
14. Autonomic symptoms	0.27*	0.17	−0.16

*$P < 0.05$ Spearman correlation coefficient rho.

participants ($N = 1305$) were assessed with the self-administered GHQ-28 items scale (Goldberg 1972, 1978, Lobo et al 1986, Goldberg & Williams 1988) identifying a cut-off score of ≥ 6 for presence and degree of anxiety and depression. Alongside this they undertook a questionnaire screening for panic spectrum (Katon et al 1987) with a cut-off of ≥ 4, and were examined for the presence of JHM using the Beighton Criteria at a score of ≥ 5. All participants who met at least one cut-off point in any of the above screening instruments were entered into the second stage of the study that comprised assessment of their SCID-DMS-III-R status by a trained psychologist.

One hundred and eighty-two subjects had JHM (13.9%), 248 (19.0%) scored for anxiety/depression; and 102 (7.8%) for panic spectrum conditions. After adjustment for age and gender, subjects with JHM were significantly more likely to suffer from panic disorder (OR = 8.19, CI 95% = 3.41–19.47), agoraphobia (OR = 5.89, CI 95% = 2.98–11.66) and social phobia (OR = 7.79 CI 95% = 2.44–24.85). No increased risk was found for simple phobia, obsessive compulsive disorder, generalized anxiety disorder, dysthymic disorder and major depression.

THE RELATIONSHIP BETWEEN ANXIETY DISORDERS AND JHS

The relationship between anxiety disorders and other medical conditions may be a consequence of a physiological manifestation of the medical illness itself, a maladaptive psychological reaction in light of the medical illness, or as an adverse effect of treatment.

With regard to JHS and anxiety, both disorders share an early age of onset, a decrease of frequency with age, a gender difference being more prevalent in females, and a familial aggregation.

The two disorders have genetic factors that are not understood and require further detailed study. Preliminary studies suggested a cytogenetic mutation in chromosome 15 in families with both disorders (Gratacós et al 2001). However these have not been replicated. Anxiety disorders and JHS certainly share an autonomic alteration (Chapter 6.1), higher anxiety sensitivity, abnormal pain perception and higher somatic sensitivity than controls.

It is proposed that the interactions between autonomic, physical and psychological disturbances are linked in a complex manor in JHS, each 'fuelling' the other (Chapter 1 – Figure 1.4).

Could they share a common genetic vulnerability? Is this relationship different from others like fibromyalgia, irritable bowel or chronic fatigue? To further our understanding of the association will require longitudinal epidemiological research, and further genetic analysis. There is also the need for further exploration of the biological aspects of anxiety and hypermobility, perhaps identifying phenotypes through neuroimaging (Chapters 3 and 5) and autonomic response, anaesthetic response and pain perception.

MANAGEMENT OF PATIENTS WITH ANXIETY AND HYPERMOBILITY SYNDROME

The management of patients with JHS and anxiety has to be a multidisciplinary or interdisciplinary approach involving the rheumatologist or pain specialist, psychiatrist, psychologist, physiotherapist and occupational therapist. Clinicians must be able to recognize the different forms of anxiety disorder and be aware of the treatment options that include analgesia, antidepressants and benzodiazepines, cognitive-behavioural therapy and physical treatments (Section 2).

PSYCHOLOGICAL TREATMENT

Patients with anxiety and distress may maintain autonomic arousal and have physical symptoms. Both anxiety and distress can induce negativity resulting in avoidance behaviour (Chapter 8). High levels of anxiety not only affect the experience of pain, but also the way in which an individual processes and recalls information (Adams et al 2006). There is general agreement that psychological approaches may be useful in the management of these patients.

From a psychological point of view these patients can be treated at different levels: 'informational discussion', psychological support, pain therapy and specific treatment of psychiatric disorders (alone or combined with pharmacologic treatment).

Informational discussion aims to provide patients with an understanding of what has occurred both in terms of their condition/illness and their anxiety disorders. For some patients this may be the most important part of treatment. Being informed gives the individual the opportunity to understand their situation, the cascade effect of anxiety and panic symptoms, the role of thoughts, conditioned fears and avoidance behaviour, and thus begin to appreciate the process of adaptive psychological mechanisms and the ways in which these can be manipulated in a positive way as part of therapy. Informational discussions can therefore provide patients with a sense of control, helping to avoid catastrophic thoughts and avoidance behaviour, and may improve compliance and adherence to different treatments.

Panic disorders with and without agoraphobia, social phobia or specific phobia can improve with cognitive-behavioural treatment (Butler et al 2006).

PHARMACOTHERAPY

Simple analgesics and anti-inflammatory drugs have a place in the management of acute soft tissue injuries and degenerative disease. The majority of patients with chronic widespread pain, however, gain little if any benefit (Chapter 7). Presumably, as with other chronic pain syndromes, this is because central pain perception is abnormal; amplified by neurophysiological, psychological and behavioural pathologies.

The clinician should also be aware of poor efficacy of local anaesthetics; found in up to 60% of patients with JHS. The mechanisms behind this are unclear (Hakim et al 2005).

Serotonergic and noradrenergic agents can be used in the context of chronic pain though for JHS there are no randomized control trials. It is speculative as to whether such agents influence central pain processing, mood and spinal column descending inhibitory pathways. Similarly, these agents may have a place in controlling autonomic disturbance of the bowel. In subjects with co-morbid pain and anxiety, benzodiazepines seem to be more effective as anxiolytic agents than analgesics; however, the decrease in anxiety may decrease somatic sensitivity and secondary the pain (Narita et al 2006).

Selective serotonin reuptake inhibitor (SSRI) antidepressants are considered as a first-choice treatment by the majority of experts (Marchesi 2008) in treating anxiety disorders such as panic disorder with or without agoraphobia, social phobia and concomitant depression. Lower starting doses may reduce the risk of stimulant side-effects in the first few days of treatment (e.g. 2.5–5 mg/day of paroxetine or fluoxetine). The therapeutic effect is seen after 14–28 days at the mean dose (20 mg/day of paroxetine or fluoxetine) and antidepressant treatment should be maintained for 12–24 months. SSRIs may inhibit the analgesic effect of tramadol and codeine through inhibition of their metabolic activation, to induce serotonin syndrome (Hersh et al 2007). Other antidepressants include imipramine and clomipramine or monoaminoxidase inhibitors. Both types of agent may induce orthostatic hypotension. Benzodiazepines may be useful for a short period of time or as acute treatment of panic disorder and are the treatment of choice when other agents have to be rapidly removed because of significant toxic side-effects such as hyponatraemia.

Beta blockade may relieve the symptoms of postural orthostatic tachycardia syndrome. Other interventions such as salt and fluid balance may be effective in orthostatic hypotension and orthostatic intolerance (Chapter 6.1).

PHYSICAL THERAPIES

Physiotherapy is often deemed unhelpful by patients with JHS. This may be because the therapist has not taken account of lax tissues, which lack the normal tensile strength. Conventional therapies may not be effective (Hakim & Ashton 2005) and methods should be adjusted (Section 2).

There is some evidence to suggest that physical exercise may help reduce symptoms of depression and anxiety disorders (Ströhle 2009). The mechanisms responsible for this improvement are not well known. There is however evidence of an increase in central noradrenaline (norepinephrine) neurotransmission (Sothman & Ismail 1984), changes in the hypothalamic adrenocortical system (Ströhle & Holsboer 2003) and the serotonin system (Dishman et al 1997) (Chapter 3). A recent study suggested that lower levels of regular exercise are associated with higher levels of anxious and depressive symptoms, but that the association was not because of any causal effect of exercise (De Moor et al 2008). In panic and phobia disorders, exercise can be used as an exposure therapy. Patients with panic disorder or panic attacks should be informed that on rare occasions exercise can give some somatic sensations that may trigger panic attacks despite the intended anxiolytic effect; in the same way that exposure to a fear situation may induce symptoms (Ströhle et al 2005). There remains a lack of systematic studies of exercise training in the management of depression and anxiety symptoms.

SUMMARY

Anxiety disorders have been associated with high rates of medically unexplained symptoms and increased utilization of healthcare resources. Moreover, anxiety disorders have been associated with functional gastrointestinal disease, cardiovascular disease, asthma, neoplasia and chronic pain. Recent studies show that anxiety disorders are also associated with JHM and JHS. The management of patients with co-morbid anxiety disorder and JHS requires a multidisciplinary approach. The nature of this clinical association is intriguing and there is a need for further epidemiological and experimental research to tease out genetic influences from environmental and maladaptive triggers.

References

Adams N, Poole H, Richardson C: Psychological approaches to chronic pain management: part 1, *J Clin Nurs* 15:290–300, 2006.

Beck AT, Steer RA: *Beck Anxiety Inventory Manual*, San Antonio, Texas, 1993, Psychological Corporation.

Bulbena A, Duró JC, Porta M, et al: Anxiety disorders in the Joint hypermobility syndrome, *Psychiatry Res* 46:59–68, 1993.

Bulbena A, Gago J, Martín-Santos R, et al: Anxiety disorder and Joint laxity: a definitive link, *Neural Psychiatry Brain Res* 11:137–140, 2004a.

Bulbena A, Agullo A, Pialhez G, et al: Is joint hypermobility related to anxiety in a nonclinical population also? *Psychosomatics* 45:432–437, 2004b.

Bulbena A, Gago J, Sperry L, et al: The relationship between frequency and intensity of fears and a collagen condition, *Depress Anxiety* 23:412–417, 2006.

Butler AC, Chapman JE, Forman EM, et al: The empirical status of cognitive-behavioural therapy: a review of meta-analyses, *Clin Psychol Rev* 26:17–31, 2006.

De Moor MHM, Boomsma DI, Stubbe JH, et al: Testing Causality in the Association Between Regular Exercise and Symptoms of Anxiety and Depression, *Am J Psychiatry* 65:897–905, 2008.

Demyttenaere K, Bruffaerts R, Lee S, et al: Mental disorders among persons with chronic back or neck pain: results from the World mental health Surveys, *Pain* 129:332–342, 2007.

Díez-Quevedo C, Rangil T, Sanchez-Planell L, et al: Validation and utility of the Patient Health Questionnaire in diagnosing mental disorders in 1003 general hospital Spanish inpatients, *Psychosom Med* 63:679–686, 2001.

Dishman RK, Renner KJ, Youngstedt SD, et al: Activity wheel running reduced escape latency and alters brain monoamine levels after foot shock, *Brain Res Bull* 42:399–406, 1997.

Ercolani M, Galvani M, Franchini C, et al: Benign joint hypermobility syndrome: psychological features and psychological symptoms in a sample pain-free at evaluation 1, *Perception Motor Skills* 107:256–356, 2008.

Gago J: *Estudio de prevalencias y de la asociación entre laxitud articular y trastornos de ansiedad en población general rural*, Tesis doctoral. Spain, 1992, Universidad Autónoma de Barcelona.

Goldberg DP: *The detection of psychiatric illness by questionnaire*, London, 1972, Oxford University Press Maudsley Monograph No 21.

Goldberg D, Williams P: *A user's guide to the GHQ*, London UK, 1988, Institute of Psychiatry.

Gratacós M, Nadal M, Martín-Santos R, et al: A polymorphic genomic duplication on human chromosome 15 is susceptibility factor for panic and phobic disorders, *Cell* 106:367–379, 2001.

Hakim AJ, Norris P, Hopper C, et al: Local Anaesthetic Failure; Does Joint Hypermobility Provide The Answer? *J R Soc Med* 98:84–85, 2005.

Hakim AJ, Ashton S: Undiagnosed, Joint Hypermobility Syndrome patients have poorer outcome than peers following chronic back pain rehabilitation, *Rheumatology* 44(3 Suppl 1):255, 2005.

Hersh EV, Pinto A, Moore PA: Adverse drug interactions involving common prescription and over-the-counter analgesic agents, *Clinical Therapy* 29 (Suppl):2477–2497, 2007.

Katon W, Vitaliano PP, Russo J, et al: Panic disorder. Spectrum of severity of somatisation, *Journal Nerve Mental Disorders* 175:12–19, 1987.

Katon WJ, Walker EA: Medically unexplained symptoms in primary care, *J Clin Psychiatry* 59 (Suppl 20):15–21, 1998.

Kessler RC, Ormel J, Demler O, et al: Co morbid mental disorders account for the role impairment of commonly occurring chronic physical disorders: results from the National Co morbidity Survey, *J Occup Environ Med* 45:1257–1266, 2003.

Kessler RC, Wang PS: The descriptive epidemiology of commonly occurring mental disorders in the United States, *Annu Rev Public Health* 29:115–129, 2008.

Kroenke K, Spitzer RL, Williams JB: The PHQ-9. Validity of a brief depression severity measure, *J Gen Intern Med* 16:606–613, 2001.

Kroenke K, Spitzer RL, Williams JB: The PHQ-15: validity of a new measure for evaluating the severity of somatic symptoms, *Psychosom Med* 64:258–266, 2002.

Lobo A, Pérez Echeverría MJ, Artal J: Validity of the scaled version of the General Health Questionnaire (GHQ-28) in Spanish population, *Psychol Med* 16:135–140, 1986.

Löwe B, Gräfe K, Zipfel S, et al: Detecting panic disorder in medical and psychosomatic outpatients. Comparative validation of the Hospital Anxiety and Depression Scale, the Patient Health Questionnaire, a screening question, and physician's diagnosis, *J Psychosom Res* 55:515–519, 2003.

Marchesi C: Pharmacological management of panic disorder, *Neuropsychiatric Disease and Treatment* 4:93–106, 2008.

Martín-Santos R: *Asociación entre laxitud articular y ansiedad*, Tesis doctoral. Spain, 1993, Universidad Autónoma de Barcelona.

Martín-Santos R, Bulbena A, Porta M, et al: Association between the joint hypermobility syndrome and panic disorder, *Am J Psychiatry* 155:1578–1583, 1998.

McHorney CA, Ware JE, Raczek AE: The MOS 36 items Short Form Health Survey (SF-36), II: psychometric and clinical test of validity in measuring physical and mental health constructs, *Med Care* 31:247–263, 1993.

McLaughlin TP, Khandker RK, Kruzikas DT, et al: Overlap of anxiety and depression in a managed care population prevalence and association with resource utilization, *J Clin Psychiatry* 67:1187–1193, 2006.

McWilliams LA, Cox BJ, Enns MW: Mood and anxiety disorders associated with chronic pain: an examination in a national representative sample, *Pain* 106:127–133, 2003.

McWilliams LA, Goodwin RD, Cox BJ: Depression and anxiety associated with three pain conditions: results from a nationally representative sample, *Pain* 111:77–83, 2004.

Narita M, Kanego C, Miyoshi K, et al: Chronic pain induced anxiety with concomitant changes in opioidergic function in the amygdala, *Neuropsychopharmacology* 31:739–750, 2006.

Norton PJ, Asmundson GJ: Anxiety sensitivity, fear, and avoidance behaviour in headache pain, *Pain* 111:218–233, 2004.

Pascual JC, Castaño J, Espluga N, et al: Somatic conditions in patients suffering from anxiety disorders, *Medicine Clinics (Barcelona)* 130:281–285, 2008.

Roy-Byrne PP, Davidson KW, Kessler RC, et al: Anxiety disorders and co morbid medical illness, *Gen Hosp Psychiatry* 30:208–225, 2008.

Sareen JS, Cox BJ, Clara I, et al: The relationship between anxiety disorders and physical disorders in the US National Co morbidity Survey, *Depress Anxiety* 21:193–202, 2005.

Sareen J, Jacobi F, Cox BJ, et al: Disability and poor quality of life associated with co morbid anxiety disorders and physical conditions, *AMA Arch Intern Med* 166:2109–2116, 2006.

Spielberg CD, Gorsuch RL, Lushene RE: *Cuestionario de ansiedad Estado-Rasgo*, Spain, 1986, Madrid TEA Editorial.

Spitzer R, Williams BW: *Structured Clinical Interview for DSM-III-R*, Patient's version. New York, USA, 1985, Biometrics Research Department. State Psychiatric Institute.

Spitzer RL, Williams JB, Gibbon M, First MB: The Structured Clinical Interview for DSM-III-R (SCID) I: History, Rationale, and Description, *Arch Gen Psychiatry* 49:624–629, 1992.

Spitzer RL, Kroenke K, Williams JB: Patient Health Questionnaire primary care study group. Validation and utility of a self-report version of PRIME-MD: the PHQ primary care study, *JAMA* 282:1737–1744, 1999.

Sothman MS, Ismail AH: Relationship between urinary catecholamine metabolites, particularly MHPG, and selected personality and physical fitness characteristics in normal subjects, *Psychosom Med* 46:523, 1984.

Smoller JW, Gardner-Schuster E, Covino J: The genetic basis of panic and phobic anxiety disorders, *Am J Med Genet C Semin Med Genet* 148:118–126, 2008.

Ströhle A, Holsboer F: Stress responsive neurohormones in depression and anxiety, *Pharmacopsychiatry* 36 (Suppl 3):207–214, 2003.

Ströhle A, Feller C, Onken M, et al: The acute antipanic activity of aerobic exercise, *Am J Psychiatry* 162:2376–2378, 2005.

Ströhle A: Physical activity, exercise, depression and anxiety disorders, *J Neural Transm* 116(6):777–784, 2009.

Tsang A, von Korff M, Lee S, et al: Common chronic pain conditions in developed and developing countries: gender and age differences and co morbidity with depression-anxiety disorders, *Pain* 9:883–981, 2008.

Wolpe J, Lang PJ: A fear schedule for use in behaviour therapy, *Behav Res Ther* 2:27–30, 1964.

Zigmond AS, Snaith RP: The Hospital Anxiety and Depression Scale, *Acta Psychiatr Scand* 67:361–370, 1983.

Chapter 5

Fibromyalgia and hypermobility

Anisur Rahman

Andrew J Holman

INTRODUCTION

Chronic musculoskeletal pain is a very common symptom. It can be conveniently divided into two categories for the purpose of epidemiological studies. Chronic widespread pain (CWP) means pain present every day for at least 3 months, in sites on both sides of the body, both above and below the waist as well as in the spinal region. Chronic regional pain (CRP) means pain present every day for at least 3 months which does not fulfil the definition of CWP. For example, pain confined to one arm or to one arm and one leg on the same side of the body. However, it is important to remember that these definitions do not separate groups that have clinically distinct illnesses. Also, individuals can move from having CWP to CRP and vice versa.

Within the definition of CWP lies the phenomenon fibromyalgia (FM) (Wolfe et al 1990). Equally, joint hypermobility syndrome (JHS) (Chapter 1) may present as widespread pain of a chronic nature, or indeed as regional pain.

Both FM and JHS are considered to be relatively common in the general population. Joint hypermobility (JHM) is very common. It is not surprising therefore that FM and JHM may occur in an individual by chance. Whether they are mutually exclusive or appear together by pathogenic association is open to debate. There has been no large-scale general population epidemiology study of either FM and JHM or FM and JHS published to date. What has emerged from several small studies is an apparent association between FM and JHM.

Perhaps most compelling in the argument that FM and JHS might share pathophysiological mechanisms are the findings of psychosocial symptoms, sensitization of the nervous system to pain and autonomic disturbance, common to both. However, it is highly plausible that these pathologies may be a consequent response to the presence of CWP rather than represent disease processes with specific mechanisms directly related to FM or JHS.

This chapter introduces CWP, then the history behind the concept of FM, and finally will examine the association between FM, JHM, JHS and autonomic dysfunction.

CHRONIC WIDESPREAD PAIN

PREVALENCE

From large population surveys the prevalence of CWP is approximately 11% and CRP 25% (Croft et al 1993, Bergman et al 2001). Bergman's community study of over 1800 people in southern Sweden over a period of 3 years demonstrated that these figures were constant over time in this population but that individual's pain patterns changed. It was noted that 76 individuals went from CRP to CWP and 64 moved in the other direction. Furthermore 222 moved from having no chronic pain to either CRP or CWP while 201 moved from CWP or CRP to no chronic pain (Bergman et al 2002).

CWP is a symptom, not a disease. That it truly is common in the general population without having identified disease or bias by focusing attention on those who seek health advice is perhaps best seen in the study carried out by Wolfe et al (1995) in Wichita, Kansas. Here, a postal questionnaire about pain was sent to households selected randomly

© 2010 Elsevier Ltd.
DOI: 10.1016/B978-0-7020-3005-5.00005-7

from a directory of addresses. Among 3000 individuals who returned data, the prevalence of CWP was 10.6% and that of CRP, 20.1%; remarkably similar to earlier studies.

Given that JHM has a population prevalence of greater than or equal to 10% one can see, even without association, that there is at least a 1 in 100 probability (1%) of identifying both CWP and JHM in any one individual by chance. Large-scale population studies would be required to identify the true degree of linkage.

Patients with CWP often have poor health and reduced quality of life. Croft et al (1993) showed strong associations between the presence of CWP and fatigue and depression. A number of other studies have looked at the factors that influence development and/or persistence of CWP (Buskila et al 2000, McBeth et al 2001a, 2001b, Bergman et al 2002) and have shown that many of these factors are psychosocial and not related to any particular organic or physical process that causes the pain. This does not mean that the pain suffered by patients with CWP is any less real and distressing than that suffered by patients with, for example, rheumatoid arthritis or osteoarthritis.

In general, it is thought that most CWP arises from soft tissues such as muscles, that otherwise appear normal on examination or scans. Thus, unlike diseases in which inflammation of a particular tissue or tissues is known to be the proximate cause of the pain there is often no physical or clear physiological cause for CWP, a phenomenon common to FM.

FIBROMYALGIA

DEVELOPING THE CONCEPT

The fact that many patients present with widespread pain apparently emanating from soft tissues, but with no specific or readily diagnosable cause, has been recognized for many years. The clinical picture has been given various names, including fibrositis. In the mid 1970s, Moldofsky et al (1975) carried out electroencephalography (EEG) readings during sleep in patients with this clinical picture, and concluded that they showed a specific pattern – the alpha-delta pattern. It was also reported that a similar pattern could be induced in healthy adults who were deprived of non-rapid-eye-movement sleep and proposed that it might result from

abnormalities in serotonin balance in the brain (Moldofsky & Scarisbrick 1976). They termed chronic pain with sleep disturbance and alpha-delta EEG pattern 'fibrositis syndrome'. Others were to use the term FM to describe such patients. There was, however, no universally accepted definition for FM, making it difficult to carry out robust prevalence studies or clinical trials.

Thus, in the late 1980s, the American College of Rheumatology (ACR) assembled a multicentre group to carry out a study to establish diagnostic criteria for FM (Wolfe et al 1990). The group reached consensus as to which clinical data should be gathered from each subject in the study including the sites at which the soft tissues should be palpated for tenderness. It emerged that two criteria were necessary to make a diagnosis with a sensitivity of 88.4% and specificity of 81.1%. These criteria were:

- CWP – as defined above
- At least 11 tender points out of 18 sites as defined on a body map (Figure 5.1).

Although other symptoms, notably sleep disturbance and fatigue were reported commonly by patients with FM, adding them to these classification criteria did not improve either specificity or sensitivity. It was also recognized that there were no blood tests, scans or histopathological findings with either specificity or sensitivity for FM.

Wolfe et al in the 1995 Kansas questionnaire study on CWP invited subjects to attend for physical examination where the number of FM tender points was assessed. Of 193 subjects examined, 25.2% of the women and 6.8% of the men had 11 or more tender points and therefore fulfilled the definition of FM. This equated to a point prevalence of 2% with a clear gender difference of 3.4% in women and 0.5% in men. It is intriguing to note that the ratio of women to men (approx. 3:1) is remarkably similar to that of JHM in the general population.

FIBROMYALGIA: THE SIZE OF THE PROBLEM

Once thought to be a nearly random assortment of unverifiable signs and symptoms, FM has emerged as a diagnosable and regrettably common disorder. It is recognized by the American College of Rheumatology (ACR), U.S. Social Security Agency, U.S. Veteran's Administration, U.S. Federal Drug Administration (FDA), European

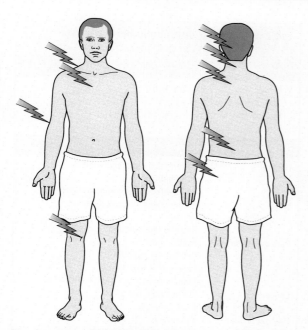

Fig. 5.1 Distribution of tender points in fibromyalgia.
There are nine sites repeated on both sides to give a
maximum score of 18.

- Occiput at the paraspinal muscle insertions of the neck
- Lower cervical spine at the inter-transverse spaces at the
  level C6–7
- Trapezius, mid way along the upper border
- Origin of supraspinatus, just above the spine of the
  scapula at its medial border
- Second rib at the costochondral junction
- Lateral humeral epicondyle, 2 cm distal from the
  epicondyles
- Lower lumbar spine
- Gluteal, in the upper inner quadrant
- Knee, medial fat pad proximal to the joint line

Reproduced with permission of the author (Hakim 2009)

Medicines Agency (EMEA) and the World Health
Organization (WHO). Given a prevalence of 2% in
the United States, 4.7% in Europe (Branco et al
2008) and increased awareness worldwide, FM is
now a major health burden for both the individual
and society at large (White et al 1999, Penrod et al
2004, Berger et al 2007, Hoffman & Dukes 2008).
In 2005, the cost of FM per patient ($10,199/year)
was nearly equal that of osteoarthritis (White
et al 2008).

In a British group of 72 patients with FM followed for a median of 4 years, 97% continued to
have symptoms of pain, tiredness and/or lethargy,
85% still had multiple tender points and 60%

felt worse at follow-up than at presentation
(Ledingham et al 1993). Half the patients had
stopped work due to their illness and 32%
described themselves as being heavily dependent.
These results are consistent with those of other
groups. Wolfe et al (1995) showed that there was
a strong correlation between FM and applications
for disability benefits, and 62% of a Swedish population with FM required such benefits (Burckhardt
et al 1994). In a large study using records from
the United Kingdom General Practice Research
Database, Hughes et al (2006) compared 2260
patients with a recorded new diagnosis of FM with
non-FM controls (ten controls per case). They
found that patients with FM had significantly
higher rates of clinical visits, prescriptions and
diagnostic tests than the control group from at least
10 years prior to the diagnosis being made.

THE ASSOCIATION WITH HYPERMOBILITY AND JOINT HYPERMOBILITY SYNDROME

In routine clinical practice, FM is usually explained
to patients as a condition in which the muscles
become tense, tender and tight due to lack of relaxation, often secondary to a poor sleep pattern and
chronic tiredness. Combining a demonstration of
tender points with an explanation that this is diagnostic for FM is a powerful approach to showing a
patient that the apparently inexplicable chronic
pain condition actually has a reasonable and well-
recognized explanation. This can reduce fear of
the unknown and enables those engaged in treatment to advise the patient about what is likely to
happen in the future. Although the pain is not
likely to disappear completely one can be clear in
advising that this syndrome does not lead to joint
destruction or deformity and that the patient is
not likely to need surgery or powerful drugs like
corticosteroids or immunosuppressants. Furthermore, as outlined in the recent EULAR guidelines
(Carville et al 2008), there are a range of different
types of treatment that can be offered to alleviate
some of the symptoms (Chapter 7).

If the pain of FM arises from tension and tenderness in muscles and soft tissues it would be reasonable to suppose that some patients with JHM
(Fitzcharles 2000) or JHS might be prone to developing FM.

To date there are no published epidemiological
studies exploring the association between FM
and JHS (by the Brighton Criteria (Chapter 1)).

However, a few small studies have addressed the issue of FM and JHM (by the Beighton Criteria (Chapter 1)), finding association significantly above that of chance in both adults and children (Gedalia et al 1993, Hudson et al 1995, Acasuso-Diaz & Collantes-Estevez 1998, Karaaslan et al 2000, Lai et al 2000, Ofluoglo et al 2006, Sendur et al 2007).

Perhaps one important component in the link between FM and JHM is deconditioning. Nearly 20 years ago it was recognized that identifying both conditions may facilitate more effective and/or greater compliance with exercise therapy, those patients recognizing the presence of FM and JHM achieving greater improvement in symptom management than non-JHM controls with FM (Goldman 1991).

AUTONOMIC DYSREGULATION: THE LINK IN FM AND JHS?

At a most basic level, a preponderance of evidence suggests that FM is the consequence of an autonomic dysregulatory state (Martinez-Lavin 2007). In terms of adaptation to stress, as well as poor maintenance of homeostasis, autonomic dysregulation permeates the FM presentation (Vaeroy et al 1998, Petzke & Clauw 2000, Raj et al 2000, Rosner et al 2000, Cohen et al 2001). Both inadequate sympathetic reactivity to new stressors (possibly resulting from a ceiling effect) (Giske et al 2008) and chronically augmented sympathetic tone (Cohen et al 2000a) are salient features of FM. Probably most importantly, patients with FM do not exhibit normal decreased sympathetic activity between 2–5 a.m. while sleeping, compared to normal controls (Martinez-Lavin et al 1998). This may contribute to fragmented stage 4 deep sleep, a leading antecedent to development of FM based on experimental human models (Moldofsky et al 1975, Moldofsky & Scarisbrick 1976, Older et al 1998, Lentz et al 1999, Roizenblatt et al 2001). Also, myriad daytime clinical autonomic dysfunctions abound, including abnormal thermoregulation, palpitations, excessive gastric acidity and irritable bowel syndrome (with consequent hypersensitivity to medications), irritable bladder, restless legs syndrome (RLS), bruxism and sleep disturbance (Table 5.1) (Martinez-Lavin & Hermosillo 2000).

Although some have attributed FM to somatization and catastrophization (Ford 1997, Hassett et al 2000, McBeth et al 2001b, Henningsen et al 2003, Rubin 2005), these behavioural observations may

Table 5.1   The autonomic nervous system: clinical considerations

Increased risk of dysautonomia	
Benign joint hypermobility (BJH)	
Obstructive sleep apnea (OSA)	
Positional cervical cord compression (PC3)	
Stress	
Dysautonomia in Fibromyalgia	
General	Abnormal thermoregulation
	Hyperhidrosis
	Aggravated autoimmune activity
Sleep	Altered sleep stage architecture
	Bruxism
	Restless legs syndrome
Cardiovascular	Palpitations
	Orthostatic hypotension
	Paroxysmal tachycardia
	Peripheral oedema (face/hands/feet)
Endocrine	Weight gain (metabolic)
	Hypoglycaemia
Gastrointestinal	Dyspepsia
	Irritable bowel syndrome
Urological	Irritable bladder (interstitial cystitis)
Psychiatric	Aggravated PTSD, anxiety, bipolar disorder

be alternatively explained, at least in part, by a hypersympathetic influence on mood. Autonomic aggravation of stress responses is not limited to somatic features alone. Heightened arousal, vigilance and fear also influence the intensity of anxiety, post-traumatic stress disorder (PTSD) and bipolar disorder (Swann et al 1991, Southwick et al 1993, Cohen et al 2000b, Cohen & Benjamin 2006). In turn, experiences of abuse, common among patients with FM (Van Houdenhove et al 2001, Castro et al 2005) may lead inexorably, in some, to hypervigilance and other long-term dysautonomic consequences. One can argue that reconstructing many psychiatric diagnoses as partial or major reflections of personal autonomic state may be reasonable.

The concept of JHS combined with FM becomes germane when considering who are most at risk for development of this dysautonomia and its many behavioural and physical consequences. Initially, the association of JHS with FM was rationalized by Fitzcharles (2000) as a painful consequence of overuse and widespread microinjury. However, an association of JHS to dysautonomia (Chapter 2 and 6.1) as an extra-articular manifestation may have broader appeal (Holman 2002, Hakim & Grahame 2004). Observation of a familial congregation of FM (Buskila & Neumann 2005) also supports a rational link to JHS, which is similarly familial. Although specific genetic markers for autonomic regulation and JHS have not yet been elucidated, tight genetic linkage of adrenergic and neurotransmitter receptor isotypes within the 'JHS gene' does have theoretical appeal. Variable penetrance and expression may also begin to explain why siblings are often, but not equally, affected by the consequences of JHS or have an identical risk of developing FM.

JHS and FM appear to predispose to greater autonomic responsiveness to appropriate sympathetic arousals: stress, fear, etc. And as a universal adaptation, cumulative or excessively intense sympathetic arousal can logically lead to more efficient arousal over time (Duke 2008). In turn, subjects may possibly react with greater vigor and duration; repetitive painful stimuli likely heighten the autonomic response over time. The autonomic nervous system winds up very well, as seen in a normal response of so-called 'flight and fight'. However, it may calm quite poorly.

Since dysautonomia and excessive arousal underlie FM, JHS subjects with a heightened capacity for autonomic arousal may also be at greater risk for one of its consequences: FM.

In this context, comorbidities able to act as dysautonomic generators become critical concerns relevant to pharmacotherapeutic choices (Chapter 7).

Beyond, psychiatric and other situational stressors able to disrupt autonomic stability and homeostasis, two specific disorders should be considered: obstructive sleep apnoea (OSA) (Leuenberger et al 2005) and positional cervical cord compression (PC3) (Holman 2008). PC3 is defined as intermittent compression of the cervical spinal cord, usually in extension, with a canal diameter less than 10 mm (normal 12–15 mm). Accurate diagnosis requires visualization of the spinal canal and cord in variable positions beyond the scope of a standard, neutral magnetic resonance image (MRI). Compression generally results from ageing of a disc and ligamentum flavum injury leading to abutment and distortion of the spinal cord while in an extended cervical position (Figure 5.2).

A direct link to JHS is unknown, but such cervical instability with intermittent cord compression following injury could possibly be more problematic in the setting of JHM or JHS.

While both OSA (Reynolds et al 2007) and cervical cord injury (Shindo et al 1997) are documented as causing significant autonomic arousals in human and animal models, PC3 is also a potential cause of widespread, referred pain (Langfitt & Elliott 1967, Elliott et al 2009). An equally concerning, yet less common correlate, would be the Chiari I malformation present in some patients with FM (Bradley & Alarcón 1999, Heffez 2002). Surgical reduction of

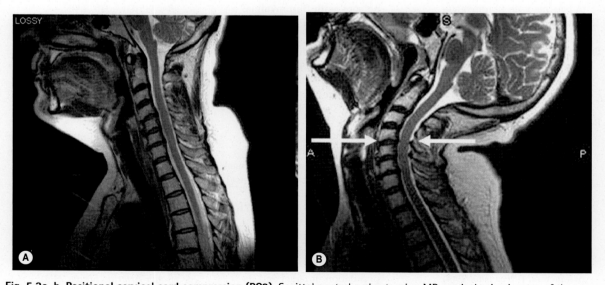

Fig. 5.2a, b Positional cervical cord compression (PC3). Sagittal neutral and extension MR cervical spine images of the same patient demonstrating cervical cord abutment at C4–5 only in extension. Note obliteration of the CSF space around the cord by positional distortion of the C4–5 disc and ligamentum flavum.

either a Chiari malformation or PC3 has led to reduced co-morbid FM-related allodynia, fatigue and dysautonomia (Heffez et al 2004, 2007). Given a 65% prevalence of PC3 among patients with FM in an initial report (Holman 2008), the potential implications for pharmacotherapeutic treatment may be considerable.

While searching for meaningful pharmacologic options to treat FM, these autonomic and anatomical issues colour the landscape. There are few effective medications able to restore, control or even reduce dysautonomia. Consequently, clinicians are often left to address the clinical endpoints of dysautonomia, including gastrointestinal, cardiovascular, psychiatric, sleep, urological and endocrine consequences. Thankfully, there are many options with considerable potential benefit documented in randomized controlled trials (RCTs) (Chapter 7).

SUMMARY

CWP is common with a prevalence of approximately 11% which is constant across different populations and in a given population over time.

It is commoner in women than men. Some patients with CWP can be said to have FM according to the ACR definition but this does not identify a distinct subgroup of patients with a specific biological explanation for their pain. The point prevalence of FM is 2%. Some patients with CWP may have JHM, though given this too has a high prevalence, this association may appear by chance. Nevertheless there are several small epidemiological surveys that demonstrate a higher preponderance of JHM in cases of FM than in controls and there are logical reasons why this may occur based on assumptions around mechanical pathologies such as muscle spasm.

There have been no published large-scale epidemiological studies looking at the association between FM and JHS. Nevertheless, given the association between JHM and FM, JHM and JHS, the commonality of functional and somatic symptoms in FM and JHS, and the display of autonomic dysregulation in FM and JHS, the argument that They're co-existence might occur as a consequence of similar pathophysiology is compelling.

References

Acasuso-Diaz M, Collantes-Estevez E: Joint hypermobility in patients with fibromyalgia syndrome, *Arthritis Care Res* 11(1):39–42, 1998.

Berger A, Dukes E, Martin S, et al: Characteristics and healthcare costs of patients with fibromyalgia syndrome, *Int J Clin Pract* 61 (9):1498–1508, 2007.

Bergman S, Herrstrom P, Hogstrom K, et al: Chronic musculoskeletal pain, prevalence rates, and sociodemographic associations in a Swedish population study, *J Rheumatol* 28(6):1369–1377, 2001.

Bergman S, Herrstrom P, Jacobsson LT, et al: Chronic widespread pain: a three year follow up of pain distribution and risk factors, *J Rheumatol* 29(4): 818–825, 2002.

Bradley LA, Alarcón GS: Is Chiari malformation associated with

increased levels of substance P and clinical symptoms in persons with fibromyalgia? *Arthritis Rheum* 42(12):2731–2732, 1999.

Branco J, Bannwarth B, Failde I, et al: Prevalence of fibromyalgia in Europe- a tip of the iceberg- results from a large-scale survey [abstract], *Arthritis Rheum* 58(9):S690, 2008.

Burckhardt CS, Mannerkorpi K, Hedenberg L, et al: A randomized, controlled clinical trial of education and physical training for women with fibromyalgia, *J Rheumatol* 21(4): 714–720, 1994.

Buskila D, Abramov G, Biton A, et al: The prevalence of pain complaints in a general population in Israel and its implications for utilization of health services, *J Rheumatol* 27(6):1521–1525, 2000.

Buskila D, Neumann L: Genetics of fibromyalgia, *Curr Pain Headache Rep* 9(5):313–315, 2005.

Carville SF, Arendt-Nielsen S, Bliddal H, et al: EULAR evidence-based recommendations for the management of fibromyalgia syndrome, *Ann Rheum Dis* 67(4): 536–541, 2008.

Castro I, Barrantes F, Tuna M, et al: Prevalence of abuse in fibromyalgia and other rheumatic disorders at a specialized clinic in rheumatic diseases in Guatemala City, *J Clin Rheumatol* 11(3): 140–145, 2005.

Cohen H, Neumann L, Shore M, et al: Autonomic dysfunction in patients with fibromyalgia: application of power spectral analysis of heart rate variability, *Semin Arthritis Rheum* 29(4): 217–227, 2000a.

Cohen H, Benjamin J, Geva AB, et al: Autonomic dysregulation in panic disorder and in post-traumatic stress disorder: application of power spectrum analysis of heart rate variability at rest and in response to recollection of trauma or panic attacks, *Psychiatry Res* 96(1):1–13, 2000b.

Cohen H, Neumann L, Shore M, et al: Abnormal sympathovagal balance in men with fibromyalgia, *J Rheumtol* 28(3):581–589, 2001.

Cohen H, Benjamin J: Power spectrum analysis and cardiovascular morbidity in anxiety disorders, *Auton Neurosci* 128(1–2):1–8, 2006.

Croft P, Rigby AS, Boswell R, et al: The prevalence of chronic widespread pain in the general population, *J Rheumtol* 20(4): 710–713, 1993.

Duke BJ: Pathogenic effects of central nervous system hyperarousal, *Med Hypotheses* 71(2):212–217, 2008.

Elliott MB, Barr AE, Clark BD, et al: High force reaching task induces widespread inflammation, increased spinal cord neurochemicals and neuropathic pain, *Neuroscience* Jan 23;158(2): 922–931, 2009.

Fitzcharles MA: Is hypermobility a factor in fibromyalgia? *J Rheumtol* 27(7):1587–1589, 2000.

Ford CV: Somatization and fashionable diagnoses: illness as a way of life, *Scand J Work Environ Health* 23(Suppl 3):7–16, 1997.

Gedalia A, Press J, Klein M, et al: Joint hypermobility and fibromyalgia in schoolchildren, *Ann Rheum Dis* 52(7):494–496, 1993.

Giske L, Vøllestad NK, Mengshoel AM, et al: Attenuated adrenergic responses to exercise in women with fibromyalgia–a controlled study, *Eur J Pain* 12(3):351–360, 2008.

Goldman JA: Hypermobility and deconditioning: important links to fibromyalgia/fibrositis, *South Med J* 84(10):1192–1196, 1991.

Hakim AJ, Grahame R: Non-musculoskeletal symptoms in joint hypermobility syndrome. Indirect evidence for autonomic dysfunction, *Rheumatology* 43(9):1194–1195, 2004.

Hakim AJ: The Musculoskeletal System. In *Chamberlains Signs and Symptoms in Clinical Medicine*, ed 13, London, 2009, Elsevier.

Hassett AL, Cone JD, Patella SJ, et al: The role of catastrophizing in the pain and depression of women with fibromyalgia syndrome, *Arthritis Rheum* 43(11):2493–2500, 2000.

Heffez DS: Surgery for fibromyalgia, *Cleve Clin J Med* 69(1):89–91, 2002.

Heffez DS, Ross RE, Shade-Zeldow Y, et al: Clinical evidence for cervical myelopathy due to Chiari malformation and spinal stenosis in a non-randomized group of patients with the diagnosis of fibromyalgia, *Eur Spine J* 13(6): 516–523, 2004.

Heffez DS, Ross RE, Shade-Zeldow Y, et al: Treatment of cervical myelopathy in patients with the fibromyalgia syndrome: outcomes and implications, *Eur Spine J* 16(9):1423–1433, 2007.

Henningsen P, Zimmermann T, Sattel H: Medically unexplained physical symptoms, anxiety, and depression: a meta-analytic review, *Psychosom Med* 65(4): 528–533, 2003.

Hoffman DL, Dukes EM: The health status burden of people with fibromyalgia: a review of studies that assessed health status with the SF-36 or the SF-12, *Int J Clin Pract* 62(1):115–126, 2008.

Holman AJ: Is hypermobility a factor in fibromyalgia? *J Rheumtol* 29(2):396–398, 2002.

Holman AJ: Positional cervical spinal cord compression and fibromyalgia: a novel comorbidity with important diagnostic and treatment implications, *J Pain* 9(7):613–622, 2008.

Hudson N, Starr MR, Esdaile JM, et al: Diagnostic associations with hypermobility in rheumatology patients, *Br J Rheumatol* 34(12): 1157–1161, 1995.

Hughes G, Martinez C, Myon E, et al: The impact of a diagnosis of fibromyalgia on health care resource use by primary care patients in the UK: an observational study based on clinical practice, *Arthritis Rheum* 54(1):177–183, 2006.

Karaaslan Y, Haznedaroglu S, Ozturk M: Joint hypermobility and primary fibromyalgia: a clinical enigma, *J Rheumtol* 27(7):1774–1776, 2000.

Lai S, Goldman JA, Child AH, et al: Fibromyalgia, hypermobility, and breast implants, *J Rheumtol* 27(9): 2237–2241, 2000.

Langfitt TW, Elliott FA: Pain in the back and legs caused by cervical spinal cord compression, *JAMA* 200(5):382–385, 1967.

Ledingham J, Doherty S, Doherty M: Primary fibromyalgia syndrome– an outcome study, *Br J Rheumatol* 32(2):139–142, 1993.

Lentz MJ, Landis CA, Rothermel J, et al: Effects of selective slow wave sleep disruption on musculoskeletal pain and fatigue in middle aged women, *J Rheumtol* 26(7):1586–1592, 1999.

Leuenberger UA, Brubaker D, Quraishi S, et al: Effects of intermittent hypoxia on sympathetic activity and blood pressure in humans, *Auton Neurosci* 121(1–2):87–93, 2005.

Martinez-Lavin M, Hermosillo AG, Rosas M, et al: Circadian studies of autonomic nervous balance in patients with fibromyalgia: a heart variability analysis, *Arthritis Rheum* 41 (11):1966–1971, 1998.

Martinez-Lavin M, Hermosillo AG: Autonomic nervous system dysfunction may explain the multisystem features of fibromyalgia, *Semin Arthritis Rheum* 29(4):197–199, 2000.

Martinez-Lavin MM: Biology and therapy of fibromyalgia. Stress, the stress response system, and fibromyalgia, *Arthritis Res Ther* 9(4):216, 2007.

McBeth J, Macfarlane GJ, Hunt IM, et al: Risk factors for persistent chronic widespread pain: a community-based study, *Rheumatology (Oxford)* 40(1): 95–101, 2001a.

McBeth J, Macfarlane GJ, Benjamin S, et al: Features of somatization predict the onset of chronic widespread pain: results of a large population-based study, *Arthritis Rheum* 44(4):940–946, 2001b.

Moldofsky H, Scarisbrick P, England R, et al: Musculosketal symptoms and non-REM sleep disturbance in patients with "fibrositis syndrome" and healthy subjects, *Psychosom Med* 37(4): 341–351, 1975.

Moldofsky H, Scarisbrick P: Induction of neurasthenic musculoskeletal pain syndrome by selective sleep stage deprivation, *Psychosom Med* 38(1):35–44, 1976.

Older SA, Battafarano DF, Danning CL, et al: The effects of delta wave sleep interruption on pain thresholds and fibromyalgia-like symptoms in healthy subjects; correlations with insulin-like growth factor I, *J Rheumatol* 25(6): 1180–1186, 1998.

Penrod JR, Bernatsky S, Adam V, et al: Health services costs and their determinants in women with fibromylagia, *J Rheumatol* 31 (7):1391–1398, 2004.

Petzke F, Clauw DJ: Sympathetic nervous system function in fibromyalgia, *Curr Rheumatol Rep* 2(2):116–123, 2000.

Raj SR, Brouillard D, Simpson CS, et al: Dysautonomia among patients with fibromyalgia; a noninvasive assessment, *J Rheumatol* 27:2660–2665, 2000.

Reynolds EB, Seda G, Ware JC, et al: Autonomic function in sleep apnea patients: increased heart rate variability except during REM sleep in obese patients, *Sleep Breath* 11(1):53–60, 2007.

Roizenblatt S, Moldofsky H, Benedito-Silva AA, et al: Alpha sleep characteristics in fibromyalgia, *Arthritis Rheum* 44(1):222–230, 2001.

Rosner I, Rozenbaum M, Naschitz JE, et al: Dysautonomia in chronic fatigue syndrome vs. fibromyalgia, *Irr Med Assoc J* 2(Suppl):23–24, 2000.

Rubin JJ: Psychosomatic pain: new insights and management strategies, *South Med J* 98(11): 1099–1110, 2005.

Sendur OF, Gurer G, Bozbas GT: The frequency of hypermobility and its relationship with clinical findings of fibromyalgia patients, *Clin Rheumatol* 26(4):485–487, 2007.

Shindo K, Tsunoda S, Shiozawa Z: Decreased sympathetic outflow to muscles in patients with cervical spondylosis, *Acta Neurol Scand* 96(4):241–246, 1997.

Southwick SM, Krystal JH, Morgan CA, et al: Abnormal noradrenergic function in posttraumatic stress disorder,

Arch Gen Psychiatry 50(4):266–274, 1993.

Swann AC, Secunda SK, Koslow SH, et al: Mania: sympathoadrenal function and clinical state, *Psychiatry Res* 37(2):195–205, 1991.

Vaeroy H, Qiao ZG, Morkrid L, et al: Altered sympathetic nervous system response in patients with fibromyalgia (fibrositis syndrome), *J Rheumatol* 16(l1):1460–1465, 1998.

Van Houdenhove B, Neerinckx E, Lysens R, et al: Victimization in chronic fatigue syndrome and fibromyalgia in tertiary care: a controlled study on prevalence and characteristics, *Psychosomatics* 42(1):21–28, 2001.

White KP, Speechley M, Harth M, et al: The London Fibromyalgia Epidemiology Study: direct health care costs of fibromyalgia syndrome in London, *Canada J Rheum* 26(4):885–889, 1999.

White LA, Birnbaum HG, Kaltenboeck A, et al: Employees with fibromyalgia: medical comorbidity, health costs and work loss, *J Occup Environ Med* 50(1):13–24, 2008.

Wolfe F, Smythe HA, Yunus MB, et al: The American College of Rheumatology 1990 criteria for the classification of fibromyalgia: report of the multicenter criteria committee, *Arthritis Rheum* 33(2):160–172, 1990.

Wolfe F, Smythe HA, Yunus MB, et al: The prevalence and characteristics of fibromyalgia in the general population, *Arthritis Rheum* 38(1):19–28, 1995.

Chapter 6

Neuromuscular physiology in joint hypermobility

6.1 Cardiovascular autonomic dysfunction and chronic fatigue in fibromyalgia and joint hypermobility syndrome

Jaime F Bravo, Gonzalo Sanhueza and Alan J Hakim

INTRODUCTION

Fatigue is a common and disabling finding in many musculoskeletal conditions including rheumatoid arthritis, systemic lupus erythematosus and fibromyalgia (FM). It is also very common, yet poorly recognized, in joint hypermobility syndrome (JHS). Pathologies associated with fatigue such as anaemia, endocrinopathies, chronic infections, malignancy, and end-organ failure should always be excluded. In the vast majority of cases of FM and JHS however, fatigue is simply an integral feature of the pain syndrome. Also, the nature of symptoms in chronic fatigue syndrome (CFS) can be identical to that of FM and JHS. All three conditions share the phenotypes of fatigue, anxiety, physical de-conditioning and poor and non-restorative sleep. Are the mechanisms leading to fatigue and pain in these conditions the same?

The autonomic nervous system (ANS) is responsible for internal homeostasis including maintenance of blood pressure, fluid and electrolyte balance, visceral function and temperature control. More recently the ANS has been considered an integral part of pain modulation driven by sympathetic dysfunction interacting with maladaptive central mechanisms within structures such as the thalamus, caudate, amygdala and hippocampus (Chapter 3). Cardiovascular autonomic dysfunction (CAD) is a common finding in CFS, FM and JHS. Research within each field has followed similar suit, utilizing investigations and therapies available in the assessment and management of primary and secondary autonomic failure. The conclusions are remarkably similar. Whilst not all individuals with fatigue have clearly defined CAD, the evidence for an association between fatigue, CAD with sympathetic over activity, and vascular de-conditioning in CFS, FM and JHS is compelling. Aside from physical differences in phenotype, these conditions may in effect be manifestations of the same thing – maladaptation of the autonomic nervous system.

In this chapter we will outline the common symptoms of fatigue and signs of CAD, review the literature for CAD in its association with CFS, FM and JHS, and discuss the therapeutic options.

FATIGUE IN JOINT HYPERMOBILITY SYNDROME

Fatigue is a common experience in JHS. In one survey of 170 adult women with JHS, 71% reported

© 2010 Elsevier Ltd.
DOI: 10.1016/B978-0-7020-3005-5.00006-9

significant fatigue that was affecting their quality of life (Hakim & Grahame 2004).

In the authors' experience the fatigue associated with JHS is often ill-understood by clinicians. The fatigue experienced by patients with JHS (and indeed FM) is not the typical tiredness one associates with post exercise or a busy day at work, but is often an over-whelming lack of energy that may appear after even the most minimal period of activity. The majority of patients may recognize that they are fine for a period of time but as the day goes on they suddenly tire and feel sleepy, as if 'the battery has run out of charge'. Many will report cold intolerance, dizziness, a fear of blackouts and poor concentration. They also complain that they cannot stand for too long as this aggravates their symptoms; both pain and fatigue. This can occur for example whilst queuing. These symptoms can be severe and lead to a poor quality of life. In children and adolescents poor concentration may lead to poor academic grades at school. Such may be the absolute desire to rest or sleep that an individual may come across to others as lazy, antisocial or perhaps even depressed. The ability to cope with the social consequences of these phenomena is compounded by the delay in or lack of diagnosis.

MEASURING FATIGUE

Several fatigue scales have been developed. These include the 'Fatigue Severity Scale' (FSS), the 'Fatigue Scale' (FS), the 'Energy/Fatigue Scale' (EFS), 'Checklist Individual Strength' (CIS), and 'Fatigue Impact Scale'. Selection of a fatigue rating score has been reviewed by Friedberg and Jason (2002); within their review several key points are noted from the literature:

- Although FSS and FS both are useful tools, the FSS may be a more accurate measure of both severity and functional disability in patients with CFS.
- The validity and consistency of the CIS have been demonstrated in healthy controls and patients with CFS and the scale has demonstrated sensitivity to change following interventions with cognitive-behavioural therapy.
- The FIS explores three domains of cognitive, physical and psychosocial functioning and as such is a useful tool when exploring impact and outcome of a wide range of associations and risks.

Jones et al (2009) have very recently examined the descriptions of fatigue within a range of chronic disease scenarios. In a retrospective review of FIS data 605 chronic disease patients and 45 normal controls were assessed by each of the three domains. The FIS appeared to be a valuable tool for comparing CFS with other disease groups.

Whilst fatigue is understood to be commonly reported in patients with JHS, it has not been examined in detail either epidemiologically or in relation to response to therapy using the validated tools described above. Interestingly, the prevalence of JHS varies in racial groups, and there is evidence to suggest similar variability in CFS (Dinos et al 2009). This is an important area for future research.

MANAGING FATIGUE

Identification and management of diseases associated with fatigue is assumed. Thereafter, there is very little published evidence to support the use of the various forms of therapy available for fatigue per se. Much is anecdotal and relates to individual successes. Nevertheless there are reasonable guiding principles. In CFS, FM and JHS, for example, the use of antidepressants, anti-anxiety drugs, sleep aids and analgesics in the general management of the condition might be expected to have some impact on the fatigue be it direct or indirect.

Lifestyle changes including pacing, changing sleep pattern, exercise, and even change of job or hours of work may help, as may behavioural therapy. These are covered in other sections of this book. Complementary therapies such as acupuncture, massage and Reiki may be beneficial.

While there is limited scientific evidence supporting the use of nutritional supplements for CFS, many doctors and patients consider them an important part of treatment. Commonly recommended supplements include Carnitine, Co-enzyme Q10 and 5-HTP. Such agents are considered to be effective in boosting the immune system, raising energy levels, and improving cognitive functioning.

Carnitine, at a dose of 500 mg twice daily, is considered to raise energy levels by increasing fat metabolism. It may also have a function in facilitating the effect of serotonin and glutamate in the central nervous system (Chapter 3). Carnitine is naturally found in red meat and poultry, fish, dairy, wheat, asparagus and avocado. The main side-effects of Carnitine include hypertension, tachycardia and fever. It may also impair thyroid function.

Co-enzyme Q10 is a powerful antioxidant required for the metabolism of adenosine triphosphate (ATP). Typically 30–90 mg is taken in two or three divided doses daily. It is slow-acting and benefit may not be realized for up to 8 weeks. Co-enzyme Q10 is found naturally in oily fish, offal and whole grains. The side effects include nausea and vomiting, diarrhoea, skin irritation, irritability, increased sensitivity to bright light and flu-like symptoms. It may also induce hypoglycaemia and hypotension.

5-HTP is directly converted to serotonin. Low serotonin is a feature of FM (Chapter 5). 5-HTP has been reported to alleviate many of the symptoms of FM. The dose range is from 50 to 500 mg a day starting at a low dose and escalating slowly. 5-HTP should not be taken with other medications that alter serotonin levels. The side effects of 5-HTP include nausea, dizziness and diarrhoea.

With all supplements it is important to remember the potential for negative interactions with other supplements and medication, that there are limited or no data on use in pregnancy and lactation, and that there is no specific dosage recommendation for CFS, FM or JHS.

SYMPTOMS, SIGNS AND INVESTIGATION OF AUTONOMIC DISTURBANCE

SYMPTOMS

The three typical findings of cardiovascular autonomic dysfunction (CAD) are orthostatic hypotension (OH), orthostatic intolerance (OI), and postural tachycardia syndrome (POTS). Patients report dizziness, light-headedness, visual blurring, tunnel vision, inattention or poor concentration and a fear of or history of 'blacking out' (syncope). In childhood and adolescence typical features include tiring easily, clumsiness and an intolerance of exercise. Because of this, it is important that paediatricians as well as adult physicians are alert to the associations. The reader will recognize that many of these symptoms also describe those reported in association with fatigue (as above) and several of the physical manifestations of JHS (Chapter 2).

Symptoms of autonomic (sympathetic) activation include palpitations, tremor, excessive sweating and anxiety (Chapter 4). Both groups of

---

> **BOX 6.1.1   Symptoms associated with autonomic dysfunction that are not specifically associated with postural change**
>
> - Flushing
> - Headaches
> - Muscle and joint pain
> - Neuropathic pain
> - Hypervigilance to bodily changes (Chapter 8)
> - Gastrointestinal dysfunction (Chapter 6.2)
> - Increased sweating

symptoms may occur transiently and immediately after standing up, and may remit spontaneously without necessarily being considered significant.

There are a number of symptoms that are not restricted to a change in posture. These are shown in Box 6.1.1.

Symptoms may be worsened by dehydration and other low-volume states such as anaemia (Table 6.1.1), high temperatures, exercise, systemic illness or prolonged bed rest. Symptoms may also fluctuate with the menstrual cycle, being at their worst during bleeding. In general this is likely to be related to blood loss and volume depletion, however in JHS sensitivity to changing levels of progesterone is recognized as a triggering factor for a number of other symptoms including pain and worsening joint stability.

As well as syncope being induced by orthostatic stressors, vasovagal syncope (VVS) may be provoked by straining, e.g. when passing urine or stool, or coughing (the Valsalva – see below), or by emotional stress.

It is not the intention of this chapter to explore pure or primary autonomic failure, multiple system atrophy or secondary autonomic failure, for example in diabetes mellitus. These have been recently reviewed in detail by Low and Benarroch (2008). However, it is important to be aware of such conditions when considering the potential cause of autonomic dysfunction in patients with CFS, FM or JHS as co-morbidity. A detailed examination is required to exclude evidence of conditions such as Parkinson disease, multiple sclerosis, syringobulbia, Guillain-Barre syndrome, transverse myelitis, diabetic neuropathy and paraneoplastic syndromes.

Likewise, as shown in Table 6.1.1, a number of medications may precipitate symptoms and a detailed history is therefore necessary.

Table 6.1.1   Clinical findings and associations with OH, OI and POTS

CONDITION	CLINICAL FINDING/DEFINITION	ASSOCIATIONS
Orthostatic Hypotension	Rapid drop in blood pressure $\geq$ 20/10 mmHg in 3 min and up to 30 min (delayed reaction) Standing intolerance	Dehydration Anaemia Extreme vasodilation e.g. heat Congestive cardiac failure **Drugs:** Diuretics ACE-inhibitors Alpha and beta blockers Tricyclic antidepressants Nitrates Calcium channel blockers Opiates Sildenafil (Viagra) Phenothiazines Hydralazine MAO inhibitors Bromocriptine Alcohol and illicit agents
Orthostatic Intolerance	Development of symptoms during standing, that disappear when lying down	Deficiency of the renin-angiotensin-aldosterone system Others as above
Postural Orthostatic Tachycardia (POTS)	> 30 bpm rise in pulse, plus symptoms of OI OR >120 beats per minute within 10 minutes of head-up tilt or standing and usually without orthostatic hypotension	Activation/hypersensitivity of sympathetic system/deconditioning

POSTURAL ORTHOSTATIC TACHYCARDIA SYNDROME

Postural orthostatic tachycardia syndrome (defined in Table 6.1.1) typically affects adults between 20–50 years of age. It is 4–5 times more common in women than men. Syncope is common and is usually of the vasovagal type. In POTS, symptoms characteristically occur after a period of standing or sitting. They may also fluctuate between acute episodes lasting just a day and chronic episodes lasting months. In addition, POTS may be accompanied by fatigue whether supine or erect, with significant negative impact on quality of life as described above (Benrud-Larson et al 2002).

The exact mechanism for POTS may remain elusive despite investigation. Low (1993) and colleagues (1995) have suggested three subgroups of the disorder: neuropathic POTS, hyperadrenergic POTS and POTS with deconditioning.

Neuropathic POTS is caused by autonomic neuropathy leading to defective peripheral vasoconstriction and excessive venous pooling in the legs during standing. It can follow a viral infection and have an autoimmune basis, suggested by autoantibodies to acetylcholine receptors found in some patients. Hyperadrenergic POTS is associated with high plasma catecholamine levels when supine or upright. Typically, standing noradrenaline (norepinephrine) levels rise over 600 pg/ml. There are individual reports of hyperadrenergic POTS associated with genetic abnormalities of catecholamine transporters and mast cell activation causing increased availability of noradrenaline in autonomic synapses (Shannon et al 2000, Robertson et al 2001, Garland et al 2002, Shibao et al 2005). These rare conditions are beyond the scope of this chapter; for a more detailed recent review of POTS and orthostatic syncope the reader is directed to Grubb (2008) and Moya and Wieling (2006) respectively.

POTS with deconditioning can follow prolonged bed rest or prolonged periods of physical inactivity leading to cardiac atrophy, reduced blood volume, and consequently reduced cardiac stroke volume.

There are no epidemiological studies of POTS; estimates of prevalence range between 170–2000/100 000. Perhaps the first descriptions of POTS date back to Beard's (1869) account of neurasthenia, and the Da Costa syndrome or irritable heart of soldiers (Da Costa 1871). As early as 1918 physicians recognized the dilemmas still present today – the heterogeneity and aetiological uncertainty of OI (Fraser & Wilson 1918, Khurana 1995).

ORTHOSTATIC HYPOTENSION AND INTOLERANCE

Clinical examination of patients with OI (defined in Table 6.1.1) will most often reveal no abnormality. After a prolonged period (which may take 30 minutes or more) a patient may begin to hyperventilate, sweat, become pale and anxious. Acrocyanosis, a dusky red/blue discoloration of the lower leg during standing may be seen. This is caused by excessive venous pooling due to increased capacitance. The legs may swell. This may be exacerbated in the collagen disorders given the excessive elasticity of the connective tissues. Orthostatic hypotension may cause considerable disability, with the potential risk of serious injury (Mathias 2007).

INVESTIGATION OF CAD

Many tests, including ECG, postural blood pressure changes, heart rate variation to deep breathing, the Valsalva manoeuvre and sustained handgrip, can all be done at the bedside or in clinic.

More detailed investigation requires a well-equipped laboratory. The findings may be subtle and dismissed clinically even though the symptoms seem profound and associated with significant morbidity. The exclusion of cardiac disease or hypotension due to drug therapy is essential (Table 6.1.1). Before planning autonomic assessment a detailed history and examination are needed.

Head–up tilt

The 'head-up tilt' is often used as the postural stimulus, especially when neurological deficit or severe hypotension makes it difficult for the patient to stand. The blood pressure and heart rate can be accurately measured using non-invasive techniques, many of which are automated and provide a printout. In autonomic failure there may be considerable variability in the basal supine levels. Typically the subject rests flat for 30 minutes and is then tilted

upright for the duration of the investigation to an angle of 60–80°. A normal response to tilting would be an increase in heart rate by 10–15 beats per minute, a rise in diastolic pressure by approximately 10 mmHg, and minimal change in systolic pressure. The abnormal responses of OH and POTS are as described in Table 6.1.1. A negative tilt test does not rule out the presence of dysautonomia, the reason being that many patients have only few symptoms. This exam is used generally for the study of syncope. It is classically informed as positive if there is presence of syncope or pre-syncope mentioning in the report, if the patient presents during the test symptoms of orthostatic intolerance or POTS. If the test reproduces the patient's symptoms, the test should be considered positive, even if there is no syncope or pre-syncope.

Heart rate variability analysis

'Heart rate variability analysis' is based on the fact that variation of heart rate is modulated by impulses from both the sympathetic or parasympathetic branches of the ANS on the sinus node of the heart. It has two domains: 'time' and 'frequency'. The 'time' domain utilizes calculations based on the R–R interval on the ECG; in particular the standard deviation of duration of R–R intervals and the percentage of adjacent R–R intervals that are greater than 50 milliseconds apart over the study period. Higher index values represent increased parasympathetic influence on the sinus node.

The 'frequency' domain uses spectral analysis. So-called 'high-frequency-band spectral power' reflects parasympathetic normal activity; this cycles rhythmically with respiration. Sympathetic activity modulates at a 'low-frequency-band spectral power', acting through arterial baroreceptors. A raised low-frequency-band to high-frequency-band ratio reflects sympathetic activity (Malik et al. Task Force of the European Society of Cardiology and the North American Society of Pacing and Electrophysiology 1996). This kind of analysis can be undertaken during tilt-testing.

Other screening tests

Other autonomic screening tests help determine the site and extent of CAD, be it cardiovagal, adrenergic, or peripheral, post-ganglionic sympathetic sudomotor denervation. These are shown in Box 6.1.2.

BOX 6.1.2   Autonomic tests used to determine the likely neurophysiological trigger of CAD

- Responses to the Valsalva manoeuvre assess sympathetic function as well as vagal function.
- Cardiac parasympathetic (vagus) activity can be assessed by heart rate responses to:
  - postural change
  - deep breathing (sinus arrhythmia)
  - hyperventilation.
- Evaluation of the postganglionic sympathetic sudomotor axon reflex using acetylcholine as a stimulus; for example the quantitative sudomotor axon reflex test (QSART) (Low et al 1983), performed at several sites including the forearm, outer thigh, inner lower leg, or the foot.

- Activation of sympathetic outflow (adrenergic function) within different afferent or central pathways is assessed by applying stimuli that raise blood pressure:
  - isometric exercise (by sustained hand grip for 3 minutes)
  - the cold pressor test (immersing the hand in ice for 90 seconds)
  - mental arithmetic (using serial-7 or -17 subtraction), activate different afferent or central pathways.

Factors contributing to orthostatic pathologies and syncope also include the response to food ingestion, exercise and carotid sinus massage.

To assess postprandial hypotension, the cardiovascular responses to a balanced liquid meal containing carbohydrate, protein and fat are measured while supine, with comparisons of the blood pressure response to head-up tilt before the meal and 45 minutes later.

To evaluate exercise-induced hypotension, responses are obtained during graded incremental supine exercise using a bicycle ergometer with measurement of postural responses before and after exercise. Many find that the tachycardia is worse during exercise; deconditioning due to lack of physical activity may complicate the disorder (Chapters 9 and 13); indeed it may be very difficult to isolate POTS as a primary autonomic dysfunction from deconditioning (Joyner & Masuki 2008). In some individuals, as with OI on prolonged standing, hyperventilation and panic attack may occur.

Thermoregulatory sweat test may be helpful in demonstrating sudomotor denervation.

Finally, in order to complete the assessment plasma catecholamine levels may be needed. Measurements are available in specialized laboratories and may be of value in certain disorders such as hyperadrenergic POTS.

AUTONOMIC DYSFUNCTION IN CHRONIC FATIGUE SYNDROME

The criteria for chronic fatigue syndrome (CFS) were proposed by Holmes et al in 1988 and then by the 'International Chronic Fatigue Syndrome Study Group' of the American Centers for Disease Control (CDC) in 1994 (Fukuda et al 1994). The 1994 criteria are those used most often in current research and diagnosis, and are shown in Box 6.1.3.

CFS is a diagnosis of exclusion; it is however also considered an over-arching term for two conditions with similar symptoms, namely myalgic encephalomyelitis (ME) and post-viral syndrome.

All other causes of chronic fatigue must be ruled out by a thorough history, assessment of mental health state (specifically excluding presence of chronic depression), physical examination, and laboratory screening for electrolyte and endocrine imbalance, and abnormal haematological indices.

The majority of symptoms that constitute the secondary criteria, with the exception of tender lymphadenopathy, are similar to those found in JHS (Chapter 1) and FM (Chapter 5). The uninitiated might therefore miss the presence of JHS or FM and 'label' a person as having CFS! Barron et al (2002), for example, found that joint hypermobility was more common in children with CFS than in healthy controls. Separating CFS from FM and JHS is not as straight forward as it might appear. Making an incomplete diagnosis is relevant not least because it may lead to the incorrect choice of physical therapy.

EVIDENCE OF AUTONOMIC DYSFUNCTION IN CFS

The association of CAD with CFS first appeared in case-reports and epidemiological studies of ME in the late 1970s (Parish 1978, Ramsay 1978). Streeten and Anderson (1992) later suggested that fatigue may be due to an inability to maintain blood

---

BOX 6.1.3   CDC 1994 Criteria for Chronic Fatigue Syndrome

Primary criteria

Persistent or relapsing chronic fatigue that is:
- New and of defined onset
- Not a result of ongoing excessive exertion
- Not substantially relieved by rest

Secondary criteria

Four or more of the following symptoms must have persisted or recurred during 6 or more consecutive months of illness and not predated the fatigue:

- Impairment in short-term memory or concentration severe enough to cause substantial reduction in previous levels of occupational, educational, social, or personal activities
- Sore throat
- Tender cervical or axillary lymph nodes
- Muscle pain
- Multi-joint pain without joint swelling or redness
- Headaches of a new type, pattern or severity
- Unrefreshing/non-restorative sleep
- Post-exertion malaise lasting more than 24 hours

---

pressure when standing. Using tilt-table technology Rowe et al (1995), Bou-Holaigah et al (1995), and Timmers et al (2002) identified a predisposition to CAD in CFS, demonstrating the presence of 'neurogenic syncope'.

Soetekouw et al (1999), recognizing that the signs of CAD in CFS can be subtle, assessed non-invasive measurements in an unselected group of 37 patients with CFS and 38 healthy controls. Blood pressure and heart rate were recorded continuously before and during forced breathing, standing up, the Valsalva manoeuvre, sustained handgrip exercise and mental arithmetic testing. At rest, there were no significant differences in blood pressure, heart rate or Valsalva ratio between the groups. However, on standing the systolic and diastolic blood pressure responses were significantly larger in CFS patients. Also, the heart rate response to mental arithmetic was found to be significantly less in the CFS group. This suggested impaired cardiac sympathetic responsiveness to mental stress. Finally, the haemodynamic responses to the hand grip exercise were lower in the CFS group than in the control group, but it was considered that this might have been attributable to lower levels of muscle exertion in the CFS patients. The findings of the study were subtle, leading to the suggestion that there were no gross alterations in cardiovascular autonomic function in CFS.

Stewart (2000) examined the nature of autonomic and vasomotor changes in symptomatic adolescents. The cohort included 22 cases of POTS, 14 of CFS with a history of orthostatic tachycardia, and ten healthy individuals and 20 cases of simple faint as controls. Stewart showed that the R–R interval on ECG and heart rate variability were decreased in the CFS and POTS patients compared with controls and remained decreased with head-up tilt. Blood pressure variability was increased in the CFS and POTS

patients compared with controls and increased further with head-up tilt. Stewart concluded that 'heart rate and blood pressure regulation in POTS and CFS patients are similar and show an attenuated efferent vagal baroreflex associated with increased vasomotor tone. The loss of beat-to-beat heart rate control may contribute to a destabilized blood pressure resulting in orthostatic intolerance. The dysautonomia of orthostatic intolerance in POTS and in chronic fatigue are similar'.

Peckerman et al (2003) also postulated that altered cardiovascular responses to mental and orthostatic stressors reported in CFS may involve changes in baroreceptor reflex functioning. Their study demonstrated that patients with CFS had a greater decline in baroreceptor reflex sensitivity during standing, although only those with severe CFS were significantly different from the controls, suggesting that classifying patients by illness severity may aid in interpreting response to CAD testing.

More recently the association between CAD and CFS has been reaffirmed (Grubb et al 2005, Newton et al 2007) and the mechanisms further described. Wyller et al (2008) showed that adolescents with CFS have increased sympathetic activity at rest with exaggerated cardiovascular responses to orthostatic stress.

Legge et al (2008) identified fatigue as a significant symptom in the presence of VVS. Fatigue was assessed in 140 sequential cases of VVS with matched controls using the FIS. The severity and type of autonomic symptoms was explored using the composite autonomic symptom scale or COMPASS (Suarez et al 1999). The conclusions were that fatigue is a significant problem in patients with VVS and that, like the observation of Peckerman et al (2003), the severity of autonomic symptoms correlated with the degree of fatigue.

The association between POTS and CFS in adolescence has also been explored by Galland et al (2008). The study concluded that CFS subjects were more susceptible to OI than controls and that the cardiovascular response predominantly manifested as POTS without hypotension. Similarly, Hoad et al (2008) showed that the maximum heart rate on standing was significantly higher in patients with CFS/ME compared with controls. Increasing fatigue was associated with increase in heart rate.

Finally, there has recently been a re-focus on cardiovascular deconditioning. Hurwitz et al (2009) examined the association between cardiac output and blood volume, lifestyle, and illness severity in CFS. Participants were subdivided into two CFS groups based on symptom severity data (severe ($N = 30$) vs. non-severe ($N = 26$)). Two healthy control groups were matched to the CFS groups. The controls were also split into subgroups on the basis of reported physical activity (sedentary ($N = 58$) vs non-sedentary ($N = 32$)). Echocardiographic measures indicated that the severe CFS participants displayed 10.2% lower cardiac volume and 25.1% lower contractility than the control groups. Deficit in 'total blood volume' in CFS explained greater than 90% of the group differences in the cardiac volume indices, and primarily within the group with severe CFS.

Newton et al (2009) examined blood pressure circadian rhythm in patients with CFS ($N = 38$), normal ($N = 120$) and fatigue ($N = 47$) controls. The fatigue controls had primary biliary cirrhosis. The study correlated blood pressure regulation with fatigue using the FIS. Lower blood pressure and exaggerated abnormal diurnal blood pressure regulation occurred in patients with CFS compared to controls.

In response to such findings Stewart (2009) has recently commented that the presence of low blood pressure, whether symptomatic or not, is 'primarily attributable to a measurable reduction in blood volume ... similar findings are observed in microgravity and bed rest de-conditioning, in forms of orthostatic intolerance, and to a lesser extent in sedentary people. The circulatory consequences of reduced cardiac output may help to account for many of the findings of the syndrome'.

AUTONOMIC DYSFUNCTION IN FIBROMYALGIA

Autonomic dysfunction is a common finding in FM and has been the source of much research over the last two decades much like that in CFS. The association between autonomic dysfunction and FM, and the historical context leading to current thinking over the last two decades has been eloquently described by Martinez-Lavin (2007). The first published study was in 1988 when Bengtsson and Bengtsson reported a controlled trial of stellate ganglion blockade, showing improvement in regional cervical pain in FM versus sham injection. Subsequently several authors published data suggesting abnormalities of sympathetic function in FM including reduced vasoconstriction to cooling (Vaeroy et al 1989), and abnormal norepinephrine response to exercise (van Denderen et al 1992).

With the advent of heart rate variability analysis and tilt-up testing a number of studies demonstrated the presence of sympathetic exaggerated responses to orthostatic stressors (Bou-Holaigah et al 1997, Martinez-Lavin et al 1997, 1998, Cohen et al 2000, 2001, Raj et al 2000, Naschitz et al 2001, Furlan et al 2005, Ulas et al 2006).

FM groups in these studies had significantly different responses to testing as compared to controls. For example Raj et al (2000) demonstrated an abnormal tilt-up test result in 64.9% cases of FM versus 21.3% of controls. However, it was also recognized that there was considerable overlap between patients and controls, reflecting the subtleness of abnormal responses of the ANS within the general population. This makes it difficult at an individual level to predict the ability of tests to demonstrate clearly definable abnormalities of the ANS in patients with FM; a phenomenon already noted above with regard to CFS.

Irritable bowel syndrome (IBS) is a common finding in FM (Chapter 5 and Chapter 6.2). Karling et al (1998) found that patients with IBS also have alterations in heart rate variability that are consistent with sympathetic overactivity. Subsequently Adeyemi et al (1999) reported deranged sympathetic response to orthostatic stress in patients with IBS and Heitkemper et al (1998) and Kooh et al (2003) have described a circadian variability to heart rate in FM that is like that seen in IBS. It is therefore perhaps not surprising, given the similar findings of autonomic dysfunction, that IBS and FM co-occur, irrespective of an assumption that IBS may be an expression of anxiety or side-effect of analgesia in FM.

Such circadian dysautonomia may also explain sleep disorder in FM. Previously it had been shown that a sympathetic surge precedes arousal or awakening in normal subjects (Otzenberger et al 1997); this finding would suggest that inappropriate sympathetic activity in FM may be responsible for excessive episodes of arousal and awakening and therefore poor sleep patterns.

All of these associations have been re-affirmed in a very recent case-control study using the COMPASS (see above) (Solano et al 2009).

Sympathetic dysfunction may lead to allodynia (Chapter 3). There is also neurophysiological evidence for central sensitization in FM (Desmueles et al 2003). Equally, sympathetic hyperactivity and increased levels of catecholamines activate primary afferent nociceptors (Sato & Perl 1991, Baron et al 1999), and sympathetic dysfunction may destabilize central pain modulation.

The conclusion is that sympathetic overactivity drives or fuels maladaption of pain, sleep, cardiovascular and bowel physiology in FM.

AUTONOMIC DYSFUNCTION IN JOINT HYPERMOBILITY SYNDROME

Patients with JHS suffer from symptoms of autonomic dysfunction in much the same way as those with CFS or FM. In the past, palpitations and atypical chest pain in hypermobile patients were thought primarily to be caused by mitral valve prolapse (Grahame et al 1981, Coghlan 1988, Mishra 1996). However, OI, most often in the form of POTS and vasovagal syncope, is much more common in patients with JHS than in the general population (Rowe et al 1999, Gazit et al 2003, Hakim & Grahame 2004, Bravo & Wolff 2008).

Gazit et al (2003) confirmed the presence of symptoms, studying 27 JHS patients with dysautonomia compared with 21 controls. Orthostatic hypotension, POTS, and uncategorized OI were found in 78% (21/27) of patients. In a study of 170 JHS patients from a specialist clinic, Hakim and Grahame (2004) indentified 41% of patients reported light-headedness and other presyncopal symptoms, 26% palpitations and shortness of breath, and 37% gastrointestinal symptoms, compared to 15%, 12% and 16% in controls, respectively. Bravo and Wolfe found dysautonomia in 23% of 230 JHS patients (2006) and later in 39.1% of 1226 patients. The prevalence of OH and OI was highest in those under age 30 years, and especially in adolescent girls. Autonomic dysfunction was present in 72% of females and 44% of males in this age group.

In one study from a specialty hypermobility clinic the presence of CAD was identified by detailed autonomic testing in symptomatic cases of JHS. Some 63% of patients had identifiable pathology (43% POTS, 14% VVS, and 6% both) (Hakim et al 2009). None were identified as having other pathologies such as anaemia or epilepsy that might explain symptoms. As such, even after detailed history and assessment, one third of symptomatic cases had no identifiable autonomic pathology; a phenomenon clearly echoing that reported in the studies of patients with CFS and FM.

TREATMENT OF CARDIOVASCULAR AUTONOMIC DYSFUNCTION

The symptoms of CAD can be successfully managed; all the more reason that they should not be missed or ignored. Management includes correcting causes of fluid loss, replacing blood and fluids, correcting endocrine deficiencies such as hypoadrenalism, and preventing vasodilatation.

NON-PHARMACOLOGICAL MANAGEMENT OF CAD

Non-pharmacological measures are a key component of management, even when drugs are used. As no single drug can effectively mimic the actions of the sympathetic nervous system, a multi-pronged approach is needed. It is important that patients should be made aware of the many factors, other than postural change, that lower blood pressure (Box 6.1.4).

Simple techniques may help reduce symptoms by either (i) increasing fluid volume in the body, or (ii) improving venous return to the heart. Good fluid balance is fundamental (Yunoszai et al 1998, Wieling et al 2002) and intake should be at least

---

BOX 6.1.4	Factors that may precipitate OH and OI and therefore to be avoided

- Rapid postural change, especially in the morning when getting out of bed
- Sitting or standing for too long in one position
- Prolonged bed rest
- Nocturnal polyuria
- Excessive straining during micturition and defaecation
- Heat
- Alcohol
- Large carbohydrate meals

2–2.5 litres a day or more. The simplest way to be sure of adequate fluid intake is the realization that the urine should become pale yellow or preferably colourless with adequate fluid intake, and that on average a person passes urine with a frequency of twice in the morning and twice in the evening. Dark urine is a sign of dehydration.

It may be necessary to increase salt intake. Studies show that salt supplementation increase plasma volume (El-Sayed & Hainsworth 1996, Claydon & Hainsworth 2004). Patients need reassurance that it is okay to increase their salt intake, as so much publicity exists around reducing salt intake for well-being and reduction of hypertension, that the message may be confusing. Isotonic drinks are recommended.

Various physical manoeuvres (Wieling et al 1993, Brignole et al 2002, Krediet et al 2002), such as leg crossing, squatting, sitting in the knee-chest position, and abdominal compression, are of value in reducing OH, as may be 'tilt training therapy' for syncope (Reybrouck et al 2002, Gajek et al 2006, Ector & Reybrouck 2007). Exercise for muscle re-conditioning is important and is the subject of much of Section 2 of this book in relation to managing the patient with JHS. Consideration should also be given to garments aimed at preventing venous pooling. These include intermittent use of lower limb elastic stockings and abdominal binders.

PHARMACOLOGICAL MANAGEMENT OF CAD

The aim is to either increase blood volume (fludrocortisone, EPO), increase vasoconstriction (midodrine, etilefrine, SSRIs), or block the effect of (nor)epinephrine (beta-blockers, disopyramide, ACE-I).

Fludrocortisone is a potent synthetic mineralocorticoid with minimal glucocorticoid effect. It encourages an increase in intra- and extravascular fluid, sensitizes vascular receptors to pressor amines, and reduces vascular wall elasticity making blood vessels more resistant to stretch. A dose of 0.1 mg daily is effective for more than 24 hours, and for this reason is useful in adolescents, because it is taken once a day and if the tablet is missed one day there is no problem. The half-life elimination in plasma is 30–35 minutes. The biological half life is 18–36 hours. Dietary salt intake must be adequate and occasionally potassium supplements

are needed to counteract the side effect of hypokalaemia. Electrolyte balance should be checked before starting the drug, in a month and then once a year. It should be noted that there are no specific trials for Fludrocortisone, or indeed any of the other agents used in management of CAD, in patients with JHS.

Midodrine is an alpha-adrenoreceptor agonist. It has an effect on arterial resistance and venous capacitance, through its active metabolite desglymidodrine. Several studies have shown it to be efficacious (Low et al 1997, Ward et al 1998, Perez-Lugones et al 2001). Midodrine is given as 2.5–10 mg 3–4 times daily and is licensed for recurrent neurogenic syncope. It is effective, but the problem is that the action lasts only 4 hours and needs to be taken several times a day. The side effects include supine hypertension, scalp tingling and urinary retention.

Selective beta-blockade with, for example bisoprolol, metoprolol or propranolol may be of value in reducing the frequency of POTS. In a recent study by Lai et al (2009) of adolescents attending the Mayo Clinic, USA, midodrine was compared to beta-blocker therapy. More patients treated with a beta-blocker reported improvement in symptoms and more attributed their improvement to their medication compared to those taking midodrine. This was in contrast to an earlier study from the Mayo Clinic in which Thieben et al (2007), reporting on 152 cases of POTS, found no differences in the symptomatic response to beta-blockers, fludrocortisone, midodrine and SSRIs, with all class of agents inducing partial symptom relief in 40–60% of patients.

Whatever the combination of the above medication required to produce the desired effect, selective targeting is often needed and is best determined under the guidance of a specialist unit. Orthostatic and postprandial hypotension may respond to L-theodihydroxyphenylserine (Droxidopa) (Freeman et al 1996, Mathias et al 2001, Goldstein 2006, Mathias 2008); acarbose also showing efficacy in postprandial hypotension (Jian & Zhou 2008), octreotide is also useful in postprandial hypotension. Orthostatic hypotension might also respond to pyridostigmine (Singer et al 2006), nocturnal polyuria and morning hypotension to desmopressin (Mathias et al 1986, Mathias & Young 2003) and POTS and hypotension to the somatostatin analogue, octreotide (Hoeldtke & Davis 1991, Smith et al 1995). Erythropoietin (Grubb & Karas 1999) may also improve blood pressure.

The drawback with erythropoietin is its cost, the need to administer by subcutaneous injection, and the need to closely monitor the red cell count.

SUMMARY

Fatigue is common in CFS, FM and JHS. In exploring the causes for fatigue identical themes related to cardiovascular autonomic dysfunction appear in the literature for each of the three conditions. Fatigue and CAD are often not considered by clinicians when assessing these patients and yet they are identifiable and several therapeutic interventions exist. Admittedly though, the signs of CAD, both clinical and laboratory, can be subtle, and there is a need to separate subpopulations of patients in order to account for physical and psychological confounders when assessing both causality and response to therapy.

The over-riding mechanisms in all three conditions are considered to be cardiovascular deconditioning, low-volume states such as dehydration, and sensitization of the sympathetic nervous system. Research suggests that sensitization is driven by an increase in peripheral levels of catecholamines, exaggerated receptor response, and complex neurogenic maladaptive changes within the midbrain. Given the latter it is highly probable that these disorders also share similar mechanisms of sympathetic modulation of pain.

Is it therefore the case that, aside from physical differences in their phenotype, the chronic fatigue and widespread pain of CFS, FM, and JHS are in fact manifestations of the same condition and a direct consequence of autonomic dysfunction?

References

Adeyemi EOA, Desai KD, Towsey M, et al: Characterization of autonomic dysfunction in patients with irritable bowel syndrome by means of heart rate variability studies, *Am J Gastroenterol* 94:816–823, 1999.

Baron R, Levine JD, Fields HR: Causalgia and reflex sympathetic dystrophy: does the sympathetic nervous system contribute to the generation of pain? *Muscle Nerve* 22:678–695, 1999.

Barron DF, Cohen BA, Geraghty MT, et al: Joint hypermobility is more common in children with chronic fatigue syndrome than in healthy controls, *J Pediatr* 141:421–425, 2002.

Beard G: Neurasthenia, or nervous exhaustion, *The Boston Medical and Surgical Journal* 217–221, 1869.

Bengtsson A, Bengtsson M: Regional sympathetic blockade in primary fibromyalgia, *Pain* 33:161–167, 1988.

Benrud-Larson LM, Dewar MS, Sandropni P, et al: Quality of life in patients with postural tachycardia syndrome, *Mayo Clin Proc* 77:531–537, 2002.

Bou-Holaigah I, Rowe PC, Kan J, et al: The relationship between neutrally mediated hypotension and the chronic fatigue syndrome, *J Am Med Assoc* 274:961–967, 1995.

Bou-Holaigah I, Calkins H, Flynn JA, et al: Provocation of hypotension and pain during upright tilt table testing in adults with fibromyalgia, *Clin Exp Rheumatol* 15:239–246, 1997.

Bravo JF, Wolfe C: Clinical study of hereditary disorders of connective tissues in a Chilean population. Joint hypermobility syndrome and vascular Ehlers-Danlos syndrome, *Arth Rheum* 54(2):515–523, 2006.

Bravo JF, Wolff C: Clinical study of dysautonomia in 1226 patients with Joint Hypermobility Syndrome, *J Clin Rheumatol* 14(4) suppl S33 (Abstract), 2008.

Brignole M, Croci F, Menozzi C, et al: Isometric arm counter-pressure maneuvers to abort impending vasovagal syncope, *Journal American College Cardiology* 40:2053–2059, 2002.

Claydon VE, Hainsworth R: Salt supplementation improves orthostatic cerebral and peripheral vascular control in patients with syncope, *Hypertension* 43:809–813, 2004.

Coghlan C: Autonomic Dysfunction in the Mitral Valve Prolapse Syndrome: The brain-heart connection and interaction. In Boudulas H, Wooley CF, editors: *Mitral valve prolapse and the mitral valve prolapse syndrome*, Mount Kisco, NY, 1988, Futura Publishing Co, pp 389–426.

Cohen H, Neumann L, Shore M, et al: Autonomic dysfunction in patients with fibromyalgia: application of power spectral analysis of heart rate variability, *Seminars Arthritis Rheumatism* 29:217–227, 2000.

Cohen H, Neumann L, Alhosshle A, et al: Abnormal sympathovagal balance in men with fibromyalgia, *J Rheumatol* 28:581–589, 2001.

Da Costa JM: On irritable heart; a clinical study of a form of functional cardiac disorder and its consequences, *Am J Med Sci* (61):18–52, 1871.

Dinos S, Khoshaba B, Ashby D, et al: A systematic review of chronic fatigue, its syndromes and ethnicity: prevalence, severity, co-morbidity and coping, *Int J Epidemiol* 38(6):1554–1570, 2009.

Desmeules JA, Cedraschi C, Rapiti E, et al: Neurophysiologic evidence of central sensitization in patients with fibromyalgia, *Arthritis Rheum* 48:1420–1429, 2003.

Ector H, Reybrouck T: Improving tolerance to upright posture: current status of tilt- training and other physical maneuvers. In Benditt DG, Brignole M, Raviele A, Wieling W, editors: *Syncope and Transient Loss of Consciousness*, Massachusetts, 2007, Blackwell, pp 72–75.

El-Sayed H, Hainsworth R: Salt supplement increases plasma volume and orthostatic tolerance in patients with unexplained syncope, *Heart* 75:134–140, 1996.

Fraser F, Wilson RM: The sympathetic nervous system and the "irritable heart of soldiers" *Br Med J* 2:27–29, 1918.

Freeman R, Young J, Landsbert L, et al: The treatment of postprandial hypotension in autonomic failure with 3,4-DL-threo-dihydroxphenylserine, *Neurology* 47:1414–1420, 1996.

Friedberg F, Jason LA: Selecting a Fatigue Rating Scale, *The CFS Research Review* (3): Autumn, 2002.

Fukuda K, Straus SE, Hickie I, et al: The chronic fatigue syndrome: a comprehensive approach to its definition and study. International Chronic Fatigue Syndrome Study Group, *Ann Intern Med* 121:953–959, 1994.

Furlan R, Colombo S, Perego F, et al: Abnormalities of cardiovascular neural control and reduced orthostatic tolerance in patients with primary fibromyalgia, *J Rheumatol* 32:1787–1793, 2005.

Gajek J, Zysko D, Halawa B, et al: Influence of tilt training on activation of the autonomic nervous system in patients with vasovagal syncope, *Acta Cardiology* 61:123–128, 2006.

Galland BC, Jackson PM, Sayers RM, et al: A matched case control study of orthostatic intolerance in children/adolescents with chronic fatigue syndrome, *Pediatr Res* 63(2):196–202, 2008.

Garland EM, Hahn MK, Ketch TP, et al: Genetic basis of clinical catecholamine disorders, *Annals New York Acadamy Science* 971:506–511, 2002.

Gazit Y, Nahir AM, Grahame R, et al: Dysautonomia in the joint hypermobility syndrome, *Am J Med* 115(1):33–40, 2003.

Goldstein DS: L-Dihydroxyphenylserine (L-DOPS): a norepinephrine prodrug, *Cardiovasc Drug Rev* 24(3–4):189–203, 2006.

Grahame R, Edwards JC, Pitcher D, et al: A clinical and echocardiographic study of patients with the hypermobility syndrome, *Ann Rheum Dis* 40:541–546, 1981.

Grubb BP, Karas B: Preliminary observation on the use of erythropoietin in the treatment of refractory postural tachycardia syndrome, *Clin Auton Res* 9(4):228, 1999.

Grubb BP, Calkins H, Rowe PC: Postural tachycardia, orthostatic intolerance, and the chronic fatigue syndrome. In Grubb BP, Olshansky B, editors: *Syncope. Mechanisms and Management*, ed 2, Massachusetts, 2005, Blackwell Futura, pp 225–244.

Grubb BP: Postural tachycardia syndrome, *Circulation* 17:2814–2817, 2008.

Hakim AJ, Grahame R: Non-musculoskeletal symptoms in joint hypermobility syndrome. Indirect evidence for autonomic dysfunction, *Rheumatology* 43:1194–1195, 2004.

Hakim AJ, Mathias C, Grahame R: Outcome of cardiovascular autonomic testing in symptomatic patients with benign joint hypermobility syndrome, *Rheumatology* 48(4):216 (Abstract), 2009.

Heitkemper M, Burr RL, Jarret M, et al: Evidence for autonomic nervous system imbalance in women with irritable bowel syndrome, *Dig Dis Sci* 43:2093–2098, 1998.

Hoad A, Spickett G, Elliott J, et al: Postural orthostatic tachycardia syndrome is an under-recognized condition in chronic fatigue syndrome, *Q J Med* 101 (12):961–965, 2008.

Hoeldtke RD, Davis KM: The orthostatic tachycardia syndrome: evaluation of autonomic function and treatment with octreotide and ergot alkaloids, *J Clin Endocrinol Metab* 73:132–139, 1991.

Holmes GP, Kaplan JE, Gantz NM, et al: Chronic fatigue syndrome: a working case definition, *Ann Intern Med* 108:387–389, 1988.

Hurwitz BE, Coryell VT, Parker M, et al: Chronic fatigue syndrome: illness severity, sedentary lifestyle, blood volume and evidence of diminished cardiac function, *Clin Sci (Lond)* Oct 19; 118(2):125–135, 2009.

Jian ZJ, Zhou BY: Efficacy and safety of acarbose in the treatment of elderly patients with postprandial hypotension, *Chin Med J (Engl)* 121:2054–2059, 2008.

Jones DE, Gray JC, Newton J: Perceived fatigue is comparable between different disease groups, *Q J Med* 102(9):617–624, 2009.

Joyner JM, Masuki Z: POTS versus deconditioning - the same or different? *Clin Auton Res* 18:300–307, 2008.

Karling R, Nyhlin H, Wiklund U, et al: Spectral analysis of heart rate variability in patients with irritable bowel syndrome, *Scand J Gastroenterol* 33:572–576, 1998.

Khurana RK: Orthostatic intolerance and orthostatic tachycardia: a heterogeneous disorder, *Clin Auton Res* 5:12–18, 1995.

Kooh M, Martínez-Lavin M, Meza S, et al: Concurrent heart rate variability and polysomnography analyses in fibromyalgia patients, Clin Exp Rheumatol 21:529–530, 2003.

Krediet CT, van Dijk N, Linzer M, et al: Management of vasovagal syncope controlling or aborting faints by leg crossing and muscle tensing, Circulation 106:1684–1689, 2002.

Lai CC, Fischer PR, Brands CK, et al: Outcomes in adolescents with postural orthostatic tachycardia syndromes treated with midodrine and beta-blockers, Pacing Clin Electrophysiol 32(2):234–238, 2009.

Legge H, Norton M, Newton JL: Fatigue is significant in vasovagal syncope and is associated with autonomic symptoms, Europace 10(9):1095–1101, 2008.

Low PA, Caskey PE, Tuck RR, et al: Quantitative sudomotor axon reflex test in normal and neuropathic subjects, Ann Neurol 14:573–580, 1983.

Low PA: Clinical evaluation of autonomic function. In Low PA, editor: Clinical Autonomic Disorders: Evaluation and Management, Boston, 1993, Little, Brown, pp 157–167.

Low PA, Opfer-Gehrking T, Textor S, et al: Postural tachycardia syndrome, Neurology 45(Suppl 5): S19–S25, 1995.

Low PA, Gilden JL, Freeman R, et al: Efficacy of midodrine vs. placebo in neurogenic orthostatic hypotension. A randomized, double-blind multicenter study, J Am Med Assoc 277:1046–1051, 1997.

Low PA, Benarroch E: Clinical autonomic disorders, ed 3, Philadelphia, 2008, Lippincott-Raven.

Malik M: Task Force of the European Society of Cardiology and the North American Society of Pacing and Electrophysiology: Heart rate variability standards of measurement, physiological interpretation, and clinical use, Circulation 93:1043–1065, 1996.

Martínez-Lavin M, Hermosillo AG, Mendoza C, et al: Orthostatic sympathetic derangement in subjects with fibromyalgia, J Rheumatol 24:714–718, 1997.

Martinez-Lavin M, Hermosillo AG, Rosas M, et al: Circadian studies of autonomic nervous balance in patients with fibromyalgia: a heart rate variability analysis, Arthritis Rheum 41:1966–1971, 1998.

Martinez-Lavin M, Hermosillo AG: Autonomic Nervous System dysfunction may explain the multisystem features of Fibromyalgia, Seminars Arthritis Rheumatism 29:197–199, 2000.

Martinez-Lavin M: Fibromyalgia as a sympathetically maintained pain syndrome, Current Pain Headache Reports 8:385–389, 2004.

Martinez-Lavin M: Biology and therapy of fibromyalgia. Stress, the stress response system, and fibromyalgia, Arth Res Ther 9(4):216, 2007.

Mathias CJ, Fosbraey P, de Costa DS, et al: Desmopressin reduces nocturnal polyuria, reverses overnight weight loss, and improves morning postural hypotension in autonomic failure, Br Med J 293:353–354, 1986.

Mathias CJ, Senard J, Braune S, et al: L-theo-dihydroxphenylserine (L-threo-DOPS; droxidopa) in the management of neurogenic orthostatic hypotension: a multi-national, multi-centre, dose-ranging study in multiple system atrophy and pure autonomic failure, Clin Auton Res 11:235–242, 2001.

Mathias CJ, Young TM: Plugging the leak – the benefits of the vasopressin-2 agonist, desmopressin in autonomic failure, Clin Auton Res 13:85–87, 2003.

Mathias C: Intolerance to upright posture in autonomic failure and the postural tachycardia syndrome: assessment and treatment strategies. In Benditt DG, Brignole M, Raviele A, Wieling W, editors: Syncope and transient loss of consciousness, Massachusetts, 2007, Blackwell, pp 67–71.

Mathias CJ: L-dihydroxyphenylserine (Droxidopa) in the treatment of orthostatic hypotension: the European experience, Clin Auton Res 18(Suppl 1):25–29, 2008.

Mishra MB, Ryan P, Atkinson P, et al: Extra-articular features of benign joint hypermobility syndrome, Br J Rheumatol 35(9):861–866, 1996.

Moya A, Wieling W: Orthostatic Syncope. In Benditt DG, Blanc JJ, Brignole M, Sutton R, editors: The evaluation and treatment of syncope, ed 2, Massachusetts, 2006, Blackwell, pp 170–184.

Naschitz JE, Rozembaum M, Rosner I, et al: Cardiovascular response to upright tilt in fibromyalgia differs from that in chronic fatigue syndrome, J Rheumatol 28:1356–1360, 2001.

Newton JL, Okonkwo O, Sutcliffe K, et al: Symptoms of autonomic dysfunction in chronic fatigue syndrome, Q J Med 100(8):519–526, 2007.

Newton JL, Sheth A, Shin J, et al: Lower ambulatory blood pressure in chronic fatigue syndrome, Psychosom Med 71(3):361–365, 2009.

Otzenberger H, Simon C, Gronfier C, et al: Temporal relationship between dynamic heart rate variability and electroencephalographic activity during sleep in man, Neurosci Lett 229:173–176, 1997.

Parish JG: Early outbreaks of epidemic neuromyasthenia, Postgrad Med J 54:711–717, 1978.

Peckerman A, LaManca JJ, Qureishi B, et al: Baroreceptor reflex and integrative stress responses in chronic fatigue syndrome, Psychosom Med 65 (5):889–895, 2003.

Perez-Lugones A, Schweikert R, Pavia S, et al: Usefulness of midodrine in patients with severe symptomatic neurocardiogenic syncope: a randomized control study, *J Cardiovasc Electrophysiol* 12:935–938, 2001.

Raj RR, Brouillard D, Simpsom CS, et al: Dysautonomia among patients with fibromyalgia: a non-invasive assessment, *J Rheumatol* 27:2660–2665, 2000.

Ramsay AM: Epidemic neuromyasthenia, *Postgrad Med J* 54:718–721, 1978.

Reybrouck T, Heidbüchel H, Van de Werf F, et al: Long-term follow-up results of tilt training therapy in patients with recurrent neurocardiogenic syncope, *Pacing Clin Electrophysiol* 25:144–146, 2002.

Robertson D, Flattem N, Tellioglu T, et al: Familial orthostatic tachycardia due to a norepinehrine transported deficiency, *Annals New York Academy Science* 940:527–543, 2001.

Rowe PC, Bou-Holaigah I, Kan JS, et al: Is neurally mediated hypotension an unrecognized cause of chronic fatigue? *Lancet* 345:623–624, 1995.

Rowe PC, Barron DF, Calkins H, et al: Orthostatic intolerance and chronic fatigue syndrome associated with Ehlers-Danlos syndrome, *J Pediatr* 135(4):494–499, 1999.

Sato J, Perl ER: Adrenergic excitation of cutaneous pain receptors induced by peripheral nerve injury, *Science* 251:1608–1610, 1991.

Shannon JR, Flattem NL, Jordan J, et al: Orthostatic intolerance and tachycardia associated with noradrenaline transporter deficiency, *N Engl J Med* 343:1008–1014, 2000.

Shibao C, Arzubiaga C, Roberts LJ 2nd, et al: Hyperadrenergic postural tachycardia syndrome in mast cell activation disorders, *Hypertension* 45:385–390, 2005.

Singer W, Sandroni P, Opfer-Gehrking TL: Pyridostigmine treatment trial in neurogenic orthostatic hypotension, *Archives Neurology* 63:513–518, 2006.

Smith GDP, Alam M, Watson LP, et al: Effects of the somatostatin analogue, octreotide, on exercise induced hypotension in human subjects with chronic sympathetic failure, *Clin Sci* 89:367–373, 1995.

Soetekouw PM, Lenders JW, Bleijenberg G, et al: Autonomic function in patients with chronic fatigue syndrome, *Clin Auton Res* 9(6):334–340, 1999.

Solano C, Martinez A, Becerril L, et al: Autonomic dysfunction in fibromyalgia assessed by the Composite Autonomic Symptoms Scale (COMPASS), *J Clin Rheumatol* 15(4):172–176, 2009.

Stewart JM: Autonomic nervous system dysfunction in adolescents with postural orthostatic tachycardia syndrome and chronic fatigue syndrome is characterized by attenuated vagal baroreflex and potentiated sympathetic vasomotion, *Pediatr Res* 48(2):218–226, 2000.

Stewart JM: Chronic fatigue syndrome: comments on deconditioning, blood volume, and resulting cardiac function, *Clin Sci (Lond)* June 18: [Epub ahead of print], 2009.

Streeten DH, Anderson GH Jr: Delayed orthostatic intolerance, *Arch Intern Med* 152:1066–1072, 1992.

Suarez GA, Opfer-Gehrking TL, Offord KP, et al: The Autonomic Symptom Profile. A new instrument to assess autonomic symptoms, *Neurology* 52:523, 1999.

Thieben MJ, Sandroni P, Sletten DM, et al: Postural orthostatic tachycardia syndrome: The Mayo clinic experience, *Mayo Clin Proc* 82(3):308–313, 2007.

Timmers H, Wieling W, Soetekouw P, et al: Hemodynamic and neurohumoral responses to head up tilt in patients with chronic fatigue syndrome, *Clin Auton Res* 12:273–280, 2002.

Ulas UH, Unlu E, Hamamcioglu K, et al: Dysautonomia in fibromyalgia syndrome: sympathetic skin responses and RR interval analysis, *Rheumatol Int* 26:383–387, 2006.

Vaeroy H, Qiao Z, Morkrid L, et al: Altered sympathetic nervous system response in patients with fibromyalgia, *J Rheumatol* 16:1460–1465, 1989.

van Denderen JC, Boersma JW, Zeinstra P, et al: Physiological effects of exhaustive physical exercise in primary fibromyalgia syndrome (PFS): is PFS a disorder of neuroendocrine reactivity? *Scand J Rheumatol* 21:35–37, 1992.

Ward CR, Gray JC, Gilroy JJ, et al: Midodrine: a role in the management of neurocardiogenic syncope, *Heart* 79:45–49, 1998.

Wieling W, van Lieshout JJ, van Leeuwen AM: Physical maneuvers that reduce postural hypotension in autonomic failure, *Clinics Autonomic Research* 3:57–65, 1993.

Wieling W, van Lieshout JJ, Hainsworth R: Extracellular fluid volume expansion in patients with posturally related syncope, *Clin Auton Res* 12:243–249, 2002.

Wooley CF: Where are the diseases of yesterday? The Da Costa syndrome, soldier's heart syndrome, effort syndrome, neurocirculatory asthenia–and the mitral valve prolapse, *Circulation* 53:749–751, 1976.

Wyller VB, Saul JP, Walloe L, et al: Sympathetic cardiovascular control during orthostatic stress and isometric exercise in adolescent chronic fatigue syndrome, *Eur J Appl Physiol* 102(6):623–632, 2008.

Yunoszai AK, Franklin WH, Chan DP, et al: Oral fluid therapy: a promising treatment for vasodepressor syncope, *Arch Pediatr Adolesc Med* 152:165–168, 1998.

6.2 Bowel dysfunction in joint hypermobility syndrome and fibromyalgia

Adam D Farmer and Qasim Aziz

INTRODUCTION

Traditional disease concepts are based on the premise that structural or biochemical abnormalities, often specific to a disorder, can be identified. However, in a substantial proportion of patients with gastrointestinal (GI) symptoms, diagnostic tests fail to identify any abnormality. Despite considerable advances in techniques such as endoscopy, GI physiology and molecular biology, structural lesions are only found in approximately 50% of patients referred for evaluation of abdominal symptoms (Koloski 2000). Unexplained GI symptoms are therefore common and frequently diagnosed as functional gastrointestinal disorders (FGID), a heterogeneous group of disorders that account for 2–5% of consultations in primary care and more than 40% of referrals to gastroenterology outpatient clinics (Sandler et al 1984).

This chapter will examine FGID, the extra-articular GI manifestations of joint hypermobility syndrome (JHS) and the overlap with fibromyalgia (FM), both in terms of psychological factors and pain as a common symptom, and reviewing the evidence for proposed pathophysiological mechanisms.

FUNCTIONAL GASTROINTESTINAL DISORDERS

FIBROMYALGIA

The term 'functional' is unhelpful in that it pertains to a disorder of function despite the absence of an identifiable structural or biochemical abnormality. It is recognized that the absence of identifiable pathologies can also lead healthcare professionals to be less likely to accept legitimate symptoms and suffering in patients (Chang et al 2006). The Rome multinational consensus sought to classify FGID defining them as 'a variable combination of chronic or recurrent gastrointestinal symptoms which are not explained by structural or biochemical abnormalities' (Drossman 2006a, 2006b). These disorders have a considerable socioeconomic impact with direct and indirect healthcare costs in the order of $34 billion in the seven largest Western economies (Chang 2004, Spiller et al 2007, Mikocka-Walus et al 2008).

Whilst many hypotheses have been proposed to explain the origin of symptoms in FGID, no single factor has achieved primacy due to the marked heterogeneity of these disorders. The increasing trend of sub-specialization within medical practice often leads to a variety of disorders being managed in isolation in super-specialized clinics despite evidence that such disorders may actually represent more generalized pathology. It is fascinating to note that FGID, JHS and FM share a remarkable number of epidemiological and clinical features (Table 6.2.1). Furthermore, two recent studies have shown that the rates of joint hypermobility are much higher in patients with FM (Sendur et al 2007) and those with unexplained GI symptoms, the latter being a group often erroneously labelled as having FGID (Farmer et al 2009). Considering these observations, it is not unreasonable to postulate that at least a proportion of patients with these disorders, currently investigated, diagnosed and managed in isolation by differing specialities, could in fact be suffering from the same multi-faceted generalized disorder.

Fibromyalgia is associated with a number of co-morbid conditions (Chapter 5) such as migraine, non-cardiac chest pain, dysmenorrhoea and irritable bowel syndrome (IBS) (Buskila & Cohen 2007). Epidemiological studies have shown that between 50–70% of patients with FM may complain of symptoms that are characteristic of functional dyspepsia or IBS (Triadafilopoulos et al 1991). Conversely, the prevalence of FM amongst IBS patients is also high, with estimates ranging from 28% to 65% (Kurland et al 2006). This has led to the suggestion that FM and IBS, where pain and psychological symptoms are prominent, may form 'disease clusters' based on common patho-aetiological factors, and nomenclature such as functional somatic disorders or central sensitization syndromes have been proposed (Wessely et al 1999, Whitehead et al 2002).

Table 6.2.1	Features common to FGID, JHS and FM		
	FUNCTIONAL GASTROINTESTINAL DISORDERS	JOINT HYPERMOBILITY SYNDROME	FIBROMYALGIA
Demographics			
Prevalence within the general population	5–17%	0.5–1.0%	6–13%
Gender	More common in females	More common in females	More common in females
Age of onset	Younger/middle age	Younger/middle age	Middle age (White 2000)
Familial Aggregation	Yes	Yes	Yes
Symptoms			
Chronic episodic pain	Yes	Yes	Yes
Headache	Yes	Yes	Yes
Diagnosis			
Validated biomarker	No	No	No
Disease Associations			
Chronic fatigue syndrome	Yes	Yes	Yes
Temporomandibular disorder	Yes	Yes	Yes
Psychiatric co-morbidity	Increased anxiety, depression and somatization	Increased anxiety and somatization	Increased anxiety, depression and cognitive difficulties
Autonomic nervous system dysfunction	Yes	Yes	Yes

Psychological factors

A recent study by Almansa et al (2009) evaluated the presence of FGID in patients with FM as well as the role of psychological factors in this relationship. In this study, 98% of patients with FM fulfilled the criteria for one or more FGID, the most common being IBS followed by functional bloating and functional abdominal pain. Furthermore, in comparison to controls, the FM group had much higher levels of psychological distress, somatization, poorer coping skills, increased anxiety and depression. This study provided evidence that FM and certain FGID, in particular IBS, may constitute part of a similar spectrum of disease.

Community-based studies have described familial patterns for psychological disorders in FM despite the fact that these psychological abnormalities may be attributed to the presence of a non-specified chronic pain disorder (Raphael et al 2004). In a cross-sectional study of a community sample of twins, Schur et al (2007) examined the inter-relationship between nine common medically unexplained conditions (FM and IBS were amongst these) and showed that the co-morbidity between these conditions in twins far exceeded that expected by chance alone. This study therefore raises the possibility that FM and FGID may share a common pathophysiological pathway that could have a genetic basis.

Pain: the ubiquitous symptom

One of the central defining features of FM and FGID is chronic pain and a growing body of work has addressed abnormalities in pain processing. Despite epidemiological and clinical similarities between FM and FGID, perceptual responses to both somatic and visceral stimuli differ between the groups of patients. FM patients characteristically exhibit somatic hyperalgesia whereas IBS patients without coexistent FM have somatic hypoalgesia (Chang et al 2000). Whether these observed alterations in sensitivity are part of a global phenomenon of generalized sensory dysfunction is controversial, as studies have reported contradictory findings (Cook et al 1987, Sarkar et al 2000, Bouin et al 2001, Verne et al 2003). Within the FGID literature, visceral pain hypersensitivity to experimental noxious stimulation is considered a germane characteristic in their pathophysiology. Mosihree et al (2007) evaluated the magnitude of visceral and somatic hyperalgesia in a group of patients with IBS vs. patients with IBS+FM vs. healthy controls. Patients with IBS+FM had greater somatic sensitivity than those with IBS only. In contrast, those with IBS only displayed greater visceral sensitivity thereby suggesting that the region of hyperalgesia is related to site of the primary pain syndrome. However, in comparison to healthy controls the patient groups displayed enhanced sensitivity to both somatic and visceral pain. These observations suggest that aberrant central processing of afferent nociceptive signalling may underlie the observed pain hypersensitivity in these disorders.

Evidence from brain imaging studies

One of the underlying mechanisms in the co-morbidity between FGID and FM that has been investigated is the aberrant CNS processing of somatic and visceral afferent nociceptive signals with a particular research effort being made in evaluating regions of the brain concerned with the processing, integration and modulation of pain, such as the anterior cingulate cortex (ACC). An elegant study by Chang et al (2003), used positron emission tomography to assess the regional cerebral blood flow (rCBF) in response to noxious visceral and somatic stimuli in a cohort of females with IBS with or without coexistent FM. They found that noxious visceral stimulation was rated as more intense than somatic stimulation in the IBS group, whereas in the IBS+FM group the converse was true. These ratings were mirrored by a greater increase in rCBF in the ACC in response to noxious visceral, but not somatic, stimuli in IBS patients. In IBS+FM patients similar increases were observed in response to noxious somatic, but not visceral, stimuli. This study provides further anatomical evidence for the importance of central structures, such as the ACC, in modulating responses to noxious sensory stimuli in both syndromes. In agreement with Mosihree et al's observations, these changes may relate to the primary pain syndrome selectively enhancing the cognitive-evaluative components of pain processing of either visceral (in IBS patients) or somatic (in IBS+FM patients) sensory inputs. On the other hand it could be suggested that the inherent differences in visceral and somatic pain in their perception and description may account for some of these differences in these two conditions.

Autonomic dysfunction as a common pathophysiological mechanism

Many important biological functions such as heart rate, metabolic rate, blood pressure and bowel function are regulated by the autonomic nervous system (ANS). Clinical symptoms suggestive of dysautonomia, such as poor sleep or syncopal episodes are common across the disorders of FGID, JHS and FM. Particular patterns of dysautonomia, specifically dysregulation of sympathetic nervous

system control of the cardiovascular system, have been described in patients with JHS (Chapter 6.1) and FM, where it is termed postural orthostatic tachycardia syndrome (POTS) (Gazit et al 2003, Staud 2008). Various types of autonomic dysfunction, involving the sympathetic division, parasympathetic division or both, have been widely reported in FGID literature (Lacy 2006), although no specific abnormality has been consistently demonstrated due to lack of homogeneity. However, it has been hypothesized that ANS dysfunction may be responsible for the anomalous viscero-visceral and viscero-somatic motor reflexes to the gut resulting in dysmotility that has been described in patients with FGID.

In the authors' experience from a tertiary referral neurogastroenterology clinic, approximately one third of patients with JHS and unexplained GI symptoms have demonstrable dysautonomia. This suggests that autonomic function tests should be performed as a matter of routine in these patients. Prospective studies are needed to determine the degree and type of dysautonomia in patients with FGID, JHS and FM to ascertain whether it represents a common pathophysiological mechanism linking these disorders.

JOINT HYPERMOBILITY

A number of studies have investigated the associations between JHS, generalized joint hypermobility (JHM) per se and visceral manifestations. Hakim and Grahame (2004) found in a cohort of 170 females with JHS, that nausea, stomach ache, diarrhoea and constipation were significantly more frequent than in an age- and sex-matched control group. The prevalence of JHM has been studied in a number of other gastrointestinal disorders such as faecal incontinence (FI), hiatus hernia (HH), slow transit constipation (STC), obstructive defecation (OD) and in GI symptoms of unexplained aetiology.

Faecal incontinence

FI is defined as the involuntary passage of faecal material through the anal canal. It is an under-reported symptom which may have a devastating impact on quality of life (QOL). FI has a community prevalence of 4.2 men and 1.7 women per 1000 between the ages of 15–64 years (Bellicini et al 2008). Risk factors for the development of FI include female gender, increasing age, poor general health and prostate disease with urinary incontinence frequently being co-existent. Jha et al, in a case control study, questioned 30 female patients with JHS and found that the prevalence of urinary and FI to be significantly higher than in healthy female controls (60% vs. 30%; $P = 0.037$, 23% vs. 0%; $P = 0.01$ respectively) (Jha et al 2007). In a recently published follow-up study by the same group, validated questionnaires evaluating symptoms of urinary and FI, were sent to members of the Hypermobility Syndrome Association (HMSA) with a confirmed diagnosis of JHS (Arunkalaivanan et al 2009); 14.9% of HMSA responders had FI with increased risk being afforded to the elderly and in those with a higher body mass index.

Constipation

Chronic constipation in adults is a common and debilitating problem that may present to a wide variety of specialist and non-specialist physicians. The Rome III definition of constipation is shown in Box 6.2.1. Whilst this definition is comprehensive, it is rather unwieldy and on this point McCallum et al define constipation as '…any patient experiencing consistent difficulty with defaecation' (McCallum et al 2009). Constipation is common with prevalence being estimated to be in the order of 12–19%, with increasing age and female gender being risk factors (Higgins & Johanson 2004).

The causes of constipation are often multifactorial but are generally cited as being due to dietary,

metabolic, neurological, painful anorectal disorders or as a side effect of prescribed medications (Chapter 6.3).

Constipation is a common complaint in patients with JHS, particularly in the paediatric population. De Kort et al (2003) questioned the parents of 89 children, aged 5–12 years, with a diagnosis of JHS and compared them with a group of healthy controls of the same age. They found that the parents of 19% of boys with JHS reported constipation in comparison to 4% of the parents of controls ($P = 0.02$). Reilley et al (2008) sought to further expand these observations and studied patients, aged 7–17 years, who had been diagnosed with STC, a form of chronic constipation that is associated with the delayed colonic passage of stool. In a group of 39 patients who had been diagnosed with STC, 15 (38%) had generalized JHM (defined as a Beighton Score of greater than or equal to 4) compared with eight (20%) healthy controls ($P = 0.06$). In a post hoc analysis by gender, 38% of STC males had JHM vs. 4% of controls. The authors conclude that generalized JHM is particularly higher in male children with STC.

Obstructed defecation

Constipation can be a manifestation of obstructive defecation (OD). Different pathophysiologies may underlie OD, and tests of anorectal function, such as proctography, play an important role in cause elucidation (e.g. mechanical or functional) in addition to directing further management. Rectal prolapse or intussusception is a recognized mechanical risk for OD and it has been established in previous studies that there is an association between rectal and genital prolapse and JHM (Norton et al 1995, Manning et al 2003). Our group has performed a prospective study designed to evaluate the link between OD and JHM (Mohammed et al 2009). The prevalence of JHM was 30% in patients presenting to our tertiary centre for physiological investigation of OD, significantly higher than the general population (Decoster et al 1997). Proctography demonstrated an obstructing mechanical cause in 71% of patients with JHM vs. 34% without ($P = 0.001$). These findings provide further evidence that the defecatory difficulties that these patients encounter may be secondary to lax gut connective tissue.

> **BOX 6.2.1   The Rome III criteria for constipation**
>
> Rome III Multinational Consensus on the Definition of Constipation
>
> Two or more of the following symptoms for at least 3 consecutive months, for 6 months prior to diagnosis
> - Straining during at least 25% of defecations
> - Lumpy or hard stool in at least 25% of defecations
> - The sensation of incomplete evacuation for at least 25% of defecations
> - The sensation of anorectal obstruction/blockage for at least 25% of defecations
> - The need to use manual maneouvres to facilitate at least 25% of defecations
> - Fewer than three bowel movements per week
> - Loose stools being rarely present without the use of laxatives

Hiatus hernia

Gastro-oesophageal reflux disease (GORD) is a common problem that is expensive to diagnose and treat in the primary and secondary care setting, with direct and indirect costs being estimated to be in the order of $14 billion in North America, of which 60% is spent on drug therapy (Shaheen et al 2006). The prevalence of GORD is increasing with important risk factors being obesity and eradication of *Helicobacter pylori*. However, an increasing body of research has focused upon transient relaxations of the lower oesophageal sphincter (LOS) and the spatial separation of the diaphragm and the LOS, a consequence of hiatus hernia (HH), as the critical mechanisms for acid reflux. The presence of a HH disrupts the anatomy and physiology of the normal antireflux mechanism. HH is associated with more severe GORD symptoms, increased prevalence and severity of reflux oesophagitis, as well as Barrett's oesophagus and oesophageal adenocarcinoma (Gordon et al 2004).

Laxity of the supporting ligamentous structure around the diaphragmatic hernia has been suggested as a potential pathophysiological factor in the development of a HH. Curci et al (2008) evaluated the peri-oesophageal ligaments in patients with GORD, with and without HH. In the group with GORD+HH, the investigators discovered subtle alterations in the elastic fibres in two of the three ligaments supporting the gastro-oesophageal junction. Al-Rawi et al assessed the prevalence of JHM in 50 patients with a confirmed HH vs. age-, sex-, parity- and body-mass-index-matched controls without HH (Al-Rawi et al 2004). The prevalence of JHM was 22% in the HH+ vs. 6% in the group without HH ($P < 0.001$). This study highlights the possibility that mechanical abnormalities in the properties of connective tissue that support the GI tract may play an integral role in the genesis of symptoms.

Unexplained gastrointestinal symptoms

We have prospectively evaluated the incidence of JHM and JHS in a cohort of 115 patients from our tertiary referral neurogastroenterology clinic (Farmer et al 2009, Zarate et al 2010). Sixty-three percent of the patients presenting to the clinic had GI symptoms without a known underlying structural, metabolic or autoimmune disorder or in the absence of a unifying diagnosis at the time of referral. Of these patients, 48% had evidence of JHM and in 61% of these a diagnosis of JHS was made. Patients with co-existent JHS and previously unexplained GI symptoms commonly experienced the symptoms of bloating, reflux, constipation and nausea. GI physiological investigations in this group of patients revealed GI dysmotility, thereby suggesting symptoms may be due to GI connective tissue laxity and therefore alterations in gut biodynamics.

A number of studies have evaluated the role of several components of the gut wall, namely the interaction between the nervous/immune system and the gut microbiota/gut mucosa. Little attention has been placed on assessing the physical and physiological characteristics of connective tissue in which many structures of the GI tract are embedded. This complex connective tissue matrix contributes significantly to the passive mechanical properties of the GI tract. Symptoms, similar to those seen in many FGID may occur due to reduced compliance, ineffective transit and dysmotility of the affected region of the GI tract. It is plausible that abnormalities in articular connective tissue laxity seen in JHS may also be present in the GI tract, leading to alterations in GI tract biomechanics, the sequelae of which potentially being FI, STC and HH. The area of GI manifestations of JHS is likely to represent a novel and fertile area for future research.

SUMMARY

Hitherto, GI tract dysfunction in JHS and FM has received scant attention despite the fact that the syndrome complexes that encompass FGID, JHS and FM share a startling number of features.

It is entirely scientifically plausible that there is a unifying pathophysiological abnormality that links them. Further work is needed to more accurately establish the epidemiology of GI symptoms in JHS and FM, as well as identifying molecular and genetic abnormalities.

As clinicians we are sometimes guilty of 'not seeing the wood from the trees'. Perhaps we need to take a step back to recognize the omnipresent connective tissue, the associations with FGID and the true impact of these symptoms on the QOL in JHS and FM patients.

References

Al-Rawi ZS, Al-Dubaikel KY, Al-Sikafi H: Joint mobility in people with hiatus hernia, *Rheumatology (Oxford)* 43:574–576, 2004.

Almansa C, Rey E, Sanchez RG, et al: Prevalence of functional gastrointestinal disorders in patients with fibromyalgia and the role of psychologic distress, *Clin Gastroenterol Hepatol* 7:438–445, 2009.

Arunkalaivanan AS, Morrison A, Jha S, et al: Prevalence of urinary and faecal incontinence among female members of the Hypermobility Syndrome Association (HMSA), *J Obstet Gynaecol* 29:126–128, 2009.

Bellicini N, Molloy PJ, Caushaj P, et al: Fecal incontinence: a review, *Dig Dis Sci* 53:41–46, 2008.

Bouin M, Meunier P, Riberdy-Poitras M, et al: Pain hypersensitivity in patients with functional gastrointestinal disorders: a gastrointestinal-specific defect or a general systemic condition? *Dig Dis Sci* 46:2542–2548, 2001.

Buskila D, Cohen H: Comorbidity of fibromyalgia and psychiatric disorders, *Curr Pain Headache Rep* 11:333–338, 2007.

Chang L, Mayer EA, Johnson T, et al: Differences in somatic perception in female patients with irritable bowel syndrome with and without fibromyalgia, *Pain* 84:297–307, 2000.

Chang L, Berman S, Mayer EA, et al: Brain responses to visceral and somatic stimuli in patients with irritable bowel syndrome with and without fibromyalgia, *Am J Gastroenterol* 98:1354–1361, 2003.

Chang L: Review article: epidemiology and quality of life in functional gastrointestinal disorders, *Aliment Pharmacol Ther* 20(Suppl 7):31–39, 2004.

Chang L, Toner BB, Fukudo S, et al: Gender, age, society, culture, and the patient's perspective in the functional gastrointestinal disorders, *Gastroenterology* 130:1435–1446, 2006.

Cook IJ, van Eeden A, Collins SM: Patients with irritable bowel syndrome have greater pain tolerance than normal subjects, *Gastroenterology* 93:727–733, 1987.

Curci JA, Melman LM, Thompson RW, et al: Elastic fiber depletion in the supporting ligaments of the gastroesophageal junction: a structural basis for the development of hiatal hernia, *J Am Coll Surg* 207:191–196, 2008.

de Kort LM, Verhulst JA, Engelbert RH, et al: Lower urinary tract dysfunction in children with generalized hypermobility of joints, *J Urol* 170:1971–1974, 2003.

Decoster LC, Vailas JC, Lindsay RH, et al: Prevalence and features of joint hypermobility among adolescent athletes, *Arch Pediatr Adolesc Med* 151:989–992, 1997.

Drossman DA: *Rome III: The functional gastrointestinal disorders*, vol xli, ed 3, McLean, VA, 2006a, Degnon Associates, p 1048.

Drossman DA: The functional gastrointestinal disorders and the Rome III process, *Gastroenterology* 130:1377–1390, 2006b.

Farmer AD, Zarate N, Knowles CH, et al: Unexplained Gastrointestinal Symptoms in Joint Hypermobility: Is Connective Tissue the Missing Link, *Neurogastroenterol Motil*, Oct 15 [Epub ahead of print], 2009.

Gazit Y, Nahir AM, Grahame R, et al: Dysautonomia in the joint hypermobility syndrome, *Am J Med* 115:33–40, 2003.

Gordon C, Kang JY, Neild PJ, et al: The role of the hiatus hernia in gastro-oesophageal reflux disease, *Aliment Pharmacol Ther* 20:719–732, 2004.

Hakim AJ, Grahame R: Non-musculoskeletal symptoms in joint hypermobility syndrome. Indirect evidence for autonomic dysfunction, *Rheumatology (Oxford)* 43:1194–1195, 2004.

Higgins PD, Johanson JF: Epidemiology of constipation in North America: a systematic review, *Am J Gastroenterol* 99:750–759, 2004.

Jha S, Arunkalaivanan AS, Situnayake RD: Prevalence of incontinence in women with benign joint hypermobility syndrome, *Int Urogynecol J Pelvic Floor Dysfunct* 18:61–64, 2007.

Koloski NA, Talley NJ, Boyce PM: The impact of functional gastrointestinal disorders on quality of life, *Am J Gastroenterol* 95:67–71, 2000.

Kurland JE, Coyle WJ, Winkler A, et al: Prevalence of irritable bowel syndrome and depression in fibromyalgia, *Dig Dis Sci* 51:454–460, 2006.

Lacy BE: IBS and autonomic nervous system responses to pain, *J Clin Gastroenterol* 40:767–768, 2006.

Manning J, Korda A, Benness C, et al: The association of obstructive defecation, lower urinary tract dysfunction and the benign joint hypermobility syndrome: a case-control study, *Int Urogynecol J Pelvic Floor Dysfunct* 14:128–132, 2003.

McCallum IJ, Ong S, Mercer-Jones M: Chronic constipation in adults, *BMJ* 338, b831, 2009.

Mikocka-Walus A, Turnbull D, Moulding N, et al: Psychological comorbidity and complexity of gastrointestinal symptoms in clinically diagnosed irritable bowel syndrome patients, *J Gastroenterol Hepatol* 23:1137–1143, 2008.

Mohammed S, Zarate N, Aziz Q, et al: New insight into the pathophysiology of obstructed defecation: the impact of joint hypermobility, *Neurogastroenterol Motil*, Abstract, 2009.

Moshiree B, Price DD, Robinson ME, et al: Thermal and visceral hypersensitivity in irritable bowel syndrome patients with and without fibromyalgia, *Clin J Pain* 23:323–330, 2007.

Norton PA, Baker JE, Sharp HC, et al: Genitourinary prolapse and joint hypermobility in women, *Obstet Gynecol* 85:225–228, 1995.

Raphael KG, Janal MN, Nayak S, et al: Familial aggregation of depression in fibromyalgia: a community-based test of alternate hypotheses, *Pain* 110:449–460, 2004.

Reilly DJ, Chase JW, Hutson JM, et al: Connective tissue disorder–a new subgroup of boys with slow transit constipation? *J Pediatr Surg* 43:1111–1114, 2008.

Sandler RS, Drossman DA, Nathan HP, et al: Symptom complaints and health care seeking behavior in subjects with bowel dysfunction, *Gastroenterology* 87:314–318, 1984.

Sarkar S, Aziz Q, Woolf CJ, et al: Contribution of central sensitisation to the development of non-cardiac chest pain, *Lancet* 356:1154–1159, 2000.

Schur EA, Afari N, Furberg H, et al: Feeling bad in more ways than one: comorbidity patterns of medically unexplained and psychiatric conditions, *J Gen Intern Med* 22:818–821, 2007.

Sendur OF, Gurer G, Bozbas GT: The frequency of hypermobility and its relationship with clinical findings of fibromyalgia patients, *Clin Rheumatol* 26:485–487, 2007.

Shaheen NJ, Hansen RA, Morgan DR, et al: The burden of gastrointestinal and liver diseases, *Am J Gastroenterol* 101:2128–2138, 2006.

Spiller R, Aziz Q, Creed F, et al: Guidelines on the irritable bowel syndrome: mechanisms and practical management, *Gut* 56:1770–1798, 2007.

Staud R: Autonomic dysfunction in fibromyalgia syndrome: postural orthostatic tachycardia, *Curr Rheumatol Rep* 10:463–466, 2008.

Triadafilopoulos G, Simms RW, Goldenberg DL: Bowel dysfunction in fibromyalgia syndrome, *Dig Dis Sci* 36:59–64, 1991.

Verne GN, Himes NC, Robinson ME, et al: Central representation of visceral and cutaneous hypersensitivity in the irritable bowel syndrome, *Pain* 103:99–110, 2003.

Wessely S, Nimnuan C, Sharpe M: Functional somatic syndromes: one or many? *Lancet* 354:936–939, 1999.

Whitehead WE, Palsson O, Jones KR: Systematic review of the comorbidity of irritable bowel syndrome with other disorders: what are the causes and implications? *Gastroenterology* 122:1140–1156, 2002.

Zarate N, Farmer AD, Grahame R, et al: Unexplained gastrointestinal symptoms and joint hypermobility: is connective tissue the missing link? *Neurogastroenterol Motil* 22(3):252–278, 2010

6.3 Gastrointestinal manifestations of opioid therapy in chronic pain syndromes

Adam D Farmer and Qasim Aziz

INTRODUCTION

It has long been recognized that opiates affect gastrointestinal (GI) motility, manifesting as constipation, nausea, bloating and occasionally even pain (Grunkemeier et al 2007). Although opioid analgesics can relieve pain effectively, and bring about improvements in quality of life (QOL), the side effects of chronic opioid administration limit their therapeutic benefit. For instance, constipation is known to occur in 15–90% of patients receiving opiates and has a negative impact on QOL (Davis 2005). These side-effects are of particular pertinence to those with chronic pain syndromes, such as joint hypermobility syndrome (JHS), fibromyalgia (FM) and functional GI disorders (FGID).

The use of opioids has increased considerably over the recent past. For instance, in the United States there was a 400% increase in the sale of methadone and oxycodone from 1997 to 2002 (Trescot et al 2006). A recent large Danish epidemiological study evaluated the long-term effects of opioids in long-term/chronic non-cancer pain (Eriksen et al 2006). The authors found that opioid treatment of long-term/chronic non-cancer pain did not significantly fulfil any of the key outcomes in terms of adequate pain relief, improved QOL or improvements in functional capacity. A recent meta-analysis of 41 trials containing 6019 patients, 7% of whom had FM, showed that opioids were more efficacious than placebo as an analgesic but had minimal effects on functional measures (Furlan et al 2006). There is evidence to suggest an over-reliance on opioids in the treatment of chronic pain, despite guidelines on the use of complementary therapies such as occupational therapy and psychological treatments (Ackerman et al 2003). Such an over-reliance may itself be counterproductive to the undesirable side-effects.

This chapter will consist of two parts. In the first, we will consider the mechanisms by which both endogenous and exogenous opioids interact with the GI tract. The second part will consider potential GI sequelae of chronic opiate use, the recently described entity of narcotic bowel syndrome (NBS), and discuss its pathophysiology and management.

OPIOID INTERACTIONS WITH THE GASTROINTESTINAL TRACT

Endogenous opioids include endorphins, dynorphins and enkephalins that act selectively at the mu, delta and kappa opioid receptor subtypes. Morphine is the most commonly used exogenous opioid which predominantly agonizes the mu receptor expressed ubiquitously throughout the peripheral and central nervous system (CNS) in addition to the GI tract (Thomas 2008).

MOLECULAR EFFECTS OF ENDOGENOUS OPIOIDS ON THE GASTROINTESTINAL TRACT

The exact role of endogenous opioids in GI tract function remains largely unknown but it is thought that they act centrally and peripherally to aid in the regulation of GI motility (Becker & Blaum 2009). Central interactions are affected through communication with the autonomic nervous system (ANS), reducing GI secretions and motility. Peripheral mechanisms operate at the level of the GI tract through opiate receptors in the enteric nervous system. For instance, isolated denervated segments of small bowel from the guinea pig demonstrated opiate-mediated slowing (Baker 2007; Van Nueten et al 1977). The mu receptor is a member of a 7-transmembrane G protein-coupled receptor, and predominant functional interactions are with the G_i/G_0 proteins causing decreased levels of intracellular cAMP in addition to a reduction in potassium and calcium conductance. The result is reduced neuronal excitability and neurotransmitter release respectively, with the sum effect of inhibition of neuronal firing, as demonstrated directly in the GI tract (De Luca & Coupar 1996). Studies in a number of animal models have shown that opiates cause relaxation of the outer longitudinal muscle and increase inner smooth muscle tone through inhibition of acetylcholine, vasoactive intestinal peptide and nitric oxide (Wood & Galligan 2004). Consequentially, peristalsis is blocked and the net opioid effect is an increase in segmental non-propulsive phasic contractions and absent or decreased propulsive migrating contractions within the colon (Ferraz et al 1995).

MOLECULAR EFFECTS OF EXOGENOUS OPIOIDS ON THE GASTROINTESTINAL TRACT

Exogenous opioids bind the mu receptors in the myenteric and submucosal plexi, facilitating 5-hydroxytryptamine (5-HT) release and activation of the 5-HT$_2$ receptor causing the release of noradrenaline (NA; norepinephrine). NA acts upon the α_2-adenoceptor to antagonize intestinal enterocytic secretion of electrolytes and fluids. In conjunction with the disruption in peristalsis, there is passive absorption of water from the luminal contents leading to harder and dryer stools, which may lead to constipation. Recently there has been interest in peripherally acting mu opioid antagonists, such as methylnaltrexone and alvimopan, which can ameliorate exogenous opioid-mediated reductions in GI secretions and motility. This class of drug represents a novel potential therapeutic option in opiate-induced bowel dysfunction.

NARCOTIC BOWEL SYNDROME

Counterintuitively, abdominal pain can be a side effect of chronic opiate therapy and when it becomes the predominant side effect, it is known as narcotic bowel syndrome (NBS). Paradoxically, there is an increase in abdominal pain despite continued or escalating dosing of opiates in an attempt to relieve the abdominal pain. Despite being recognized as a clinical entity over 25 years ago, there is a limited evidence base with respect to its management (Sandgren et al 1984).

NBS is characterized by chronic or intermittent colicky abdominal pain or discomfort that worsens after the narcotic effects of opiates wear off. Over time, and as a result of tachyphylaxis, the pain-free periods become shorter in duration despite increasing doses of opiates. Escalating the opiate dosage only compounds the effect on pain sensitivity and further reduces GI secretion and motility.

However, given the profound analgesic effects of opiates it is somewhat baffling to accept the argument that opiates can provoke the very pain that they are treating. Evidence from a number of recently published studies has shown that pain may be dynamically modulated by the CNS, peripheral neural and opioid pathways which inhibit, as well as facilitate, pain perception (Grunkemeier et al 2007). Moreover, chronic opiate use induces neuroplastic changes that paradoxically enhance hyperalgesia and give rise to tolerance. It has been proposed that there are at least three putative mechanisms that may lead to pro-nociceptive opiate effects:

● bimodal opioid dysregulation
● abnormalities in counter-regulatory mechanisms
● and glial activation.

BIMODAL OPIOID REGULATORY SYSTEM

Bimodal refers to the excitatory and inhibitory modulation of the sensory neuron action by opiates. Preferential activation of these excitatory pathways may, over time, lead to opiate tolerance and pain augmentation. These excitatory effects of opiates have been seldom recognized due to the inhibitory effects that opioids have when administered in analgesically active (high) concentrations. These effects are mediated through G$_s$ receptor activation at the dorsal root ganglia. Through chronic opiate administration, the G$_s$ receptor becomes super-sensitized resulting in tolerance and ultimately hyperalgesia (Crain & Shen 2000). These observations provide rationale for concomitant administration of low-dose opiate antagonists, such as methylnaltrexone and alvimopan, in preventing G$_s$ receptor-mediated super-sensitivity, thereby enhancing exogenous opioid-mediated analgesia but at lower doses (Lobmaier et al 2008).

COUNTER-REGULATORY MECHANISMS

Dynorphin, an endogenous opiate, when released at the level of the spinal cord is thought to increase the release of excitatory neurotransmitters from the primary afferents thereby causing amplification of the afferent sensory signal. Evidence for this pro-nociceptive role comes from observations that dynorphin is increased in chronic pain states and that pain behaviours in animals are attenuated following the administration of dynorphin antagonists (Bian et al 1999, Vanderah et al 2000). Chronic opiate use leads to up-regulation of dynorphin production at the spinal dorsal horn, which induces further hyperalgesia. By blocking this effect hyperalgesia is reduced, analgesia is restored and opiate tolerance is prevented (Nichols et al 1997).

GLIAL ACTIVATION AND OPIOID FACILITATION

Activation of spinal cord glia is a novel mechanism that has been demonstrated to be involved in pain amplification in chronic pain states. Spinal dorsal horn glia can be activated in response to a number of factors including inflammation, infection, opiates, peripheral injury and in response to central signals allowing for the possibility that the central effects of stress may facilitate pain at a peripheral level (Milligan et al 2008). It is interesting to note that glial cells express receptors for a number of pro-inflammatory cytokines such as interleukin-1, interleukin-6 and tumour necrosis factor-α, as well as having the ability, when activated, to release mediators such as nitric oxide, prostaglandins and excitatory amino acids, all of which can enhance pain transmission and further drive neuropathic pain (Watkins et al 2001). Exogenous opiates, binding directly to the mu receptor, cause the activation of glia with the concomitant release of pro-inflammatory cytokines, thereby accelerating this process. Glia, in response to the release of inflammatory mediators, may activate neurons through a novel chemokine, known as fractalkine, mediated mechanism (Watkins et al 2005).

These mechanisms provide important evidence for the concept of opiate-induced hyperalgesia. Translational pharmacological studies are now warranted to support these proposed mechanisms and their targeted effects in humans.

MANAGEMENT OF NARCOTIC BOWEL SYNDROME

There is no consensus on the absolute management of NBS, but central to a successful outcome, and a cornerstone of treatment, is the physician–patient relationship, as each party may approach therapy with contrasting agendas. The physician's agenda is to withdraw the use of the counterproductive opiate therapy in order to potentially improve the patient's symptoms. However, from the patient's perspective opiate withdrawal or restriction may bring into question the legitimacy of their symptoms, issues regarding addiction or an overly paternalistic approach from the physician. In this respect, the physician must acknowledge the validity of the patient's symptoms and engage and respond to the patient's concerns, providing reassurance wherever possible. The patient will need a degree of willingness and determination to succeed within a set of realistic and achievable goals. Treatment plans should be discussed with other parties such as allied healthcare professionals and the patient's family members. The management is considerably more complicated than following a simple opiate-withdrawal protocol. Whereas the preparatory phase for treatment may be undertaken as an outpatient, an opiate-withdrawal programme undertaken in secondary or tertiary care under the supervision of an experienced specialist may be preferable.

TREATMENT MODALITIES

The specific goals involve the initiation of treatments that minimize the immediate withdrawal effects of opiates in addition to treating psychological co-morbidities whilst achieving pain control for the underlying pathology. The time frame that is needed for a successful opiate-withdrawal programme is extremely variable but those who have had longer durations and higher doses of opiates often require a more prolonged period of graded withdrawal. The typical period needed for full detoxification is 3–10 days. Grunkemeier et al (2007) advocate switching the offending opiate for an equivalent dose of a medium-to-long-acting opioid, such as methadone, and then decreasing the dose of this by 10–33% per day. A divided daily dose should be used so as to limit large variations in plasma concentrations and thereby avoid rebound pain during trough levels. When rapid withdrawal regimens are used, patients need to be closely monitored for:

● orthostatic hypotension
● syncope
● urinary retention
● cardiac dysrhythmia.

Concomitant medications can be commenced during the opiate withdrawal phase for variable periods to treat coexisting anxiety, psychological co-morbidity and provide long-term central analgesia. Typical agents include antidepressants, benzodiazepines and clonidine. Figure 6.3.1 summarizes the pharmacological approaches to opiate withdrawal.

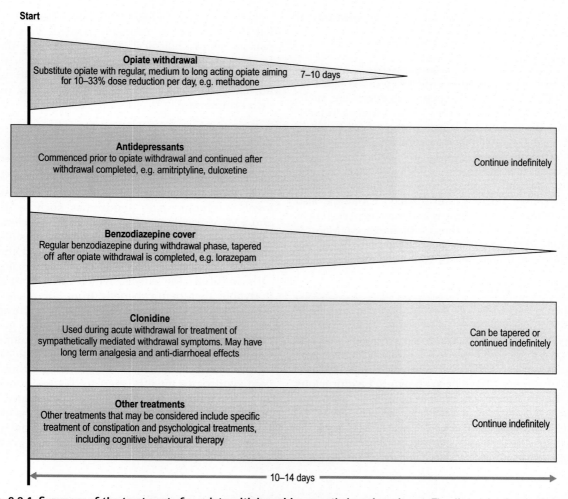

Fig. 6.3.1 Summary of the treatments for opiate withdrawal in narcotic bowel syndrome. The diagnosis of narcotic bowel syndrome needs to be made and a therapeutic doctor–patient relationship established before treatment can commence

ANTIDEPRESSANTS

Antidepressants should be commenced prior to opiate withdrawal and may be continued indefinitely, although clinical benefit may not be tangible for a number of weeks. Tricyclic antidepressants, e.g. amitriptyline, are the treatment of choice due to their beneficial noradrenergically mediated analgesic effects. However, tolerance is limited often by anticholinergic (constipation, blurred vision, dry mouth) and histaminergic (somnolence) side effects. Alternatives include the serotonin-noradrenergic reuptake inhibitors, such as duloxetine, which provide long-term analgesia and antidepressant activity with improved GI tolerance.

BENZODIAZEPINES

Medium- and long-acting benzodiazepines, such as lorazepam or clonazepam, may be helpful in anxiety reduction associated with the acute phase of opiate withdrawal and may be given throughout the withdrawal period. During the weaning period, benzodiazepines have a particular role in the prevention of sympathetically mediated side effects. Benzodiazepines may themselves be weaned after opiate withdrawal has been completed.

CLONIDINE

Clonidine is an α-2 adrenergic receptor agonist with central and peripheral action. CNS effects are mediated in the 'anxiety centre' – the locus caerulus – whilst the peripheral effects in the GI tract are via decreasing acetylcholine release, thereby reducing the strength and frequency of colonic motor contractions. It is also highly effective in reducing the sympathetically mediated opiate-withdrawal effects of sweating, flushing and anxiety. Clonidine also has central analgesic effects and may increase transit times in the GI tract in those with diarrhoea (Mann & Shinkle 1998). Clonidine may be tapered after opiate withdrawal is complete or continued long term.

OTHER TREATMENTS

Patients may develop constipation during opiate withdrawal and in the absence of GI obstruction may be treated with laxatives. Although there is no convincing evidence for recommending one particular type of cathartic over another, polyethylene glycol solutions have been shown to be efficacious in the treatment of chronic idiopathic constipation (Di Palma et al 2007). As discussed earlier, novel mu opioid receptor antagonists, such as methylnaltrexone and alvimopan, may have benefit in the management of opioid-induced constipation.

Long-term psychological support after the initial detoxification is invariably needed. Educating patients in psychological strategies allowing them to manage their chronic pain, such as relaxation techniques, aids symptom management and empowers patients to achieve a sense of control over their symptoms.

SUMMARY

Opiates have become one of the most commonly prescribed analgesics, particularly in management of chronic pain syndromes such as JHS and FM. Molecular mechanisms reinforce clinical observations that opioids have a major physiological role in gut motility and secretion and these actions account for many of the pharmacologically induced side effects, which often limit the derivable therapeutic benefit from this class of medication. NBS is a sequelae of chronic escalating opiate administration and there is good experimental evidence to support the counterintuitive notion of opiate-mediated hyperalgesia. In this respect, clinicians who manage chronic pain syndromes must be alert to this easily overlooked diagnosis. Research is now warranted to further explore the molecular mechanisms that underlie this paradox as well as identifying the most efficacious withdrawal regimens in the treatment of NBS.

References

Ackerman SJ, Mordin M, Reblando J, et al: Patient-reported utilization patterns of fentanyl transdermal system and oxycodone hydrochloride controlled-release among patients with chronic nonmalignant pain, *J Manag Care Pharm* 9:223–231, 2003.

Baker DE: Loperamide: a pharmacological review, *Rev Gastroenterol Disord* 7(Suppl 3): S11–S18, 2007.

Becker G, Blum HE: Novel opioid antagonists for opioid-induced bowel dysfunction and postoperative ileus, *Lancet* 373(9670):1198–1206, 2009.

Bian D, Ossipov MH, Ibrahim M, et al: Loss of antiallodynic and antinociceptive spinal/ supraspinal morphine synergy in nerve-injured rats: restoration by MK-801 or dynorphin antiserum, *Brain Res* 831:55–63, 1999.

Crain SM, Shen KF: Antagonists of excitatory opioid receptor functions enhance morphine's analgesic potency and attenuate opioid tolerance/dependence liability, *Pain* 84:121–131, 2000.

Davis MP: The opioid bowel syndrome: a review of pathophysiology and treatment, *J Opioid Manag* 1:153–161, 2005.

De Luca A, Coupar IM: Insights into opioid action in the intestinal tract, *Pharmacol Ther* 69:103–115, 1996.

Di Palma JA, Cleveland MV, McGowan J, et al: An open-label study of chronic polyethylene glycol laxative use in chronic constipation, *Aliment Pharmacol Ther* 25:703–708, 2007.

Eriksen J, Sjogren P, Bruera E, et al: Critical issues on opioids in chronic non-cancer pain: an epidemiological study, *Pain* 125:172–179, 2006.

Ferraz AA, Cowles VE, Condon RE, et al: Opioid and nonopioid analgesic drug effects on colon contractions in monkeys, *Dig Dis Sci* 40:1417–1419, 1995.

Furlan AD, Sandoval JA, Mailis-Gagnon A, et al: Opioids for chronic noncancer pain: a meta-analysis of effectiveness and side effects, *CMAJ* 174:1589–1594, 2006.

Grunkemeier DM, Cassara JE, Dalton CB, et al: The narcotic bowel syndrome: clinical features, pathophysiology, and management, *Clin Gastroenterol Hepatol* 5:1126–1139, 2007. quiz 1121–1122.

Lobmaier P, Kornor H, Kunoe N, et al: Sustained-release naltrexone for opioid dependence, *Cochrane Database Syst Rev* 2008. CD006140.

Mann NS, Shinkle JM: Effect of clonidine on gastrointestinal transit time, *Hepatogastroenterology* 45:1023–1025, 1998.

Milligan ED, Sloane EM, Watkins LR: Glia in pathological pain: a role for fractalkine, *J Neuroimmunol* 198:113–120, 2008.

Nichols ML, Lopez Y, Ossipov MH, et al: Enhancement of the antiallodynic and antinociceptive efficacy of spinal morphine by antisera to dynorphin A (1–13) or MK-801 in a nerve-ligation model of peripheral neuropathy, *Pain* 69:317–322, 1997.

Sandgren JE, McPhee MS, Greenberger NJ: Narcotic bowel syndrome treated with clonidine. Resolution of abdominal pain and intestinal pseudo-obstruction, *Ann Intern Med* 101:331–334, 1984.

Thomas J: Opioid-induced bowel dysfunction, *J Pain Symptom Manage* 35:103–113, 2008.

Trescot AM, Boswell MV, Atluri SL, et al: Opioid guidelines in the management of chronic non-cancer pain, *Pain Physician* 9:1–39, 2006.

Van Nueten JM, Van Ree JM, Vanhoutte PM: Inhibition by met-enkephalin of peristaltic activity in the guinea pig ileum, and its reversal by naloxone, *Eur J Pharmacol* 41:341–342, 1977.

Vanderah TW, Gardell LR, Burgess SE, et al: Dynorphin promotes abnormal pain and spinal opioid antinociceptive tolerance, *J Neurosci* 20:7074–7079, 2000.

Watkins LR, Milligan ED, Maier SF: Glial activation: a driving force for pathological pain, *Trends Neurosci* 24:450–455, 2001.

Watkins LR, Hutchinson MR, Johnston IN, et al: Glia: novel counter-regulators of opioid analgesia, *Trends Neurosci* 28:661–669, 2005.

Wood JD, Galligan JJ: Function of opioids in the enteric nervous system, *Neurogastroenterol Motil* 16(Suppl 2):17–28, 2004.

6.4   Proprioceptive dysfunction in JHS and its management

William R Ferrell and Peter W Ferrell

INTRODUCTION

On questioning patients with joint hypermobility syndrome (JHS) about their symptoms and experiences, it is very frequently the case that they describe themselves as being 'clumsy' and/or having relatively poor balance. These patients were often good at gymnastics during their early school years, presumably as a consequence of the advantage gained from being hypermobile, although often not at activities requiring a good sense of balance. These clinical features are invariably present from childhood, with clumsiness and poor coordination being frequently reported in hypermobile children (48% and 36% respectively) (Adib et al 2005).

Postural control is complex, involving afferent input from a variety of sensory receptors, including proprioceptors in muscles, articular and periarticular structures, vestibular receptors, cutaneous receptors and, importantly, visual receptors. All these receptors provide sensory feedback to the central nervous system, to correct postural deviations from the centre of gravity (sway) by recruitment of motor units in specific muscles, both in terms of the numbers of motor units activated and their discharge frequencies. Bridging the afferent and efferent pathways are integrating centres, important among these being the basal ganglia and cerebellum. Proprioceptors play a significant role in maintaining balance as shown by the Romberg test, which is negative in a healthy individual who can maintain balance when standing upright with the feet together and the eyes closed. Under these conditions, sensory feedback from proprioceptors enables maintenance of balance despite absence of visual input. However, the visual pathways also play an important role in maintaining balance. This is illustrated in subjects with a positive Romberg test (exaggerated swaying and/or loss of balance once the eyes are closed), as such individuals can maintain balance with the eyes open, the input from visual receptors compensating for the loss of proprioceptive feedback. The importance of the integrating centres is clear from patients with cerebellar dysfunction in whom swaying and/or loss of

balance whilst attempting the Romberg test occurs even with the eyes open. Finally, an abnormality of the efferent pathways, stroke for example, can obviously also result in loss of balance, in this case primarily due to inadequate control of α-motoneurons innervating muscles which control posture.

As JHS patients do not exhibit any significant alteration of visual function, the cause of their 'clumsiness' could arise from other factors, but of these, motor dysfunction is unlikely, since the majority of patients have normal power (though pain can limit the generation of full power).

Cerebellar dysfunction is also unlikely, because these patients do not show evidence of ataxia or other characteristic features of cerebellar disease and, when performed, the Romberg test with eyes open is normal. However, no comprehensive testing of balance in JHS patients has yet been described in the literature, leaving deficiency of proprioceptive feedback as the most likely cause of 'clumsiness'. Only one study has attempted to investigate balance in the context of joint hypermobility, and although greater use of distal joints to maintain balance (ankle strategy) was observed in hypermobile subjects, there was no overall impairment of postural stability (Røgind et al 2003). Unfortunately, the Brighton Criteria were not employed and therefore the extent of inclusion of JHS patients is unknown.

PROPRIOCEPTION AND ITS MEASUREMENT

The term proprioception is often rather loosely used, compared to the original definition. It was first coined by Sir Charles Sherrington (1906), who suggested that this 'sixth' sense arose from receptors in the 'deep field' (i.e. muscle and joint mechanoreceptors), as a consequence of the actions of the organism, and resulted in the perception of joint and body movement as well as position of the body or body segments in space. Strictly speaking, the original definition of proprioception only refers to active movements, but it is now generally accepted to include passive movements as well. This term encompasses two separate sensations: joint kinaesthesia (awareness of movement) and joint position sense (awareness of position). Although likely to arise from the same types of sensory receptors, as both velocity and positional information can be encoded by specific mechanoreceptors in joints (Ruffini endings) (Boyd & Robert 1953) and muscles (muscle spindles) (Matthews 1964), these are nevertheless separate sensations. It has been demonstrated that healthy subjects can still detect a change in joint position even when very slow displacement velocities are used ($\leq 2^\circ \text{min}^{-1}$), which are below the threshold for movement detection (Clark et al 1985). In other words, when asked if the joint is moving during very slow joint displacements, subjects deny being able to detect movement, but after the displacement is completed and the joint now at a new position, they can correctly detect that its position has changed (Clark et al 1985).

The standard procedure used in everyday clinical practice for testing proprioceptive sensations arising from peripheral joints is a very blunt tool and will only detect gross abnormalities, which often accompany other sensory abnormalities as part of a neurological disease process. More refined and sensitive methods are required to detect subtler alterations of proprioception, although there are a number of potential pitfalls with such protocols.

The Romberg test is a well-known clinical procedure which can provide an indication of disturbance of proprioceptive feedback. Although this test is positive in patients with abnormalities of peripheral or central proprioceptive pathways, vestibular disturbances can also yield a positive result. The test also requires normal muscle power and coordination, and is therefore also evaluating these other modalities. To obtain more definitive information about sensations arising from peripheral proprioceptors, testing procedures have been developed involving displacement of individual limbs, either actively or passively.

The commonest method for assessing joint kinaesthesia involves a threshold detection paradigm where a joint is rotated in one plane, usually by means of a motorized system under computer control, with the subject halting the motor once the displacement is detected. The angular displacement which occurs prior to detection (the threshold angle) provides an indication of proprioceptive acuity (Hall et al 1994); the smaller this angle, the greater the acuity. However, rapid displacements are easily detected with this procedure, even in subjects with generalized sensory impairment,

so the displacement velocity should be kept relatively low ($<1^\circ \sec^{-1}$) to improve discrimination. Another factor is that the reaction time of the subject can become a significant confounder at high displacement velocities. This threshold method for testing joint kinaesthesia is most accurately performed with the requirement for the subject to correctly identify the *direction* of displacement before halting joint rotation, as detection simply of a displacement having occurred could arise from non-proprioceptive mechanoreceptors in skin.

The testing of joint position sense can involve a position-matching paradigm, which consists of displacement of one joint and the subject required to match this with the contralateral joint, either actively or passively. A potential problem with active displacement of the matching limb by the subject is that this involves motor commands and is therefore an assessment of both sensory and motor function. An additional issue is that in very many studies, joint displacement velocities were employed which were substantially above the threshold for movement detection (2°min^{-1}), so detection of the final position reached could have been computed by the central nervous system using the velocity/time relationship. The only way to truly assess position sense requires the use of extremely slow joint displacements which are imperceptible to the subject.

An alternative protocol is the reproduction angle, which involves displacement of a given joint to a particular position. The joint is then returned to the starting position and the subject is required to reproduce the initial displacement as accurately as possible, either actively or passively. Although it has been reported that the ability of healthy subjects to match knee joint angle from memory is as good as active positioning using the opposite leg (Horch et al 1975), any observed decrement in performance in a clinical study could result from impairment of memory or cognitive function as opposed to reduction of proprioceptive feedback per se. Again, all studies using this paradigm invariably employed displacement velocities which are well above the threshold for movement detection.

JOINT INSTABILITY AND PROPRIOCEPTION

Hypermobility can in some cases be extreme, resulting in substantial joint instability which can be accompanied by dislocation. It is therefore possible that lesser degrees of hypermobility could result in some degree of joint instability, raising the question whether unstable joints exhibit impaired proprioception. Joint instability occurs in many orthopaedic conditions, of which the most studied involves rupture of the anterior cruciate ligament (ACL). After such injury, the knee joint becomes unstable with resulting pain and decreased function and such joints can develop early osteoarthritic changes. Many studies have been performed on patient groups to assess functional deficit and associated factors after ACL injuries. Of the latter, proprioception has been shown to be decreased after ACL injury, comparisons being made with a control group of subjects with normal joint function in some studies (Fridén et al 1996) and with the contralateral leg being used as an 'internal control' in others (Borsa et al 1997). Although the latter approach has merit in terms of statistical robustness by reducing the well-known biological variability between subjects, it is uncertain whether contralateral limb biomechanics might have been altered by injury to the ipsilateral limb and consequently affected proprioception in the 'control' joint. Although one study found little difference between the uninjured knee compared to healthy controls (Barrack et al 1989), a subsequent study in a larger cohort of patients and controls found that unilateral ACL deficit is associated with significantly reduced proprioception in the uninjured knee compared to an external control group (Reider et al 2003). Despite such methodological limitations, all of these studies observed proprioceptive impairment in the injured knee using a paradigm involving the threshold to detect passive movement, rotating the knee at a slow angular velocity ($0.5° \ sec^{-1}$) into flexion and extension from different starting positions. This testing procedure is similar to that described earlier, although in these studies of ACL deficient joints, patients were only required to respond when motion was detected and did not have to indicate the direction of movement. As indicated previously, this represents a significant limitation to the testing procedure as subject confirmation of the directional displacement requires greater proprioceptive sensitivity and offers greater specificity.

To further investigate the link between joint instability and proprioception, symptomatic and asymptomatic patients with ACL injury were compared, with greater impairment of proprioception found in those with severe symptoms, such as

sensations of instability and episodes of the knee 'giving way' (Roberts et al 1999). It was also observed that the asymptomatic group did not differ significantly from the uninjured control group (presumably because threshold measurements in the asymptomatic group showed substantial variability), suggesting a relationship between proprioception and perception of joint function. Subsequent work by the same research group linked joint laxity, muscle strength and proprioception to functional outcome (using a single-legged hop test) and subjective outcome. These results showed increased laxity (measured using the KT-1000 arthrometer) and reduced proprioception to have a significant effect on function (Roberts et al 2007).

Kennedy et al (1982) were the first to suggest that loss of proprioception after ACL injury could contribute to progressive joint instability due to loss of stabilizing reflexes originating from mechanoreceptors in the cruciate ligaments. Barrack et al (1989) found a significant correlation between increased threshold to detect movement and joint laxity, but no difference between acute and chronic cases of ACL injury. If impairment of proprioception was solely due to increasing joint laxity, it would not be expected to occur acutely but become progressively worse with increasing joint instability. This supports the concept that following the initial injury, there is loss of knee proprioception and that this is a cause, rather than an effect of progressive joint laxity thereafter (Barrack et al 1989). This also supports previous perceptions that proprioceptive deficit can significantly impact on the development of further joint laxity resulting in poorer functional outcomes. Such observations have clear relevance to patients with JHS where instability may be less pronounced than with ACL rupture but functional impairment can be comparable, perhaps due to proprioceptive deficiency.

PROPRIOCEPTION IN JHS

Against the backdrop of joints rendered unstable through trauma showing impaired proprioception, the question then arises as to whether hypermobile joints exhibit altered proprioception. Evidence for disturbed proprioception in JHS was first obtained by examination of the finger joints (Mallik et al 1994), where it was observed that the ability of adult

JHS patients to detect the position of the proximal interphalangeal joint of the index finger was impaired compared to normomobile subjects. This employed a novel methodology which permits testing position sense at a single joint by requiring subjects to visually align a finger silhouette, coaxial with the joint, to the perceived position of the unseen finger using proprioceptive feedback (Ferrell & Craske 1992). This approach has the advantage of avoiding potential 'doubling' of the matching error using the contralateral joint, as visual acuity is substantially more precise than proprioceptive acuity.

Subsequently, using a threshold detection paradigm (Fig. 6.4.1) it was found that knee joint kinaesthesia was impaired in a group of JHS patients compared to an age- and sex-matched control group (Hall et al 1995) although there was no correlation between the degree of proprioceptive impairment and the Beighton hypermobility score. Using a reproduction angle testing procedure, impairment of knee joint proprioception has recently been confirmed in a larger group of JHS patients compared to an age- and sex-matched control group (Sahin et al 2008a).

A complication of using such psychophysical testing procedures is that whilst any decrement in proprioceptive performance could arise through some form of deficiency of peripherally located proprioceptors, any abnormality in central neural pathways conveying proprioceptive information could yield similar deficits, as would any cognitive impairment. However, there is evidence for peripherally originating proprioceptive dysfunction in JHS, as it has been observed that segmental musculoskeletal reflexes are impaired in a significant proportion of these patients (Ferrell et al 2007). This study involved recording electromyographic activity in quadriceps femoris in response to weak electrical stimulation of the common peroneal nerve (Fig 6.4.2). By stimulus-triggered averaging it is possible to detect facilitation of quadriceps motoneurones, which is modulated by knee joint position.

In healthy subjects the reflex is invariably present, its magnitude being greatest at full extension of the knee and diminishing on movement into flexion. However, this reflex was absent in almost half of the JHS patients tested (Ferrell et al 2007). In those patients where the reflex was present, although it diminished on movement into flexion, similar to normomobile subjects, it also progressively reduced in amplitude on movement into *hyperextended* positions. This observation is

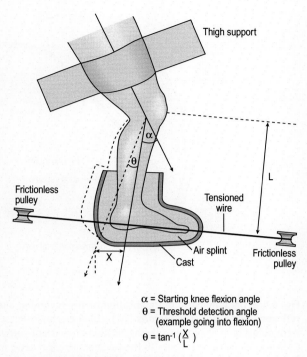

α = Starting knee flexion angle
θ = Threshold detection angle
(example going into flexion)
$\theta = \tan^{-1}\left(\dfrac{X}{L}\right)$

Fig. 6.4.1 Apparatus used to assess knee joint proprioception using the threshold detection paradigm.
A specially designed rig was used to displace the knee at a constant angular velocity of $0.4°$ s^{-1}. Subjects lay on their contralateral side to the limb being tested on an examination couch, the test limb being supported proximal to the knee by a support bar. The ankle and foot of the test limb were immobilized by an air splint and attached to the rig via a half female plaster cast. Tensioned wires running over virtually frictionless pulleys attached the cast to a stepper motor and gearbox. The weight of the distal portion of the limb was taken by the rig ensuring no active muscle contraction was required to maintain the test limb in position. Strapping proximal to the knee kept other body motions to a minimum, ensuring movement occurred only about the knee joint. The motor speed and direction was computer controlled. Subjects were instructed to stop the motor via a handset once they could detect that a movement had occurred *and* knew its direction. From the effective limb length (L) and the linear displacement (X), the angular displacement (θ) can be calculated. *Figure reproduced from Hall et al (1995), with permission*

interesting in the context of the common description by JHS patients of the knee suddenly 'giving way', particularly on stairs. Normally, facilitation of extensor motoneurones on full extension during walking would assist with bracing the joint prior to heel strike, but with hypermobility of the knee,

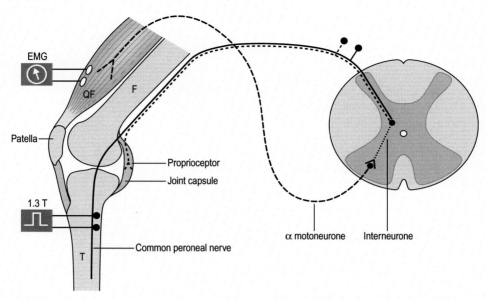

Fig. 6.4.2 Diagrammatic representation of the recording and stimulation arrangements for eliciting musculoskeletal reflexes from quadriceps femoris (QF). Using electrodes attached to the skin surface, electromyographic (EMG) recordings were obtained in response to the application of constant current rectangular pulses. These were delivered transcutaneously at 1 Hz via monopolar electrodes to the common peroneal nerve at the level of the fibular neck at 1.3 times the motor threshold. This was sufficient to cause a minor twitch of the anterior tibial muscles accompanied by a mild tapping sensation. The recorded signal was processed by post-stimulus time averaging (60 pulses), and segmental reflex responses typically occurred within 20–40 ms of the stimulus. Moving the knee to different positions altered proprioceptive feedback to spinal reflex pathways, resulting in modulation of the reflex response. F = femur; P = patella; T = tibia. *Figure reproduced from Ferrell et al (2007), with permission*

this facilitation progressively diminishes the greater the displacement into the hyperextended range, increasing the probability of the joint 'giving way'. That there is likely to be a relationship between reflex dysfunction and the sensation of the knee 'giving way' is suggested by a recent study of patients with anterior cruciate ligament rupture, where the medium latency stretch reflex response was 30% longer in patients with 'giving way' symptoms compared to a group with the same injury but without such symptoms (Melnyk et al 2007).

Proprioceptive dysfunction has recently been demonstrated in children (aged 9–13 years) diagnosed with JHS where, compared to healthy age-matched controls, the JHS group showed consistently greater threshold detection and reproduction angles (Fatoye et al 2008, 2009), suggesting impairment of kinaesthesia and position sense respectively. These findings suggest that JHS is associated with impaired proprioception acuity in childhood and could account for delayed motor development which is known to be associated with hypermobility in infants (Jaffe et al 1988, Tirosh et al 1991). This concept is supported by the experimental observation that motor coordination is crucially dependent on proprioceptive feedback (Sainburg et al 1993). Recent work tends to confirm this suggestion, since it has been shown that JHS is five times more common in children diagnosed with developmental coordination disorder compared to a control group (Kirby & Davies 2007).

Intuitively, in the context of proprioceptive dysfunction it would be expected that balance would be adversely affected in JHS patients, which would be consistent with patient descriptions of 'clumsiness'. However, based on unpublished data generated previously in a group of 18 JHS patients (Ferrell et al 2004), balance and proprioception were in fact found to be weakly correlated ($r = 0.24$).

This may relate to the fact that balance is not solely dependent on proprioceptive feedback, but requires in addition both adequate integration of such feedback in the higher motor centres and accurate temporal and spatial output to alpha motoneurones. This emphasizes the need for formal testing of balance in JHS patients compared to control subjects. This has not been systematically investigated to date, although limited observations suggest that when appropriately challenged, JHS patients are less able to maintain balance than healthy normomobile subjects. Although the Romberg test is negative in JHS patients, there is sometimes a tendency to greater swaying than in control subjects but without loss of balance. However, when required to stand on one leg, JHS patients tend to perform less well than normomobile subjects. Interestingly, anecdotal observations indicate that asymptomatic hypermobile subjects are comparable to normomobile individuals, suggesting that hypermobility per se may not be the causative factor for impaired balance in JHS patients, but rather that there is an associated neurophysiological dysfunction in JHS. To some extent this is supported by the discovery of dysautonomia in some of these patients, characterized by dysregulation of the control of the cardiovascular system by the sympathetic nervous system, in the presence of normal parasympathetic function of the heart (Gazit et al 2003) (Chapter 6.1). Thus, in addition to abnormality of the peripheral somatic nervous system, characterized by proprioceptive dysfunction, there may also exist an abnormality of the autonomic nervous system in JHS patients, suggesting more widespread, but subtle, neurologic dysfunction.

MANAGEMENT OF PROPRIOCEPTIVE DYSFUNCTION IN JHS

In a survey of UK consultant rheumatologists, physiotherapy was considered to be an effective form of management for many JHS patients (Grahame & Bird 2001). Physiotherapy management for these patients has been well defined and the following key principles identified (see Section 2):

- Improving joint stability by means of joint-stabilizing exercises
- Avoiding end-of-range joint positions which could be potentially damaging
- Reversing muscle deconditioning which accompanies muscle disuse

- Through appropriate aerobic exercise, enhance fitness and stamina
- Improve core stability
- Manage chronic pain by pacing and coping strategies
- Encouraging self-management and empowerment
- Improving proprioception by employing appropriate exercises.

The rationale for physiotherapeutic intervention in JHS comes from literature indicating that institution of appropriate exercises is beneficial in patients with unstable joints, even when this has occurred following injury (Keays et al 2006). Interestingly, in this study it was observed that a home-based exercise programme not only improved quadriceps muscle strength and balance in patients with deficiency of the anterior cruciate ligament, but instrumented assessment of passive stability of the knee was also improved.

In JHS patients there is some evidence to indicate improvement of symptoms following physiotherapeutic intervention. A 6-week training regimen designed to stabilize hyperlax joints showed improvement in the ability to perform daily tasks and reduced knee hypermobility (Barton & Bird 1996). However, any benefits obtained with the exercise programme receded once this was stopped. In another study, a retrospective analysis of children (2–14 years) with JHS indicated that following a 6-week programme of home-based exercises, symptoms improved in about two thirds of children and 15% became asymptomatic (Kerr et al 2000).

As there is clear evidence for impairment of proprioception in JHS, the question arises as to the evidence available for its improvement by appropriate physiotherapeutic intervention. It was observed in an earlier study that joint position sense in subjects with functionally unstable ankles was unaffected following an exercise programme designed to improve proprioception (Bernier & Perrin 1998). However, this may have been due to the limitations of the methodology employed, as the reproduction angle paradigm was used, and the passive test performed at $5° \sec^{-1}$ which, as described earlier, is well above the threshold for movement detection. In a recent study of JHS patients using a cross-over design, Ferrell et al (2004) investigated whether performance of home-based exercises could lead to an improvement in knee joint proprioception, balance, musculoskeletal pain (using a visual analog scale), hamstring and quadriceps muscle strength and quality of life. A group of JHS patients were examined on three occasions, 8 weeks apart, and the above parameters assessed. Between the first and second set of measurements no specific intervention was undertaken and there was no significant alteration in any of these parameters. However, following an 8-week programme of progressive closed chain kinetic exercises combined with practice on a balance board, significant improvement was detected in all of these, particularly proprioception and balance (Fig. 6.4.3). The improvement in muscle strength following the exercise programme is valuable, since weakness of the quadriceps muscle group has been documented in JHS patients, compared to an age- and sex-matched control group (Sahin et al 2008b). The physiotherapy regimen employed in this study consisted of progressive increase in the number of sessions involving practice on a balance board, closed kinetic chain exercises (squat, plié, bridging, side lunge, front lunge) and a static hamstring exercise. Closed kinetic chain exercises were employed because they are considered to be safer, more specific, and more functional than open kinetic chain exercises (Snyder-Mackler 1996). Closed kinetic chain exercises are thought to increase knee joint stability by facilitating muscle co-contraction, recruiting hamstrings and quadriceps simultaneously, and so place less strain on the ligaments of the knee (Henning et al 1985). In addition, such exercises may also facilitate the discharge of knee joint proprioceptors by increasing intra-articular

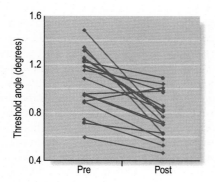

Fig. 6.4.3 Effect of an exercise programme on proprioception and balance in JHS patients. Threshold detection angle before and after the eight week exercise programme. Decrease in magnitude equates to improved proprioceptive acuity. *Figure reproduced from Ferrell et al 2004, with permission*

pressure, thereby stimulating Ruffini nerve endings in the fibrous part of the joint capsule, which are sensitive to changes in intracapsular fluid volume (Wood & Ferrell 1984). These mechanoreceptive nerve endings have been shown to encode information about joint position and angular velocity, in terms of their static and dynamic discharge characteristics (Boyd & Robert 1953, Boyd 1954).

A recognized limitation of the study by Ferrell et al (2004) was the lack of a contemporaneous untreated (non-exercised) control group of JHS patients, which would have permitted evaluation of the effect of 'attention', although this was mitigated to some extent by the cross-over design of the investigation. However, a recent study undertaken in Turkey, involving comparison of a group of JHS patients undertaking an exercise regimen with a parallel JHS control group, has corroborated a number of these findings (Sahin et al 2008a). Prior to intervention there was no difference in knee joint proprioception, knee joint pain (VAS) and functional status (AIMS-2) between the two groups, but after undergoing an 8-week period of exercises designed to improve proprioception, the exercise group showed enhancement of proprioception, reduction in pain scores and improvement in functional status, whereas the control group did not. Together such studies provide strong evidence for the value of physiotherapy in managing the pain and reduced quality of life associated with JHS. Although these aspects are of great importance to patients, it is interesting to note that parameters such as proprioception, which are less amenable to the psychological status of the individual, are also improved by such intervention. Perhaps even more striking is that segmental reflex function, which is even less amenable to influence by cognitive factors, is also affected by appropriate exercises (Ferrell et al 2007). As described earlier, musculoskeletal reflexes could not be elicited in almost half of the JHS patients tested, but following an 8-week programme of progressive closed kinetic chain exercises, these were now elicited in all patients. The experimental procedure used for this study, involving only a segmental reflex pathway, provides a more objective assessment of proprioceptive and motor function. The results from this study therefore suggest that this change in reflex function is unlikely to be a phenomenon involving the higher centres of the nervous system, but may involve facilitation of segmental spinal interneuronal pathways leading to improved motoneuron activation. Thus, changes in neuronal function may occur even at the spinal level as a consequence of undertaking an exercise programme, suggesting considerable plasticity in spinal circuitry.

SUMMARY

These observations provide a sound scientific basis for the physiotherapeutic management of JHS, but much remains to be discovered about the nature of the condition and how best it might be managed.

In particular, anecdotal evidence suggests that asymptomatic hypermobile individuals appear to have relatively normal balance and coordination, and therefore presumably normal proprioceptive function. However, formal assessment of proprioception or balance in this group is important to undertake because should this prove to be similar to normomobile individuals, it would suggest that JHS patients may have a subtle form of neurological dysfunction affecting the somatic and autonomic nervous systems, which clearly warrants further investigation.

References

Adib N, Davies K, Grahame R, et al: Joint hypermobility syndrome in childhood. A not so benign multisystem disorder? *Rheumatology* 44:744–750, 2005.

Barrack RL, Skinner HB, Buckley SL: Proprioception in the anterior cruciate deficient knee, *Am J Sports Med* 17:1–6, 1989.

Barton LM, Bird HA: Improving pain by the stabilization of hyperlax joints, *J Orthop Rheumatol* 9:46–51, 1996.

Bernier JN, Perrin DH: Effect of coordination training on proprioception of the functionally unstable ankle, *J Orthop Sports Phys Ther* 27:264–275, 1998.

Borsa PA, Lephart SM, Irrgang JJ, et al: The effects of joint position and direction of joint motion on proprioceptive sensibility in anterior cruciate ligament-deficient athletes, *Am J Sports Med* 25:336–340, 1997.

Boyd IA, Robert TDM: Proprioceptive discharges from stretch-receptors in the knee-joint of the cat, *J Physiol* 122:38–58, 1953.

Boyd IA: The histological structure of the receptors in the knee-joint of the cat correlated with their physiological response, *J Physiol* 124:476–488, 1954.

Clark FJ, Burgess RC, Chapin JW, et al: Role of intramuscular receptors in the awareness of limb position, *J Neurophysiol* 54:1529–1540, 1985.

Fatoye FA, Palmer ST, Macmillan F, et al: Repeatability of joint proprioception and muscle torque assessment in healthy children and in children diagnosed with hypermobility syndrome, *Musculoskeletal Care* 6:108–123, 2008.

Fatoye FA, Palmer ST, Macmillan F, et al: Proprioception and muscle torque deficits in children with hypermobility syndrome, *Rheumatology* 48:152–157, 2009.

Ferrell WR, Craske B: Contribution of joint and muscle afferents to position sense at the human proximal interphalangeal joint, *Exp Physiol* 77:331–342, 1992.

Ferrell WR, Tennant N, Sturrock RD, et al: Proprioceptive enhancement ameliorates symptoms in the joint hypermobility syndrome, *Arthritis Rheum* 50:3323–3328, 2004.

Ferrell WR, Tennant N, Baxendale RH, et al: Musculoskeletal reflex function in the joint hypermobility syndrome, *Arthritis Care Res* 57:1329–1333, 2007.

Fridén T, Roberts D, Zätterström R, et al: Proprioception in the nearly extended knee. Measurements of position and movement in healthy individuals and in symptomatic anterior cruciate ligament injured patients, *Knee Surg Sports Traumatol Arthrosc* 4:217–224, 1996.

Gazit Y, Nahir AM, Grahame R, et al: Dysautonomia in the joint hypermobility syndrome, *Am J Med* 115:35–40, 2003.

Grahame R, Bird HA: British consultant rheumatologists' perceptions about the hypermobility syndrome: a national survey, *Rheumatology* 40:559–562, 2001.

Hall MG, Ferrell WR, Baxendale RH, et al: Knee joint proprioception: threshold detection levels in healthy young subjects, *Neuro-Orthopedics* 15:81–90, 1994.

Hall MG, Ferrell WR, Sturrock RD, et al: The effect of the hypermobility syndrome on knee joint proprioception, *Br J Rheumatol* 34:121–125, 1995.

Henning C, Lynch M, Glick K: An in vivo strain gauge study of elongation of the anterior cruciate ligament, *Am J Sports Med* 13:22–26, 1985.

Horch KW, Clark FJ, Burgess PR: Awareness of knee joint angle under static conditions, *J Neurophysiol* 38:1436–1447, 1975.

Jaffe M, Tirosh E, Cohen A, et al: Joint mobility and motor development, *Arch Dis Child* 63:159–161, 1988.

Keays SL, Bullock-Saxton JE, Newcombe P, et al: The effectiveness of a pre-operative home-based physiotherapy programme for chronic anterior cruciate ligament deficiency, *Physiother Res Int* 11:204–218, 2006.

Kennedy JC, Alexander IJ, Hayes KC: Nerve supply of the human knee and its functional importance, *Am J Sports Med* 10:329–335, 1982.

Kerr A, Macmillan CE, Uttley WS, et al: Physiotherapy for children with hypermobility syndrome, *Physiotherapy* 86:313–317, 2000.

Kirby A, Davies R: Developmental Coordination Disorder and Joint Hypermobility Syndrome – over lapping disorders? Implications for research and clinical practice, *Child Care Health Dev* 33:513–519, 2007.

Mallik AK, Ferrell WR, McDonald A, et al: Impaired proprioceptive acuity at the proximal interphalangeal joint in patients with the hypermobility syndrome, *Br J Rheumatol* 33:631–637, 1994.

Matthews PBC: Muscle spindles and their motor control, *Physiology Review* 44:219–288, 1964.

Melnyk M, Faist M, Gothner M, et al: Changes in stretch reflex excitability are related to "giving way" symptoms in patients with anterior cruciate ligament rupture, *J Neurophysiol* 97:474–480, 2007.

Reider B, Arcand MA, Diehl LH, et al: Proprioception of the knee before and after anterior cruciate ligament reconstruction, *Arthroscopy* 19:2–12, 2003.

Roberts D, Fridén T, Zätterström R, et al: Proprioception in people with anterior cruciate ligament-deficient knees: comparison of symptomatic and asymptomatic patients, *J Orthop Sports Phys Ther* 29:587–594, 1999.

Roberts D, Ageberg E, Andersson G, et al: Clinical measurements of proprioception, muscle strength and laxity in relation to function in the ACL-injured knee, *Knee Surg Sports Traumatol Arthros* 15:9–16, 2007.

Røgind H, Lykkegaard JJ, Bliddal H, et al: Postural sway in normal subjects aged 20–70 years, *Clin Physiol Funct Imaging* 23:171–176, 2003.

Sahin N, Baskent A, Cakmak A, et al: Evaluation of knee proprioception and effects of proprioception exercise in patients with benign joint hypermobility syndrome, *Rheumatol Int* 28:995–1000, 2008a.

Sahin N, Baskent A, Ugurlu H, et al: Isokinetic evaluation of knee extensor/flexor muscle strength in patients with hypermobility syndrome, *Rheumatol Int* 28:643–648, 2008b.

Sainburg RL, Poizner H, Ghez C: Loss of proprioception produces deficits in interjoint coordination, *J Neurophysio* 70:2136–2147, 1993.

Sherrington CS: *The Integrative Action of the Nervous System*, New Haven, 1906, Yale University Press.

Snyder-Mackler L: Scientific rationale and physiological basis for the use of closed kinetic chain exercises in the lower extremity, *Journal of Sport Rehabilitation* 5:2–12, 1996.

Tirosh E, Jaffe M, Marmur R, et al: Prognosis of motor development and joint hypermobility, *Arch Dis Child* 66:931–933, 1991.

Wood L, Ferrell WR: The response of slowly adapting articular mechanoreceptors in the cat knee joint to alterations in intra-articular volume, *Ann Rheum Dis* 43:327–332, 1984.

Section 2

Therapy

Chapter 7

Pharmacotherapy

7.1 Pharmacotherapy in fibromyalgia

Andrew J Holman

INTRODUCTION

The symptoms in fibromyalgia (FM) and their complex associations with psychological and autonomic dysfunction are discussed in Chapter 5. Understanding this landscape and its components expressed in each individual is fundamental to rationalizing the use of pharmacotherapeutic interventions.

This chapter specifically discusses the options and evidence available in the management of FM. It complements Chapter 7.2 where Howard Bird discusses the role of these agents in joint hypermobility syndrome (JHS) where the principles for utilizing such therapies might be considered the same as for FM, but where evidence from randomized controlled trials (RCTs) is lacking.

TRADITIONAL MEDICATIONS

Pharmacotherapeutic choices may be divided into off-label, older therapies discovered through trial and error with clinical benefits occasionally supported by RCTs and newer medications promoted by recent publications as well as pharmaceutical companies. Until 2007, no medication was approved by the Federal Drug Administration (FDA), European Medicines Agency (EMEA) for treatment of FM. Left to their wits, clinicians generally rationalized medication choice by various treatment objectives linked to drug effects with which they were already familiar. Analgesics, anticonvulsants, sedative hypnotics, antipsychotics, antidepressants and similar options have been widely utilized.

TRICYCLIC AND OTHER ANTIDEPRESSANTS

Amitriptyline

For many, amitriptyline has been a mainstay and often first-line agent used to treat FM. The RCT evidence for its popularity arises from a handful of supportive studies between 1986 and 1994 (Carette et al 1986, Goldenberg et al 1986, Jaeschke et al 1991). While doses ranging from 10–50 mg at bedtime for 2–9 weeks demonstrated significant pain reduction, Carrette reported no benefit with 30 mg at bedtime over a 24-week period (Carette et al 1994). Further supportive evidence, however, was found in a fluoxetine-amitriptyline, four-arm, 6-week, cross-over study in 1996 by Goldenberg (Goldenberg et al 1996). Either agent alone decreased pain and fatigue better than placebo, but their combination significantly reduced the Fibromyalgia Impact Questionnaire (FIQ) by 34% (Box 7.1.1).

Arguably, the FIQ has become the preeminent FM assessment tool evaluating pain, function, fatigue, depression, anxiety and work functions (Burckhardt et al 1991). While in need of some

© 2010 Elsevier Ltd.
DOI: 10.1016/B978-0-7020-3005-5.00010-0

BOX 7.1.1   Fibromyalgia Impact Questionnaire (FIQ) domains

Ten-item function score for activities of daily living

How many days did you feel good? (0–7)
How many days did you miss work because of FM? (0–7)
Visual analog 10 cm scale (none [0] to overwhelming [10]) for
    Pain at work
    Pain severity
    Daily fatigue
    Morning fatigue
    Stiffness
    Anxiety
    Depression

(Burckhardt et al 1991)

---

updating (Bennett 2005), it remains ostensibly a mandatory inclusion in any FM study or application for regulatory approval for a new FM treatment option. Meta-analyses of amitriptyline demonstrated even stronger evidence for its inclusion into the FM armamentarium, yet the overall benefits were modest (Arnold & Keck 2000, O'Malley et al 2000, Nishishinya et al 2008). Clinical responses ranged from 25–37% benefit, but while sleep, fatigue and pain improved, tender point score did not. Comparing amitriptyline to other types of antidepressant has been attempted, but evidence is weak. Only one study has been conducted with nortriptyline; it was found to be ineffective (Heymann et al 2001).

Cyclobenzaprine

Although often considered a muscle relaxant, cyclobenzaprine is structurally a tricyclic moiety, and has demonstrated similar reduction of FM pain (30%) in several trials (Bennett et al 1988, Quimby et al 1989, Hamaty et al 1989). All RCTs were dosed at 30 mg per day over 4–12 weeks, but again, Carette found inefficacy at 24 weeks (Carette et al 1994). This study comparing amitriptyline, cyclobenzaprine and placebo yielded a benefit at 6 and 12 weeks, but not at 24 weeks. However, a meta-analysis endorsed the efficacy of cyclobenzaprine for treatment of FM (Tofferi et al 2004). Even very low doses (1–4 mg) at bedtime have demonstrated some analgesic efficacy and have improved sleep stage architecture (Modolfsky 2002).

Selective serotonin reuptake inhibitors

Contrary to the Goldenberg crossover study with amitriptyline, the selective serotonin reuptake inhibitor (SSRI) fluoxetine at a dose of 20 mg each morning was not superior to placebo after 6 weeks (Wolfe et al 1994). Yet, in another study allowing flexible dosing $\leq$ 80 mg/d, statistically significant efficacy was evident (Arnold et al 2002). Not unexpectedly, depression sub-score of the FIQ contributed to overall FIQ score improvement, but pain and fatigue were also reduced compared to placebo, even after correcting for depression score. Again, tender-point (TP) score did not improve, and this observation has become a theme in FM research. To date, RCTs have only rarely recorded a statistically significant improvement in TP score, which is intriguing given that TPs are the hallmark clinical diagnostic sign of FM.

Other SSRIs have been assessed in RCTs, including a report of sertraline (50 mg) attaining equivalent efficacy with amitriptyline (25 mg) (Celiker & Cagavi 2000). Üçeyler et al (2008) conducted an exhaustive review of antidepressant studies in FM concluding multi-outcome efficacy for amitriptyline (25–50 mg/d), fluoxetine (20–40 mg/d), sertraline (50 mg/d) and paroxetine (20 mg/d) (Patkar et al 2007) but not for citalopram (20–40 mg/d) (Nørregaard et al 1995). Unfortunately for SSRIs as a group, mean pain reduction and mean improved quality of life was only 18% and 16%, respectively, after correcting for placebo effect. Therefore, such options are unlikely to achieve substantial clinical benefits or meaningful remission for most FM patients.

MUSCLE RELAXANTS, NON-STEROIDAL ANTI-INFLAMMATORIES, OPIOIDS AND OTHER ANALGESICS

Muscle relaxants and benzodiazepines

The muscle relaxant, carisoprodol, has been found to reduce FM pain in one trial dosed at 1200 mg/d for 8 weeks (Vaerøy et al 1989). Unlike other muscle relaxants, carisoprodol is metabolized to an anxiolytic, meprobamate, a potential drug of abuse (Bailey & Briggs 2002) and is associated with teratogenicity (Timmermann et al 2008) and increased road traffic accidents (Logan et al 2000). This reduces clinical confidence given concern for addictive risk and tolerance, yet its muscle-relaxant properties are considerable. Comorbid positional cervical spinal cord compression (PC3) has been documented in 65% of patients with FM in a recent pilot study using flexion–extension cervical spinal magnetic resonance imaging. Theoretically, this combination of FM and PC3 may be more amenable to treatment with this agent given the benefit of some anxiolytics (benzodiazepines) for spinal cord irritability among patients with cervical spinal cord injury (Merritt 1981, Dahm et al 1989, Winkler et al 1997).

An open trial of two benzodiazepines, lorazepam or clonazepam (2 mg at bedtime), among 202 patients with FM demonstrated widespread and considerable reduction in pain over 2 weeks (Holman 1998) sustained for 49% of subjects at 52 weeks without dose escalation or abuse (Holman 1999). Both agents also decrease symptoms of restless leg syndrome (RLS), found to be more common among patients with FM (34% vs. 2% controls) (Yunus & Aldag 1996), and may reduce cervical spinal cord irritability (Fenollosa et al 1993). Studies with other benzodiazepines have yielded mixed findings. Alprazolam (0.5–3.0 mg/d) for 6 weeks was ineffective (Russell et al 1991), while temazepam (15–30 mg at bedtime) for 12 weeks was beneficial (Hench et al 1989). Neither agent reduces RLS or spinal cord irritability, but temazepam may influence sleep deficit in FM.

NSAIDs, steroids and opiates

Non-steroidal anti-inflammatory drugs (NSAIDs), including naproxen (Goldenberg et al 1986) and ibuprofen (Yunus et al 1989), as well as corticosteroids (Clark et al 1985) have been uniformly ineffective in FM RCTs. Tramadol, a centrally acting analgesic with combined mu-opioid activity and inhibition of serotonin/norepinephrine reuptake, has been studied in three RCTs (Biasi et al 1998, Russell et al 2000, Bennett et al 2003). A variety of pain measures improved statistically with good tolerability. In an interesting design based on time to study withdrawal for inefficacy over 91 days with 315 subjects, those in the tramadol arm were less likely to withdraw for any reason (48% [tramadol] vs. 62% [placebo]) and noted better pain relief and improved FIQ scores. Most common adverse effects (AE) were nausea (20%) and constipation (15%). Tizanidine, an alpha-2 receptor antagonist useful for reduction of muscular spasticity, has also been beneficial and reduces cerebrospinal fluid (CSF) neuroamines and

substance P levels in patients with FM (4–24 mg/day) (Russell et al 2002).

Curiously, there have been no opioid RCTs in patients with FM. Nevertheless, their use is not uncommon, yet clinicians may assume inefficacy without justification. And, as understanding of cervical spinal cord research expands into a reappraisal of chronic widespread pain (CWP) and FM (Chapter 5), clinicians may eventually discover a less biased and more evidence-based approach to narcotic usage.

NEWER MEDICATIONS

With the advent of recent FDA approval of medications indicated for the treatment of FM, many reviews have been recently published. Pharmaceutical industry support of most and ongoing advertisement campaigns simultaneously highlight the importance of FM to the uninitiated, but can also adversely burden clinicians searching for independent, unbiased information. Fair comparisons are essential, and a reasonable rationale explaining clinical responses to these medications adds credibility and confidence.

HYPNOTICS

Although abnormal sleep stage architecture, non-restorative sleep and fatigue remain fundamental elements of FM, sedative hypnotics have been remarkably unhelpful. Many options reduce abnormal sleep indirectly, but generally, traditional hypnotics fail to reduce pain and TPs. The zolpidem RCT provides an illustrative example (Moldofsky et al 1996). As an agent that increases stage 2 sleep, FM subjects noted improved sleep duration and decreased sleep latency, but not reduced pain and fatigue. Interestingly, pioneering studies inducing FM findings occurred with auditory arousal from deeper and more restorative stage 4 sleep (Chapter 5). Therefore, addressing stage 2 sleep appears to be an inadequate ambition.

Sodium oxybate

To date, only one commercial compound induces stage 4 sleep: sodium oxybate (Lapierre et al 1990). This agent is FDA approved for treatment of narcolepsy with cataplexy and is a naturally occurring CNS metabolite found in the hippocampus and basal ganglia (Snead 3rd & Liu 1984). Given its potential as a drug of abuse and its ease of non-commercial manufacture, it is highly regulated and available in the US only through a central pharmacy or in the UK on a case-by-case basis. Nevertheless, Scharf et al (2003) initially conducted a double-blind cross-over trial over 1 month with a 2-week wash out period. A total of 18 subjects completed the trial dosed at 6.0 g at bedtime (two divided doses, 4 hours apart) and were monitored by polysomnogram (PSG), tender point index and subjective measures of improvement in daily diaries. A variety of pain and fatigue scores improved by 29–33% in the active arm compared with 6–10% in the placebo arm ($P < 0.005$). Tender point score decreased by 8.4 points with sodium oxybate compared with an increase of 0.4 points in the placebo arm ($P = 0.008$). PSG measures of inappropriate CNS arousal, including alpha wave intrusion, sleep latency and rapid eye movement (REM) sleep decreased with treatment, while stage 3 and 4 slow-wave sleep increased compared with placebo ($P < 0.005$).

In a second study, 188 subjects were randomized (1:1:1) to placebo and sodium oxybate doses of 4.5 g and 6.0 g in divided nightly doses (Russell et al 2005). Outcomes were more challenging and included a triple outcome measure of $\geq 20\%$ improved 10 cm visual analogue pain (PVAS), $\geq 20\%$ improved total FIQ, and either 'much better' or 'very much better' on patient global impression of change (PGIC). This triple primary outcome was achieved by 13% receiving placebo, 35% receiving 4.5 g ($P = 0.005$) and 27% receiving 6.0 g ($P = 0.05$) doses. Dose response was lacking possibly due to greater early withdrawal from overly rapid initial dose escalation in the 6.0 g arm and the use of a categorical outcome variable. Based on four PSG evaluations per subject, sleep quality measures also improved, including increased stage 4 sleep (Moldofsky & Alvarez-Horine 2008). The most common adverse events (AEs) were nausea and dizziness.

A large phase 3 trial designed for application to the FDA for approval for use in FM was reported by Jazz Pharmaceuticals (Palo Alto, CA, USA) (2008) as successful with details to follow. Although sodium oxybate does not directly address dysautonomia or have a known cervical spinal cord effect, it directly induces stage 4 sleep, which may begin to explain its clinical benefit

in FM. Further research will be required to determine how this agent will be incorporated into the host of new options available to clinicians and combination trials are underway.

ANTICONVULSANTS

As a class, anticonvulsants have been considered a mainstay for treatment of many types of pain. Most have not been evaluated in FM RCTs, but two have: gabapentin and pregabalin. Initially, the rationale of incorporating an anticonvulsant into an FM regimen relates to its effect of potentially modulating neuronal hyperexcitability (Cohen & Abdi 2002). Both gabapentin and pregabalin are structural analogues of γ-aminobutyric acid (GABA), which has been found to reduce allodynia in experimental chronic pain models (Gee et al 1996, Bian et al 2006). Because GABA influences α_2-δ receptor control of calcium channels leading to decreased neuronal hyperexcitation, the mechanism of action of gabapentin and pregabalin has been thought to be related (Baillie & Power 2006). As FM research begins to delineate the nature of central sensitization (Yunus 2007), use of these agents for treatment of FM seems ever more reasonable.

Gabapentin

Gabapentin has been evaluated in an FM RCT reported by Arnold et al (2007). In this 12-week RCT, 1800 mg per day of gabapentin was compared to placebo in 150 age/gender-matched subjects. Using the Brief Pain Inventory (BPI) on a 0–10 scale, gabapentin reduced pain by a difference of –0.92 [95%CI = –1.75, –0.71] compared with controls ($P = 0.015$). However, given the mean baseline pain score of 5.8, the relative benefit reflected only a 16% reduction in pain. Mean FIQ benefit was –8.4 ($P = 0.001$), or an 18% improvement. The most common AEs include dizziness, somnolence, oedema, light-headedness and weight gain.

Pregabalin

The first medication to achieve FDA approval for treatment of FM was pregabalin, an analogue of gabapentin with greater target affinity at the α_2-δ receptor. Initially, in an 8-week study, three pregabalin doses (150 mg/d, 300 mg/d and 450 mg/d) and placebo were randomized (1:1:1:1) to 529 patients (Crofford et al 2005). Mean baseline pain score was 7 (range: 1[no pain]–10[worst pain]) for a group comprised of 90% women with a mean FM duration of 8 years. All patients discontinued concomitant medications and 77% completed the trial. Improvement was noted in all active arms as early as week 2, and was sustained through week 8. Maximum pain benefit relative to placebo (in the 450 mg arm) was moderate (−0.93 [1–11 scale]), while the degree of statistical significance ($P = 0.0009$) likely reflected an ample study size.

Additional RCTs assessed up to 600 mg/d, but pain reduction was again modest (−0.66 [$P = 0.007$]) (Mease et al 2008a). With both studies, response was consistent, but equivalent to a 13% and 9% reduction in pain from baseline, respectively. Lower doses in the initial study (150 mg and 300 mg) were not statistically superior to placebo, but enlarging the second study to 748 subjects enhanced statistical validity of benefit associated with the 300 mg arm in the second study (−0.43 [0–10 scale]; $P = 0.0449$). In the first study, 29% of subjects achieved a ≥50% reduction in pain compared to 13% receiving placebo ($P = 0.003$). A non-significant difference in 'responders' defined as ≥ 30% reduced pain was reported for the 300 mg (43%), 450 mg (43%), 600 mg (44%) and placebo (35%) in the second study. Still, secondary outcomes favoured pregabalin over placebo, including assessments of sleep, patient assessment of global change, and several other domains of quality of life. Important AEs were dose related and included dizziness, somnolence, weight gain and dry mouth. The rationale for selection of pregabalin as an FM option beyond its FDA approval include its consistent, albeit modest response, improvement in secondary outcomes, and its mechanism of action, which may further implicate a spinal cord concern. Positional cervical cord compression (PC3) imbedded in the FM presentation could be aggravated by enhanced range of motion prevalent among patients with JHS. Although not yet studied, this dysautonomic concern may be responsive to pregabalin, since pregabalin is already specifically approved by the EMEA for treatment of central, cervical spinal pain in Europe (Pfizer Inc 2006). Further studies are required to evaluate whether pain reduction in the pregabalin FM RCTs is due to an effect on comorbid PC3 embedded within FM or due to an effect on FM itself.

MIXED SEROTONIN–NORADRENALINE REUPTAKE INHIBITORS (SNRI)

Increasing complexity of antidepressant mechanisms of action has fuelled even greater interest and reliance on their role as FM therapeutic options. Recently, their function as antidepressants has been augmented to also include that of a legitimate analgesic. The first SNRI to be approved by the FDA for treatment of FM in 2008 was duloxetine, with a second, milnacipran approved in 2009. Although milnacipran favours reuptake inhibition of norepinephrine (NE) over serotonin (5-HT), duloxetine is more balanced and does not interact with opioid, muscarinic, histamine-1, α_1-adrenergic, dopamine, 5-HT1A, 5-HT1B, 5-HT1D, 5-HT2A or 5-HT3C receptors (Arnold et al 2004). Duloxetine has significant analgesic properties as well, documented by reduced pain behaviour in animal models compared to venlafaxine, amitriptyline or desipramine (Iyengar et al 2002). Its mechanism of action in animal models and in humans with FM is unknown, but augmented descending inhibition of pain through the spinal cord is a prominent hypothesis (Millan 2002).

Duloxetine

Of five important duloxetine RCTs, two pivotal trials secured the FDA indication for treatment of FM. Earlier, an initial proof of concept trial randomized 207 patients (1:1) to 60 mg/d and placebo for 12 weeks (Arnold et al 2004). Interestingly, it did not achieve its dual primary outcomes: FIQ total score (treatment difference −5.53 [$P = 0.027$]) and FIQ 0–10 pain VAS subscore (treatment difference −0.63 cm [$P = 0.13$]). But, further sub-analysis revealed that treatment response in the 22 men unexpectedly favoured placebo over duloxetine. Also, a secondary measure of pain, the Brief Pain Inventory (BPI) did achieve statistical significance. Consequently, a second 12-week trial of 354 patients eliminated men and employed the BFI as the primary outcome (Arnold et al 2005). Subjects were randomized (1:1:1) to 60 mg daily, 60 mg twice per day and placebo. Pain decreased significantly using the BPI ($P < 0.001$) and was independent of mood. Reduction of pain by ≥ 50% was achieved by 41% receiving 60 mg, 41% receiving 120 mg and 23% receiving placebo ($P = 0.003$).

In a third study by Russell et al (2008), and the second pivotal study submitted for FDA review, 520 subjects (5% men and 25% with major depressive disorder [MDD]) were randomized to duloxetine doses of 25 mg, 60 mg, 120 mg and placebo. Pain reduction was significant overall as well as greater for those with MDD, but did not distinguish 60 mg from the 120 mg dose. Adverse events and premature discontinuation were dose-dependent. In a fourth study by Chappell et al (2007) of non-responders to 60 mg were randomized to either continuation of 60 mg or an increased dose of 120 mg/d. By 60 weeks, treatment at 120 mg was no more likely to achieve >30% reduced pain than continuing the 60 mg/d dosage.

Safety was reported from two prior RTC extensions and was a primary endpoint of a fifth recent study of over 60 weeks (Chappell et al 2008). Important safety concerns with duloxetine in FM trials have been nausea, headache, insomnia, dizziness and constipation as well as concern raised over hepatic failure, hyponatraemia and orthostatic hypotension.

Of note, all antidepressants as a class, including duloxetine, carry a label warning from the FDA highlighting an increased risk of suicide, especially among children and young adults. Neither duloxetine nor milnacipran is approved for use among children. In terms of potential drug interactions, some analgesics commonly used by patients with FM require a cautionary note. Tramadol, previously reviewed, should not be co-administered with duloxetine given the risk of developing serotonin syndrome. And, through cytochrome P450 enzyme system interactions, duloxetine may prolong effects of methadone, oxycodone and propoxyphene, but not fentanyl, codeine and morphine.

Polypharmacy is a commonly employed strategy in FM, since no treatment is sufficiently effective. Nevertheless, cautious appraisal and reappraisal of patient safety, tolerability and efficacy remains fundamental.

Milnacipran

Recently, milnacipran also successfully competed for FDA approval as a treatment of FM. An initial proof of concept trial of milnacipran dosed 100 mg/d, 100 mg twice per day and placebo randomized 125 patients (3:3:2) and defined its primary outcome as either $\geq 30\%$ or $\geq 50\%$ reduction in pain at 12 weeks (Gendreau et al 2005). Only the 100 mg twice per day dose achieved a statistically significant outcome of $\geq 50\%$ decreased pain

compared to placebo (37% [100 mg twice a day; $P = 0.04$], 22% [100 mg daily; $P = 0.55$], 14% placebo). Other pain assessments, including Gracely pain scores, demonstrated a significant benefit, yet the 10 cm VAS pain scale did not ($P = 0.595$).

Two subsequent and much larger 3-month studies, documented efficacy for both the 100 mg daily and 100 mg twice per day dosing (P value range = 0.004—0.025) (Mease et al 2008b, Clauw et al 2008). These studies ($N = 888$ and $N = 1196$) used a composite outcome defined as $\geq 30\%$ pain reduction combined with a rating of 'much improved' and 'very much improved' on the PGIC, somewhat similar to the sodium oxybate trials. Secondary outcomes, including the FIQ total score and Multi-Dimensional Fatigue Inventory (MFI) also improved significantly. A third large study randomized 884 patients to 100 mg twice daily and placebo (1:1) for 12 weeks to demonstrate efficacy with the same composite outcome ($P = 0.003$) as well as significant improvement in FIQ ($P = 0.015$) and other secondary measures (Short Form 36 Health Survey, MFI, and FIQ subscores) (Branco et al 2008). Important AEs included nausea, headache, constipation, hyperhidrosis, hot flushes, dizziness, palpitations, dry mouth and hypertension.

DOPAMINE AGONISTS

Over 15 years ago, Russell et al reported a relative decrease in biogenic amines, including dopamine, in the cerebrospinal fluid (CSF) of patients with FM compared with age/gender-matched controls (Russell et al 1992). More recently, in a controlled study, Wood et al (2007) reported relatively deficient dopaminergic neurotransmission in the limbic system, particularly at the hippocampus. Current discussion continues as to whether this relates to the pain augmentation phenomenon or the dysautonomic balance of FM, since the hippocampus affects both functions (Chapter 3). Interestingly, the hippocampus is responsible for attenuation of autonomic arousal (Drevets et al 2008, Emad et al 2008). If its failure to generate an adequate dopaminergic signal to decreased excessive autonomic arousal (especially at night) predominates, then its autonomic role in FM may be fundamental.

Second-generation dopamine agonists (DAs), including pramipexole and ropinirole, were originally devised to treat Parkinson's disease and were later found to be effective treatments for RLS

(Lin et al 1998, Trinkwalder 2006). They have enhanced specificity for dopamine 2 and 3 receptors (D_2, D_3), with no significant effect on other dopamine receptors (D_1, D_4, D_5), 5-HT, acetylcholine, histamine, muscarinic, opioid, α_1-adrenergic or β-adrenergic receptors (Dziedzicka-Wasylewska et al 2001). Of note, the greatest concentration of $D_{2,3}$ receptors is in the limbic system and at the hippocampus, specifically (Okubo et al 1999). Therefore, a clinical effect in FM could theoretically be related to re-establishing hippocampal dampening of the autonomic arousal fragmenting stage 4 sleep.

Pramipexole

Consideration of pramipexole as an FM treatment option comes from three studies: an initial report of 166 subjects (Holman 2003), a small multicentre study (Holman et al 2004), and one RCT (Holman & Myers 2005). The RCT randomized 60 patients (2:1) to either a gradual fixed-dose escalation to 4.5 mg at bedtime over 14 weeks or placebo. As a unique feature, concomitant medications, including narcotics use (50%), and disabled patients (30%) were accepted. Traditionally, all FM RCTs exclude those disabled as well as nearly all concomitant medications. Also, two important comorbidities independently able to cause significant autonomic arousal were exclusion criteria: OSA and PC3. Since DAs were hypothesized to act by restoring normal autonomic tone through hippocampal dampening of brainstem arousal during sleep, other independent autonomic arousals (OSA and PC3) were considered overly confounding. Both obstructive sleep apnoea and PC3 could theoretically interfere with the beneficial DA mechanism of action in FM. The threshold of $\geq$ 50% reduced pain was achieved by 42% of subjects in the active arm compared with 14% in the placebo arm ($P = 0.008$). Other outcomes, including measures of pain, fatigue, global outcome, FIQ and PGIC, were similarly significant.

Ropinirole

A small RCT of ropinirole (20 active, 10 placebo) employing a fixed-dose escalation over 14 weeks to 8 mg at bedtime, did not demonstrate a statistical benefit (Holman 2004). Forty-five percent of the active subjects and 30% of the placebo subjects achieved $\geq$ 50% reduced pain ($P = 0.31$).

A new extended-release ropinirole trial by GlaxoSmithKline (2008) was also unsuccessful in Europe, but lack of exclusion of OSA and PC3 may have affected results. Also, the ropinirole doses tested in all of these studies were 66–80% lower than the equivalent dosage strength used in the pramipexole trial. A pramipexole dose of 4.5 mg equates to a ropinirole dose of 24 mg (5:1). Since DAs act as autoreceptors at low concentrations and act to restore dopaminergic neurotransmission only at high concentration (Dziedzicka-Wasylewska et al 2001), peak dose is more important to produce a positive clinical outcome than duration of DA exposure.

EUROPEAN LEAGUE AGAINST RHEUMATISM (EULAR) RECOMMENDATIONS

Until recently, consensus recommendations in FM based on RCTs were unthinkable. Yet, over the past few years, there has been an explosion of FM RCTs and a surge in clinical interest. The European League Against Rheumatism (EULAR) published the first FM consensus recommendations in 2007 from a multidisciplinary task force review of 146 trials (Carville et al 2008). And, although clinicians will find variable patient response and tolerability requiring flexibility when prescribing pharmacotherapeutic options, comparisons are currently reasonable based on the response threshold of $\geq$ 50% pain reduction (Table 7.1.1).

While the FDA has approved pregabalin, duloxetine and milnacipran for treatment of FM, the EULAR recommendations highlight a multidisciplinary approach that also includes education and non-pharmacotherapeutic options. In terms of pharmacotherapy, however, they recommended tramadol for management of pain, but not narcotics 'based mainly on expert opinion due to insufficient data' (McClean 2000, Goldenberg et al 2004, Baker & Barkhuizen 2005). They recommended consideration of amitriptyline, fluoxetine, duloxetine, milnacipran, moclobemide and pirlindole. In addition, tropisetron, pramipexole and pregabalin were felt to reduce pain and 'should be considered for treatment of fibromyalgia'.

Unfortunately, there have been no comparator trials, and arguably this most important concept in FM pharmacotherapy i.e. combination therapy, was not addressed by the EULAR group.

Table 7.1.1	Comparison of recently published randomized, placebo–controlled trials for treatment of fibromyalgia			
MEDICATION (WITH REFERENCE)		SUBJECTS WITH > 50% PAIN REDUCTION (%)		P VALUE
	N/dose/duration	Active arm	Placebo arm	
Pregabalin (1)	(528 pts/450 mg/8 wks)	29%	11%	0.001
Pregabalin**(2)	(748 pts/600mg/13 wks)	44%*	35%*	0.007
Gabapentin*(3)	(150 pts,1200-2400 mg/12 wks)	51%**	31%**	0.015
Milnacipran (4)	(125 pts/200 mg/12 wks)	37%	14%	0.04
Duloxetine (5)	(207 pts/120 mg/12 wks)	28%	17%	0.06
Duloxetine (6)	(354 pts/120 mg/12 wks)	41%	23%	0.003
S Oxybate*(7)	(188 pts/4.5-6g/8 wks)	28-30%*	15%*	<0.01
Pramipexole (8)	(60 pts/4.5 mg/14 wks)	42%	14%	0.008

*reported as 20% decreased (0-10cm) VAS pain.
**reported as 30% decreased BPI pain.
1 – Crofford et al 2005
2 – Mease et al 2008a
3 – Arnold et al 2007
4 – Gendreau et al 2005
5 – Arnold et al 2004
6 – Arnold et al 2005
7 – Russell et al 2005
8 – Holman & Myers 2005

Clinicians will need to continue to monitor patients most carefully as these therapies are integrated into a thoughtful approach to FM management. Combination treatments have been and will most likely continue to be omnipresent in the FM clinical experience (Mease & Seymour 2008).

The old adage of 'start low; go slow' remains as important as any formal trial.

References

Arnold LM, Keck PE: Antidepressant treatment of fibromyalgia: a meta-analysis and review, Psychosomatics 41:104–113, 2000.

Arnold LM, Hess EV, Hudson JI, et al: A randomized, placebo-controlled, double-blind, flexible-dose study of fluoxetine in the treatment of women with fibromyalgia, Am J Med 112:191–197, 2002.

Arnold LM, Lu Y, Crofford LJ, et al: A double-blind multicenter trial comparing duloxetine to placebo in the treatment of fibromyalgia with and without major depressive disorder, Arthritis Rheum 50(9):2974–2984, 2004.

Arnold LM, Rosen A, Pritchett YL, et al: A randomized, double-blind, placebo-controlled trial of duloxetine in the treatment of women with fibromyalgia with and without major depressive disorder, Pain 119(1–3):5–15, 2005.

Arnold LM, Goldenberg DL, Stanford SB, et al: Gabapentin in the treatment of fibromyalgia: a randomized, double-blind, placebo-controlled, multicenter trial, Arthritis Rheum 56(4):1336–1344, 2007.

Bailey DN, Briggs JR: Carisoprodol an unrecognized drug of abuse, Am J Clin Pathol 117(3):396–400, 2002.

Baillie JK, Power I: The mechanism of action of gabapentin in neuropathic pain, Curr Opin Investig Drugs 7(1):33–39, 2006.

Baker K, Barkhuizen A: Pharmacologic treatment of fibromyalgia, Curr Pain & Headache Reports 9:301–306, 2005.

Bennett RM, Gatter RA, Campbell SM, et al: A comparison of cyclobenzaprine and placebo in the management of fibrositis: a double-blind, controlled study, Arthritis Rheum 31:1535–1542, 1988.

Bennett RM, Kamin M, Karin R, et al: Tramadol and acetaminophen combination tablets in the treatment of fibromyalgia pain, Am J Med 114:537–545, 2003.

Bennett R: The Fibromyalgia Impact Questionnaire (FIQ): a review of its development, current version, operating characteristics and uses,

Clin Exp Rheumatol 23(5 Suppl 39): S154–S162, 2005.

Bian F, Li Z, Offord J: Calcium channel alpha(2)-delta type 1 subunit is the major binding protein for pregabalin in neocortex, hippocampus, amygdala, and spinal cord: an ex vivo autoradiographic study in alpha(2)-delta type 1 genetically modified mice, *Brain Res* 1075:68–80, 2006.

Biasi G, Manca S, Manganelli S, et al: Tramadol in the fibromyalgia syndrome: a controlled trial versus placebo, *Int J Clin Pharmacol Res* 18:13–19, 1998.

Branco JC, Perrot S, Bragee G, et al: *Milnacipran for the treatment of fibromyalgia syndrome: a European multi-center, randomized, double-blind, placebo-controlled trial [abstract THU0365]*, Presented at the European League Against Rheumatism, Paris, France, 2008, Annual European Congress of Rheumatology.

Burckhardt CS, Clark SR, Bennett RM: The fibromyalgia impact questionnaire: development and validation, *J Rheum* 18(5):728–733, 1991.

Carette S, McCain GA, Bell DA, et al: Evaluation of amitriptyline in primary fibrositis, *Arthritis Rheum* 29:655–659, 1986.

Carette S, Bell MJ, Reynolds WJ, et al: Comparison of amitriptyline, cyclobenzaprine, and placebo in the treatment of fibromyalgia. A randomized, double-blind clinical trial, *Arthritis Rheum* 37(1):32–40, 1994.

Carville SF, Arendt-Nielsen S, Bliddal H, et al: EULAR evidenced based recommendations for the management of fibromyalgia syndrome, *Ann Rheum Dis* 67(4):536–541, 2008.

Celiker R, Cagavi Z: Comparison of amitriptyline and sertraline in the treatment of fibromyalgia syndrome [abstract], *Arthritis Rheum* 43:S332, 2000.

Chappell A, Bradley L, Wiltse C, et al: Duloxetine 60–120 mg versus placebo in the treatment of fibromyalgia syndrome [abstract], *Arthritis Rheum* 56(9):S609, 2007.

Chappell AS, Littlejohn J, Kajdasz D, et al: *A 1-year safety and efficacy study of duloxetine in patients with fibromyalgia [abstract THU0370]*, Presented at the European League Against Rheumatism, Paris, France, 2008, Annual European Congress of Rheumatology.

Clark S, Tindall E, Bennett RM: A double blind crossover trial of prednisone versus placebo in the treatment of fibrositis, *J Rheum* 12(5):980–983, 1985.

Clauw DJ, Mease P, Palmer RH, et al: *Milnacipran for the treatment of fibromyalgia syndrome: a 15-week, randomized, double-blind, placebo-controlled trial [abstract THU0366]*, Presented at the European League Against Rheumatism, Paris, France, 2008, Annual European Congress of Rheumatology.

Cohen S, Abdi S: Central pain, *Curr Opin Anaesthesiol* 15(5):575–581, 2002.

Crofford LJ, Rowbotham MC, Mease PJ, et al: Pregabalin 1008–105 Study Group: Pregabalin for the treatment of fibromyalgia syndrome: results of a randomized, double-blind, placebo-controlled trial, *Arthritis Rheum* 52(4):1264–1273, 2005.

Dahm LS, Beric A, Dimitrijevic MR, et al: Direct spinal effect of a benzodiazepine (midazolam) on spasticity in man, *Stereotact Funct Neurosurg* 53(2):85–94, 1989.

Drevets WC, Price JL, Furey ML: Brain structural and functional abnormalities in mood disorders: implications for neurocircuitry models of depression, *Brain Struct Funct* 213(1–2):93–118, 2008.

Dziedzicka-Wasylewska M, Ferrari F, Johnson RD, et al: Mechanisms of action of pramipexole: effects of receptors, *Rev Contemp Pharmacother* 12:1–31, 2001.

Emad Y, Ragab Y, Zeinhom F, et al: Hippocampus dysfunction may explain symptoms of fibromyalgia syndrome. A study with single-voxel magnetic resonance spectroscopy, *J Rheum Jul* 35(7): 1371–1377, 2008.

Fenollosa P, Pallares J, Cervera J, et al: Chronic pain in the spinal cord injured: statistical approach and pharmacological treatment, *Paraplegia* 31(11): 722–729, 1993.

Gee NS, Brown JP, Dissanayake VU, et al: The novel anticonvulsant drug, gabapentin (neurontin), binds to the α_2-δ subunit of a calcium channel, *J Biol Chem* 271:5768–5776, 1996.

Gendreau RM, Thorn MD, Gendreau JF, et al: Efficacy of Milnacipran in patients with fibromyalgia, *J Rheum* 32:1975–1985, 2005.

GlaxoSmithKline. Requip (ropinirole) corporate document: "A randomized, double-blind, placebo-controlled, parallel group study to investigate the safety and efficacy of controlled-release ropinirole", *GlaxoSmithKline*, http://www.gsk-clinicalstudyregister.com/files/pdf/21016.pdf. (accessed November 2008).

Goldenberg DL, Felson DT, Dinerman HA: Randomized, controlled trial of amitriptyline and naproxen in the treatment of patients with fibromyalgia, *Arthritis Rheum* 29:1371–1377, 1986.

Goldenberg D, Mayskiy M, Mossey C, et al: A randomized, double-blind crossover trial of fluoxetine and amitriptyline for the treatment of fibromyalgia, *Arthritis Rheum* 39(11):1852–1859, 1996.

Goldenberg DL, Burckhardt C, Crofford L: Management of fibromyalgia syndrome, *JAMA* 292(19):2388–2395, 2004.

Hamaty D, Valentine JL, Howard R, et al: The plasma endorphin, prostaglandin and catecholamine profile of patients with fibrositis treated with cyclobenzaprine and placebo: a 5-month study, *J Rheumatol Suppl* 19:164–168, 1989.

Hench PK, Cohen R, Mitler MM: Fibromyalgia: effects of amitriptyline, temazepam and placebo on pain and sleep [abstract], *Arthritis Rheum* 32:S47, 1989.

Heymann RE, Helfenstein M, Feldman D: A double-blind, randomized, controlled study of amitriptyline, nortriptyline and placebo in patients with fibromyalgia. An analysis of outcome measures, *Clin Exp Rheumatol* 19(6):697–702, 2001.

Holman AJ: Effect of Lorazepam on Pain Score for Refractory Fibromyalgia [abstract], *Arthritis Rheum* 41(9):S259, 1998.

Holman AJ: Safety and Efficacy of Lorazepam for Fibromyalgia after One Year [abstract], *Arthritis Rheum* 42(9):S152, 1999.

Holman AJ: Pramipexole and fibromyalgia: promise and precaution. [letter], *J Rheum* 30(12):2733, 2003.

Holman AJ: Treatment of Fibromyalgia with the Dopamine Agonist Ropinirole: a 14-week Double-blind, Pilot, Randomized Controlled Trial with 14-week Blinded Extension, *Arthritis Rheum* 50(Suppl 9):S698, 2004.

Holman AJ, Neiman RA, Ettlinger RE: Preliminary efficacy of the dopamine agonist, pramipexole for fibromyalgia: the first, open label, multicenter experience, *J Musculoskeletal Pain* 12(1):69–74, 2004.

Holman AJ, Myers RR: A randomized, double-blind, placebo-controlled trial of pramipexole, a dopamine agonist, in patients with fibromyalgia receiving concomitant medications, *Arthritis Rheum* 52(8):2495–2505, 2005.

Iyengar S, Ahmad L, Simmons RM: Efficacy of the selective serotonin and norepinephrine reuptake inhibitor duloxetine in the formalin model of persistent pain, *Bio Psychiatry* 51(Suppl 8):75S–76S, 2002.

Jazz Pharmaceuticals, Inc., Palo Alto, CA, press release, 2008, http://www.jazzpharma.com/news.php?id=84.

Jaeschke R, Adachi J, Guyatt G, et al: Clinical usefulness of amitriptyline in fibromyalgia: the results of 23 N-of-1 randomized controlled trials, *J Rheum* 18(3):447–451, 1991.

Lapierre O, Montplaisir J, Lamarre M, et al: The effect of gamma-hydroxybutyrate on nocturnal and diurnal sleep of normal subjects: further considerations on REM sleep-triggering mechanisms, *Sleep* 13(1):24–30, 1990.

Lin SC, Kaplan J, Burger CD, et al: Effect of pramipexole in treatment of resistant restless legs syndrome, *Mayo Clin Proc* 73(6):497–500, 1998.

Logan BK, Case GA, Gordon AM: Carisoprodol, meprobamate, and driving impairment, *J Forensic Sci* 45(3):619–623, 2000.

McClean G: Does intravenous lidocaine reduce fibromyalgia pain?: a randomized, double-blind, placebo-controlled cross-over study, *Pain Clinic* 12:181–185, 2000.

Mease PJ, Russell IJ, Arnold LM, et al: A randomized, double-blind, placebo-controlled, phase III trial of pregabalin in the treatment of patients with fibromyalgia, *J Rheum* 35(3):502–514, 2008a.

Mease P, Clauw DJ, Palmer RH, et al: *Milnacipran efficacy and safety in the treatment of fibromyalgia syndrome [abstract THU0379]*, Presented at the European League Against Rheumatism, Paris, France, 2008b, Annual European Congress of Rheumatology.

Mease PJ, Seymour K: Fibromyalgia: should the treatment paradigm be monotherapy or combination therapy? *Curr Pain & Headache Reports* 12:399–405, 2008.

Merritt JL: Management of spasticity in spinal cord injury, *Mayo Clin Proc* 56(10):614–622, 1981.

Millan MJ: Descending control of pain, *Prog Neurobiol* 66:355–474, 2002.

Moldofsky H, Lue FA, Mously C, Roth-Schechter B, Reynolds WJ: The effect of zolpidem in patients with fibromyalgia: a dose ranging, double-blind, placebo-controlled, modified crossover study, *J. Rheum* 23:529–533, 1996.

Moldofsky H: A double-blind, randomized, parallel study of very-low dose cyclobenzaprine compared to placebo in subjects with fibromyalgia [abstract], *Arthritis Rheum* 46:S614, 2002.

Moldofksy H, Alvarez-Horine S: *Effect of sodium oxybate on sleep physiology and sleep-related symptoms in fibromyalgia [abstract THU0381]*, Presented at the European League Against Rheumatism, Paris, France, 2008, Annual European Congress of Rheumatology.

Nishishinya B, Urrútia G, Walitt B, et al: Amitriptyline in the treatment of fibromyalgia: a systematic review of its efficacy, *Rheumatology (Oxford)* 47(12):1741–1746, 2008.

Nørregaard J, Volkmann H, Danneskiold-Samsøe B: A randomized controlled trial of citalopram in the treatment of fibromyalgia, *Pain* 61(3):445–449, 1995.

Okubo Y, Olsson H, Ito H, et al: PET mapping of extrastriatal D2-like dopamine receptors in the human brain using an anatomic standardization technique and [11C]FLB 457, *Neuroimage* 10(6):666–674, 1999.

O'Malley PG, Balden E, Tompkins G, et al: Treatment of fibromyalgia with antidepressants, *J Gen Intern Med* 15:659–666, 2000.

Patkar AA, Masand PS, Krulewicz S, et al: A randomized, controlled, trial of controlled release paroxetine in fibromyalgia, *Am J Med* 120(5):448–454, 2007.

Pfizer Press release, Pfizer, Inc. NY, September 19, 2006, http://www.docguide.com/news/content.nsf/news/852571020057CCF6852571EE000FDE49.

Quimby LG, Gratwick GM, Whitney CD, et al: A randomized trial of cyclobenzaprine for the treatment of fibromyalgia, *J Rheumatol Suppl* 19:140–143, 1989.

Russell IJ, Fletcher EM, Michalek JE, et al: Treatment of primary fibrositis/fibromyalgia syndrome with ibuprofen and alprazolam. A double-blind, placebo-controlled study, *Arthritis Rheum* 34(5):552–560, 1991.

Russell IJ, Vaeroy H, Javors M, et al: Cerebrospinal fluid biogenic amine metabolites in fibromyalgia/fibrositis syndrome and rheumatoid arthritis, *Arthritis Rheum* 35(5):550–556, 1992.

Russell J, Kamin M, Bennett R: Efficacy of tramadol in treatment of pain in fibromyalgia, *J Clin Rheumatol* 6:250–257, 2000.

Russell IJ, Michalek JE, Xiao Y, et al: Therapy with a central alpha-2 agonist (Tizanidine) decreases cerebral spinal substance P, and may reduce serum hyaluronic acid as it improves clinical symptoms of the fibromyalgia syndrome [abstract], *Arthritis Rheum* 46:S614, 2002.

Russell IJ, Bennett RM, Michalek JE: Sodium oxybate relieves pain and improves sleep in fibromyalgia syndrome [FMS]: a randomized, double-blind, placebo-controlled, multi-center clinical trial. [abstract], *Arthritis Rheum* 52(12):L30, 2005.

Russell IJ, Mease PJ, Smith TR, et al: Efficacy and safety of duloxetine for treatment of fibromyalgia in patients with and without major depressive disorder: results from a 6-month, randomized, double-blind, placebo-controlled, fixed-dose trial, *Pain* 136(3):432–444, 2008.

Scharf MB, Baumann M, Berkowitz DV: The effects of sodium oxybate on clinical symptoms and sleep patterns in patients with fibromyalgia, *J Rheum* 30(5):1070–1074, 2003.

Snead OC 3rd, Liu CC: Gamma-hydroxybutyric acid binding sites in rat and human brain synaptosomal membranes, *Biochem Pharmacol* 33(16):2587–2590, 1984.

Timmermann G, Acs N, Bánhidy F, et al: A study of teratogenic and fetotoxic effects of large doses of meprobamate used for a suicide attempt by 42 pregnant women, *Toxicol Ind Health* 24(1–2):97–107, 2008.

Tofferi JK, Jackson JL, O'Malley PG: Treatment of fibromyalgia with cyclobenzaprine: A meta-analysis, *Arthritis Rheum* 51(1):9–13, 2004.

Trenkwalder C: The weight of evidence for repinirole in restless leg syndrome, *European Journal of Neurology* 13:21–30, 2006.

Üçeyler N, Häuser W, Sommer C: A systematic review on the effectiveness of treatment with antidepressants in fibromyalgia syndrome, *Arthritis Rheum* 59(9):1279–1298, 2008.

Vaerøy H, Abrahamsen A, Førre O, et al: Treatment of fibromyalgia (fibrositis syndrome): a parallel double blind trial with carisoprodol, paracetamol and caffeine (Somadril comp) versus placebo, *Clin Rheumatol* 8(2):245–250, 1989.

Winkler T, Sharma HS, Stålberg E, et al: Benzodiazepine receptors influence spinal cord evoked potentials and edema following trauma to the rat spinal cord, *Acta Neurochir Suppl* 70:216–219, 1997.

Wolfe F, Cathey MA, Hawley DJ: A double-blind placebo controlled trial of fluoxetine in fibromyalgia, *Scand J Rheumatol* 23:255–259, 1994.

Wood PB, Patterson JC, Sunderland JJ, et al: Reduced presynaptic dopamine activity in fibromyalgia syndrome demonstrated with positron emission tomography: a pilot study, *J Pain* 8(1):51–58, 2007.

Yunus MB, Masi AT, Aldag JC: Short term effects of ibuprofen in primary fibromyalgia syndrome: a double blind, placebo controlled trial, *J Rheum* 16(4):527–532, 1989.

Yunus M, Aldag J: Restless legs syndrome and leg cramps in fibromyalgia syndrome: a controlled study, *BMJ* 312:1339, 1996.

Yunus MB: Role of central sensitization in symptoms beyond muscle pain, and the evaluation of a patient with widespread pain, *Best Pract Res Clin Rheumatol* 21(3):481–497, 2007.

7.2 Pharmacotherapy in joint hypermobility syndrome

Howard A Bird

INTRODUCTION

The pharmacotherapeutics of fibromyalgia (FM), autonomic dysfunction, and functional bowel disorders are dealt with in Section 1 and Chapter 7.1, respectively. Given many of the features of chronic widespread pain are similar in FM and joint hypermobility syndrome (JHS) and that the conditions may co-exist, pharmacological interventions that impact on the sensitization and central neuropathic pain mechanisms in FM may be of some relevance to JHS and potentially to regional pain syndromes related to hypermobility.

Unlike in FM, there is a dearth of formal clinical trials of analgesics and other drugs in JHS. In part, this reflects absence of diagnostic criteria over and above the 1973 Beighton hypermobility criteria, albeit more recently redressed by the 1998 Brighton Criteria (Chapter 1).

Ultimately, pain in joint hypermobility may be dependent upon diverse factors including tendonopathies, subluxation and dislocation, the shape of the articulating surfaces, neuromuscular tone, proprioception, peripheral and central sensitization, and physiological factors (Chapter 2). Drug management is best modified towards each of these separate contributing causes.

The drugs discussed in this chapter represent a didactic choice based on experience in the management of patients with JHS. Drug treatment is no substitute for persevering with applied physical rehabilitation and behavioural therapies as appropriate.

ANALGESICS

However effective physiotherapy might be and however effectively life's daily activities might be paced, analgesics are still often necessary.

PARACETAMOL AND CODEINE

Worldwide, paracetamol (acetaminophen) as perhaps the weakest but safest analgesic is available over the counter in many countries. Even if prescribed up to a maximum dose of 4.0 g/day (as 1.0 g q.d.s.) it is often ineffective in JHS aside from acute minor soft tissue trauma, and more general common pains such as headache/migraine. Nevertheless it should probably always be tried first.

UK practice allows access to compound generic analgesics of which co-codamol (paracetamol with codeine) and co-dydramol (paracetamol with dihydrocodeine) can be prescribed. The argument for these combinations is that standard paracetamol dosage is boosted by a small admixture of a more potent opiate-like drug, reducing the side effects from this compound. With both components having similar half-lives, there is likely to be synergy with safety. Co-codamol, which tends to constipate, is probably the first choice; co-dydramol (where the dihydrocodeine is more prone to cause central nervous system side effects) is second. Co-proxamol (a low dose of dextropropoxyphene with paracetamol) is in the process of being withdrawn in the UK, at the time of writing only available by special arrangement, because of concern over safety. Significant difference in half-life between the two components sometimes led to unintentional overdosing with the dextropropoxyphene given its longer half-life. There is also evidence that when the drug was used for suicide attempts the side effects from the dextropropoxyphene rendered these more likely to be successful than when other compound analgesics were used instead. The euphoric lift provided by dextropropoxyphene, which seemed of particular benefit in patients with chronic joint pain, was thereby deprived to the arthritic community (Miller et al 1970).

MEPTAZINOL AND TRAMADOL

If paracetamol and codeine-based analgesics are not helpful Meptazinol at 800 mg/day in divided doses, and then to Tramadol may be efficacious. Tramadol is a weak opioid agonist that inhibits the reuptake of both serotonin and noradrenaline (norepinephrine) at the level of the dorsal horns

(Biasi et al 1988). It may be effective in JHS and FM because of its dual mechanism of action, though use is limited because of side effects. The maximum recommended dose is 400 mg/day in divided doses.

ANALGESIC HALF–LIFE

Table 7.2.1 shows the half-life of common analgesics. This should be discussed with the patient in the knowledge that maximum therapeutic effect will be obtained at or just before the time of the half-life, very little therapeutic benefit still obtained after twice the half-life. Drugs of short half-life are suited to 'as-required' dosing, which is of particular value in managing painful events that only occur at certain times of day.

Given the relatively short half-life of certain compounds it is not unusual for patients to experience an 'on–off' effect to their pain control and to describe the apparent limited efficacy at night. Some patients may perceive this as their analgesic 'not working' whereas in fact it is behaving exactly as might be predicted from the half-life. Assuming there is actual pain relief, it is often helpful to convert the compound to a slow-release version, smoothing out the peaks and troughs in pain relief and giving better coverage over night.

OPIATE PATCHES

If compound generic analgesics alone have failed to relieve pain, consideration should be given to adding a second complementary drug with a different mechanism of action. In some cases, even when one or two further such drugs have been added, pain will persist. Consideration could then be given to topical opiate applications, of which two are marketed at present in the UK. These are applied to the skin. There should therefore be caution in those patients with fragile skin where skin tearing may make their use difficult or impossible.

Some patients develop localized sensitivity as well. Providing none of these apply, buprenorphine (available as the oral preparation of Temgesic and the proprietary preparations BuTrans and Transtec) or fentanyl (available as a non-proprietary patch or as the proprietary Durogesic DTrans) could be tried. Both have recently been reformulated in their patch preparation to allow wider variety of dosing.

The lowest recommended dose should be used first and titrated upwards towards the maximum allowed sequentially with close attention to the patient's symptoms. If the dose that gives benefit starts to produce side effects, the dose might be titrated one step lower with a second milder drug added alongside.

NSAIDs AND STEROIDS

Rationally, anti-inflammatory agents might be best restricted to the relief of episodes of inflammation as occur clinically when mechanical events or even a subluxation causes an episode of traumatic tendonitis or synovitis within a joint, recognized by the patient by the experience of stiffness and swelling as much as pain (Forrest & Brooks 1988).

Although corticosteroids represent the drug of supreme anti-inflammatory effect, amongst the side effects of these is reduction of total collagen content in the capsule of joints, which can add to the magnitude of hypermobility as well as adding to the easy bruising of skin. For this reason oral and intra-articular steroids have little place in the routine management of hypermobile patients. If oral steroids are indicated for a concomitant disease, the dose used should be the lowest compatible with the control of the other disease.

NSAIDs are therefore the anti-inflammatory agents of choice. Practise favours the giving of these by mouth since the transcutaneous route of application does not circumvent side effects, including gastrointestinal irritation. This group of drugs can be classified either by chemical structure (which has implications for side effects), by half-life (which is of the most practical use) or by pharmacological action (which also has implications for side effects).

The initial prototype was aspirin and all other members of the group are distantly related to this drug (Preston et al 1989). Aspirin and its analogues are no longer marketed as anti-inflammatory agents, though in much lower doses that avoid

Table 7.2.1	Half-life of common analgesics
	HOURS
Paracetamol	2
Pentazocine	2
Codeine	3
Dihydrocodeine	3
Dextropropoxyphene	12

side effects aspirin has a cardioprotective effect. Phenylbutazone and analogues, with their propensity for bone marrow failure, are no longer in use. Indometacin, arguably a 'stronger' drug, tends to cause too much fluid retention and central nervous system side effects for routine use though several of its watered-down analogues remain in the pharmacopoeia.

The majority of NSAIDs available, however, are close relatives of ibuprofen, which has no effect on the bone marrow, modest effect on the gastrointestinal tract and kidney, and sometimes causes a rash (Brooks & Day 1991). Oxicams are a group deliberately developed to provide a much longer half-life and the most recent group, the coxibs, have side effects on the cardiovascular system. In the view of this author, morbidity from these is extremely modest compared to the significantly reduced risk of more serious gastrointestinal events.

If a drug from one of these groups consistently causes side effects, it makes sense to try a drug from a separate pharmacological group.

Those NSAIDs currently available in the UK are listed in order of half-life in Table 7.2.2. The wide variation in half-life is unusual in a class of drugs with such similar pharmacological effect and carries the advantage of wide practical choice of drug in relation to the patient's requirements. Thus, if swelling in a hypermobile joint only

Table 7.2.2	Half-life of common NSAIDs
	HOURS
Diclofenac	2
Ketoprofen	2
Ibuprofen	2
Mefenamic acid	4
Flurbiprofen	4
Aspirin	5
Acemetacin	5
Tolmetin	6
Sulindac	7
Fenoprofen	9
Diflunisal	10
Fenbufen	10
Indomethacin	12
Naproxen	17
Azapropazone	20
Tenoxicam	45
Piroxicam	48

occurs at certain times of day (e.g. after a morning shopping trip or after an evening session in the gym), anti-inflammatory protection can be provided by a single dose of a drug of short half-life just before the precipitating biomechanical event. For the more persistent swelling that may accompany a major dislocation, for which dosing over a period of up to one week might be required, a drug with a longer half-life might be selected. As always, the lowest possible dose, carefully titrated against the patient's symptoms and needs, is the safest.

The major pharmacological variation is between those drugs that are traditionally felt to be exclusive inhibitors of cyclo-oxygenase-1 (COX-1 inhibitors) and the recently introduced group of drugs that selectively inhibit cyclo-oxygenase-2 (COX-2 inhibitors) (FitzGerald & Patrono 2001). Since COX-1 is a constitutive ('protective') enzyme, the use of a highly selective COX-2 inhibitor implies improved protection. Increasing use of highly selective COX-2 inhibitors has led to the realization that there is a small but appreciable cardiovascular risk. For this reason, several drugs from the group have been withdrawn or have not been developed. Celecoxib and etoricoxib both remain available in the UK, however, the former is perhaps preferred because of the tendency of etoricoxib to cause hypertension (Silverstein et al 2000). It is the view of this author that if an NSAID is required long term, the greater expense and slight risk of cardiovascular problems (estimated in some series to be one extra minor event for every 400 patient years of treatment when compared to conventional NSAIDs) are more than justified in view of the greater gastrointestinal protection that these drugs undoubtedly afford, the risk of haematemesis even more critical in the hypermobile patient who might have fragile blood vessel walls and therefore a greater propensity to bleeding (CSM update 1986).

ANTIDEPRESSANTS

The use of this group of drugs as a single nocturnal dose, at a dose much lower than that required to remedy a classical depression, may be of value in the management of pain from hypermobility syndrome. That this group of drugs is often also effective in FM provides one of the strongest arguments for a clear relationship between the mechanisms that drive pain. It is possible that the benefit to pain relief during the day may in part result from the undoubted hypnotic properties of some of these drugs, allowing the patient to sleep relatively undisturbed. They are perhaps most rationally used when sleep is disturbed by pain but are invariably worth a trial as an adjunct to ineffective analgesics and are probably safer than adding in NSAIDs in this situation.

Amitriptyline in doses titrated typically between 10–150 mg is often used though many develop side effects at doses that provide ineffective analgesia (Carrette et al 1994). It seems unlikely that there is a specific abnormality of drug metabolism in JHS, raising the possibility of increased sensitivity at the end organ. The symptoms of side effects are often typical of those manifested through the autonomic nervous system.

Dosulepin (dothiepin) also has proven efficacy (Caruso et al 1987), though perhaps not as good as amitriptyline but with less of a propensity to side effects. Cyclobenzaprine is available in the USA but not in Europe. It is possible that these drugs affect neurogenic amines in the brain.

Claims for efficacy have also been made for serotonin-uptake inhibitors (Wolfe et al 1994), including fluoxetine, paroxetine and sertraline.

An important clue as to the mechanisms leading to pain comes from the enhanced benefit when low doses of these drugs are used in combination, implying that more than one neurotransmitter may be involved and that both need to be blocked simultaneously (Arnold et al 2000, O'Malley et al 2000). Venlafaxine is efficacious (Dwight et al 1998). This drug inhibits serotonin and noradrenaline (norepinephrine) uptake. When drugs are used in combination (notably amitriptyline as a tricyclic with fluoxetine as a selective serotonin reuptake inhibitor) the benefit is enhanced. There have also been recent claims for benefit from trobisetron (Papadopoulous et al 2000), a serotonin antagonist.

Intriguingly, monoamine-oxidase inhibitors, also effective in depression, are not of value in JHS (Hannonen et al 1998).

In the case of each of these drugs, titration against symptoms should be gradual with close attention to side effects. The patient may accept the side effects that occur during sleep though the tachycardia can summate with autonomic abnormalities sometimes found in JHS and FM, and a dry mouth the following day can be inconvenient.

ANTIEPILEPTICS

Empirically, drugs from this group are sometimes prescribed in the management of JHS with neuropathic pain. It is possible that carbomazepine and tegretol both sometimes relieve pain, though since the evidence base for this is slim, their use is perhaps best restricted to situations when a variety of antidepressants have been tried and found to be ineffective.

Two drugs, gabapentin (Huckle 2004) and pregabalin (Lauria-Horner & Pohl 2003), are more frequently encountered. Both are licensed for the treatment of neuropathic pain and pregabalin is licensed for the treatment of generalized anxiety disorder. A variety of side effects can be encountered, some of them suspiciously close to autonomic abnormalities, and the unexplained dizziness and vasodilatation both raise the possibility of a subtle relaxant effect on collagen, which might be a disadvantage in patients with JHS.

Of even more concern are those drugs licensed for the management of status epilepticus, such as diazepam, lorazepam and midazolam. The possible rationale for considering this group of drugs is to relieve the undoubted muscle spasm that occurs in some of the most severely afflicted hypermobile patients. The relaxant effect of these drugs, however, renders them unsuitable for use in the vast majority of these patients; indeed the opposite might be found that joint symptoms in the hypermobile individual improve significantly when these drugs are gradually and carefully withdrawn.

TOPICAL APPLICATIONS

A variety of different drug classes are formulated for transcutaneous delivery (Bird 2008). Factors to be considered include the speed and reliability with which the drug actually passes through the skin (which is essentially a protective barrier), whether the drug has been formulated with vasodilators, which enhance absorption, and the level of plasma concentration and the speed with which this is obtained. Once absorbed, the rules of half-life apply and although there may be some localization in the area below the skin over which the drug is applied, this is limited. It is unrealistic to argue, for example, that if a drug is placed over a painful knee the majority of drug absorbed will be localized within that knee joint. It will be distributed rapidly around the body and systemic side effects will therefore not be avoided, a point that is often forgotten.

Hypermobile patients are susceptible to peripheral vasospasm, even Raynaud's, and there is an impression of an even wider variability of absorption (enhanced when vasodilated; reduced when vasoconstricted) in hypermobile patients compared to normals.

The psychological benefits from 'applying the drug just where it is needed' should not be ignored however. Just as a red placebo tablet provides better placebo effect than a white one, many patients derive satisfaction, perhaps therefore benefit, from assiduously applying the drug where they feel it is needed. Opinions polarize, however. Some consider this time-consuming and messy and when the drug has a natural colour, there is sometimes staining of the overlying clothes. Preparations formulated with fragrance are amongst the most popular.

A variety of proprietary 'over the counter' preparations are available, described as 'rubefacients'. Sometimes these contain a mild analgesic, sometimes an astringent. The chances that these would be effective where paracetamol and compound generic analgesics have been tried and discarded are slim.

The use of topical NSAIDs may be slightly more logical but systemic side effects, including gastrointestinal side effects, will not be avoided and therapeutic localization will remain modest.

Capsaicin may offer the most potential in this group (Schmader 2002). In high strength, this is licensed for the symptomatic relief of post-herpetic neuralgia after the healing of lesions and also for the relief of painful diabetic neuropathy. In hypermobility, it probably acts mainly as a counter-irritant though it is also licensed for the symptomatic relief of osteoarthritis. A major problem, especially in the elderly, is the severe irritation encountered when it is accidentally smeared on mucus membranes, including the lips and conjunctiva. Hand-washing after use needs to be meticulous and the drug is sometimes marketed under the banner of 'the pain that helps you'. However, these reservations apart, there may be a role for its use especially if it allows the dose of oral analgesic to be reduced.

HORMONES

Clinicians treating hypermobile patients are becoming increasingly aware of the extent to which the hormonal environment can influence the pain from hypermobile joints. The reason for this is not entirely clear but many female patients attest to the way in which within a normal menstrual cycle, there is deterioration in symptoms in the few days prior to menstruation when the cycle is progesterone dominated. Some describe increased pain, others a little swelling. Perhaps even more to the point is that some claim 'clumsiness' or 'lack of coordination' suggesting a neurological mechanism as much as a relaxation of the joint capsule. By contrast, symptoms are often at their best when the normal menstrual cycle is at maximal oestrogen dominance.

The mechanism for the deterioration of hypermobile joints during a first and second pregnancy, less so in the third and subsequent pregnancies, is probably for similar reasons, the deterioration normally persisting until breastfeeding is completed and implying a role for prolactin and analogues.

It follows that the choice of oral contraceptive might be an influential factor and clinical experience suggests that this is the case. Many patients notice a marked deterioration in joint symptoms within a few weeks of the introduction of the Mirena coil with its significant progestogen (levonorgesterel) reservoir, even though release is controlled and modest. Symptoms often improve when the coil is removed. Parenteral progestogen-only contraceptives (Depo-Provera, noristerat) and the implant, Implanon, all tend to exacerbate symptoms within a short period of their introduction. Progestogen-only oral contraceptives (cerazette, femulen, micronor, norgeston and noriday) all seem to be more likely to exacerbate symptoms than a combined oral contraceptive pill where, by implication, the oestrogen component may give a protective effect.

There also seems to be a variation in the response of joints between the different progestogen analogues that are used in the formulation of combined pills. Yasmin (drospirenone; an analogue of spironolactone for which there is a specific warning in Scotland) also seems more problematic than most. The highest dose of oestrogen component that can be tolerated is likely to be protective for the joint and, if symptoms are exacerbated by the introduction of a new contraceptive, an alternative contraceptive following the analysis above should be tried, at least for a trial period.

In general, HRT seems to be protective though the gynaecological indications for an early hysterectomy also need to be taken into account. Patients with endometriosis or polycystic ovary syndrome seem to experience deterioration in their joints at the onset of these gynaecological conditions.

There is also a strong impression that patients with hormonal abnormalities or the need for hormonal modification of a concomitant medical condition may encounter problems. This might include the use of anti-oestrogen (clomifene) and the use of male sex hormones and antagonists, e.g. in the treatment of prostatic conditions.

FUTURE TRENDS

As the pathophysiological mechanisms accounting for pain pathways are unravelled it is likely that precise matching of drug therapy to the many variant causes may become more refined. It also remains a possibility that new drug families will be identified. The most effective analgesics in Western medicine at present are invariably derived from opiates. Cannabinoids represent an alternative group of drugs, distinctive though distantly related, tending to have properties that are mildly euphoric rather than mildly depressant, as with opioids. It has previously been shown, at a time when drug availability was less restricted than at present, that arthritic pain is better relieved with appetite suppressants with a stimulant property than appetite depressants with more depressive properties, independently of any weight loss achieved (Bird et al 1987). The slight euphoric lift of dextropropoxyphene, which seemed to make it so much more effective than codeine or dihydrocodeine in the management of arthritic pain comes to mind. Certain cannabinoids also have properties in the relief of muscle spasm, which can occur in some of the most extreme variants of hypermobility syndromes and is probably the reason that they are used by patients with multiple sclerosis.

The role of cytokines may also be relevant in the management of some types of FM though it is unlikely that pro-inflammatory cytokine manipulation would be relevant in a group of conditions that were essentially inherited (Bird 2007). This does not apply, however, to cytokines relevant to growth and although Marfan syndrome is only distantly related to JHS, the theoretical attraction of modifying levels of TGF beta, such that production of abnormal collagen might be increased to give collagen that was once again essentially 'strong' represents an exciting prospect for the future, at least in a subset of hypermobile patients. The modification of cytokine effect downstream at the end organ, with conventional and therefore less expensive drugs, also excites interest. The current trials of losartan, an antihypertensive that seems to be effective in modifying the rate of aneurysm progression independently of any antihypertensive effect, come to mind. Perhaps these represent better and more cost-effective research prospects than a search for candidate genes since, even if these were identified and were ubiquitous in a heterogeneous hypermobile population, chromosome modification is unlikely to be imminently available.

Finally, there may be opportunities in the future to influence peripheral sodium and other ligand–ion channel mechanisms.

SUMMARY

The majority of patients will have tried painkillers of one sort or another. To help with further management it is fundamentally important to ascertain which ones have been taken and also why they were stopped. Did it not work at all? Were there side-effects and if so what? Was the patient worried about becoming dependent on a drug and therefore did not take it or perhaps took it less often than might be considered effective?

Before abandoning an analgesic as unhelpful it is therefore important to find out the frequency and maximum dose tried, and whether there was any relief that then wore off.

A number of patients will say their painkiller did not work but on further questioning one discovers that either (a) they did not take enough, frequently enough, or (b) the drug actually worked for a few hours and then wore off (editors' opinion) (Hakim 2009). The latter would be expected given the pharmacokinetics of most agents. Converting the painkiller to a long-acting slow-release formula may reduce the 'on–off' effect controlling, for example, nocturnal and early morning relief of pain by giving such formulation before going to bed.

References

Arnold LM, Keck PE Jr, Welge JA: Antidepressant Treatment of Fibromyalgia. A Meta-Analysis and Review, *Psychosomatics* 41(2):104–113, 2000.

Biasi G, Manca S, Manganelli S, et al: Tramadol in the fibromyalgia syndrome: A controlled clinical trial versus placebo, *Int J Clin Pharmacol Res* 18(1):13–19, 1988.

Bird HA, Wright V, le Gallez P, et al: A controlled study of two psychotropic agents for the relief of pain in osteoarthrosis, *Br Med J* 295(6612):1521–1522, 1987.

Bird HA: Speculative trends in the future drug treatment of fibromyalgia, *Future Rheumatol* 2(3):271–277, 2007.

Bird HA: There's the rub, *Arthritis Today* 141, 2008.

Brooks PM, Day RO: Nonsteroidal antiinflammatory drugs – differences and similarities, *N Engl J Med* 324(24):1716–1725, 1991.

Carrette S, Bell MJ, Reynolds WJ, et al: Comparison of Amitriptyline, Cyclobenzaprine, and Placebo in the Treatment of Fibromyalgia, *Arthritis Rheum* 37(1):32–40, 1994.

Caruso I, Sarzi Puttini PC, Boccassini L: Double-blind study of dothiepin versus placebo in the treatment of primary fibromyalgia syndrome, *J Int Med Res* 15:154–159, 1987.

CSM Update: Non-steroidal and anti-inflammatory drugs and serious gastrointestinal adverse reactions - 1, *Br Med J* 292(6520):614, 1986.

Dwight MM, Arnold LM, O'Brien H, et al: An Open Clinical Trial of Venlafaxine Treatment of Fibromyalgia, *Psychosomatics* 39(1):14–17, 1998.

FitzGerald GA, Patrono C: The Coxibs, Selective Inhibitors of Cyclooxygenase-2, *N Engl J Med* 345(6):433–442, 2001.

Forrest M, Brooks PM: Mechanism of action of non-steroidal anti-rheumatic drugs, *Baillière's Clinical Rheumatology* 2(2):275–294, 1988.

Hakim AJ: The Musculoskeletal System in *Chamberlain's Symptoms and Signs in Clinical Medicine* 13, Elsevier, London, 2009.

Hannonen P, Malminiemi K, Yli-Kettula U, et al: A randomized, double-blind, placebo-controlled study of moclobemide and amitriptyline in the treatment of fibromyalgia in females without psychiatric disorder, *Rheumatol* 37(12):1279–1286, 1998.

Huckle R: Pregabalin (Pfizer), *Curr Opin Investig Drugs* 5(1):82–89, 2004.

Lauria-Horner BA, Pohl RB: Pregabalin: a new anxiolytic, *Expert Opin Investig Drugs* 12(4):663–672, 2003.

Miller RR, Feingold A, Paxinos J: Propoxyphene hydrochloride. A critical review, *JAMA* 213(6):996–1006, 1970.

O'Malley PG, Balden E, Tomkins G, et al: Treatment of Fibromyalgia with Antidepressants: A Meta-analysis, *J Gen Intern Med* 15(9):659–666, 2000.

Papadopoulous IA, Georgiou PE, Katsimbri PP, et al: Treatment of Fibromyalgia with Tropisetron, a 5HT$_3$ Serotonin Antagonist: A Pilot Study, *Clin Rheumatol* 19(1):6–8, 2000.

Preston SJ, Arnold MH, Beller EM, et al: Comparative analgesic and anti-inflammatory properties of sodium salicylate and acetylsalicylic acid (aspirin) in rheumatoid arthritis, *Br J Clin Pharmacol* 27(5):607–611, 1989.

Schmader KE: Epidemiology and Impact on Quality of Life of Postherpetic Neuralgia and Painful Diabetic Neuropathy, *Clin J Pain* 18(6):350–354, 2002.

Silverstein FE, Faich G, Goldstein JL, et al: Gastrointestinal Toxicity With Celecoxib vs Nonsteroidal Anti-inflammatory Drugs for Osteoarthritis and Rheumatoid Arthritis: The CLASS study: A Randomized Controlled Trial, *J Am Med Assoc* 284(10):1247–1255, 2000.

Wolfe F, Cathey MA, Hawley DJ: A Double-Blind Placebo Controlled Trial of Fluoxetine in Fibromyalgia, *Scand J Rheumatol* 23(5):255–259, 1994.

Chapter 8

Pain management and cognitive behavioural therapy

H Clare Daniel

INTRODUCTION

Cognitive behavioural interventions are psychologically based therapies that aim to reduce distress. In the context of health conditions such as chronic pain these interventions enable people to develop psychological and physical strategies that help them to manage the condition and its physical and psychological consequences (Moorey & Greer 2002, Quarmby et al 2006, Hutton 2008). They are one of the most effective interventions for reducing the impact of chronic pain (Morley et al 1999).

This chapter will discuss why people with pain suffer; why cognitive behavioural interventions are important in chronic pain; describe the content of these interventions and address some issues that need to be considered when working with people with joint hypermobility syndrome (JHS) or fibromyalgia (FM).

WHY PEOPLE WITH PAIN SUFFER

Chronic pain is defined as pain that has lasted for more than 3 months (The International Association for the Study of Pain 2003). When pain is long term the secondary biological, psychological and social effects of the condition can begin to play a significant role in the increase and maintenance of many difficulties (Turk & Monarch 2002). These difficulties can be extremely wide ranging:

- Distress relating to their experience of the healthcare system
  - Have been told different things by different people about the cause of their pain
  - Have been offered a variety of treatments; some of which may have helped but many have not helped
- Lack of understanding about their pain
  - Confusion about its cause
  - Concerns about increasing damage
  - Not knowing the best way forward for them and their pain
- Medication
  - Tried many different types, many of which only take the edge off the pain
  - Experienced many side effects
- Fitness
  - Reduction in fitness
  - Weak muscles
  - Stiff joints (despite being hypermobile)
- Friends and family
  - Reduction in social life
  - Loss of contact with friends
  - Increased isolation
  - Difficulties in sex life due to pain, fatigue, worry, misunderstandings
- Work
  - Difficult to fulfil role at work due to pain
  - Experience that managers/colleagues do not understand
  - Reduction on working hours or stopped working
- Sleep and fatigue
  - Hard to initiate sleep
  - Wake during the night
  - Feeling tired and fatigued throughout the day

© 2010 Elsevier Ltd.
DOI: 10.1016/B978-0-7020-3005-5.00012-4

- Sleep during the day, but unable to sleep at night
- Mood
  - Depression or low mood
  - Fear, anxiety, worry and concerns
  - Guilt about being unable to fulfil their role as, for example, a parent, a partner, a colleague, the 'bread winner'
  - Feeling unable to achieve anything
  - Feeling hopeless about their situation
  - Feeling unable to cope during times of increased pain
  - Frustration about the pain interfering with many aspects of life.

THE HISTORY OF CHRONIC PAIN MODELS

To understand the complexity of chronic pain and its effects one needs to look beyond the original models of pain such as that proposed by Descartes in the 17th century. This was a dualistic model suggesting that pain perception was purely physical and did not involve psychological factors. The model proposed that a direct, unbroken pathway exists between peripheral pain receptors and specific brain centres and that pain is always a result of damage. The intensity of pain is considered proportional to the amount of damage and psychological processes are not involved in this pathway or in pain perception.

This dualistic model of pain was used until developments in scientific research and clinical observations gathered evidence to refute its reality. Some of the evidence lies in the following observations:

- Pain can continue to be experienced if the pain 'pathway' is cut. For example, people can experience phantom limb pain following the amputation of a painful limb.
- The physical changes that are seen on X-rays and scans are not proportional to the pain experienced. The results of X-rays and scans of people who report pain can be normal. Conversely, people who do not report pain can have abnormal X-rays and scans.
- Reports of pain are influenced by cognitive and psychological processes such as attention, emotions and beliefs about pain.

Developments in psychophysical and functional magnetic resonance imaging (fMRI) research have helped increase our understanding of the neural correlates of the pain experience and the role of psychological processes in the experience of pain. Imaging studies have shown that despite giving identical external noxious stimuli to a range of participants their reports of pain intensity varied (Coghill et al 2003). fMRI results show that reports of pain intensity do not correlate with stimulus intensity but with the degree of cortical activation in several brain regions that are not only important in pain processing but also cognitive processes. Participants who rated the noxious stimuli as very painful showed greater and more frequent activation of the following areas:

- Primary somatosensory cortex (thought to be involved in pain localization processing)
- Anterior cingulate cortex (thought to be involved in motivation and goal-oriented cognitive processes)
- Prefrontal cortex (associated with the affective component of pain and contributes to providing the negative emotional valence to the pain experience).

For a more in-depth discussion about psychological factors and pain the reader is directed to Chapter 3 and also Wall (2000) and Melzack (2001). Suggesting that psychological factors influence our experience of and responses to pain is not the same as saying that pain is psychological; rather it is the recognition that physical and psychological factors play a role in the processing and perception of physical symptoms.

In addition to biological and psychological factors influencing pain perception, it is now understood that social factors also play a role (Morris 1993, Frank 1997, Carr et al 2005). We do not live in isolation but within systems such as the family, work, healthcare, friendships and society. A variety of beliefs, messages, rules, stories and narratives exist within these systems, all of which influence our own beliefs and behaviour. The messages and information that we hear about illness and coping play a significant role in the perception of illness and the way in which the illness impacts on our lives.

Using the dualistic model to understand health conditions is now considered to be outdated and unhelpful (Sharpe & Williams 2002). It can result in patients' pain being unhelpfully labelled as psychogenic or even if they are not told this explicitly patients are very sensitive to the possibility that a clinician believes that someone's pain is psychological. Many of those suffering from JHS or FM have had this experience. This results in anger, frustration and a feeling of being disbelieved (Gurley-Green 2001) (see Prologue).

Those who have moved away from using the dualistic model now use a biopsychosocial framework (Engel 1977) to help them and the patient understand their condition and the effects that it is having on them and their lives.

The biopyschosocial model highlights the dynamic interaction between biological, psychological and social factors in all health conditions for everyone. The degree to which each of these factors plays a role will differ between individuals but this is seen as normal rather than pathological. This model has been applied to pain (Main & Williams 2002, Waddell 2004) and has placed psychological and social factors firmly in the realm of pain research and practice (Linton 2000).

COGNITIVE BEHAVIOURAL THERAPY

Medical interventions can be helpful for some but not all people with chronic pain. Research has suggested that even if these interventions reduce the pain by 30% this does not necessarily result in an improvement in the quality of people's lives because the secondary psychological and physical effects of pain remain (Dworkin et al 2003). The absence of a cure for everyone with chronic pain has led to the development of psychologically based interventions. The cognitive behavioural model is a psychological model that is used to understand and address people's distress. It was developed by Beck (1976) and its application to a range of difficulties is now supported by the National Institute for Health and Clinical Excellence (NICE) (2007).

The central tenet of the model is that our thoughts, emotions, behaviour and bodily sensations influence one another (Fig. 8.1).

The model hypothesizes that it is our interpretation of the situations that we are in that is one of the main precursors of distress. If a number of people are in the same situation it is very likely that they will have different thoughts about the situation and therefore experience different emotions and will respond to the situation in different ways. People's interpretations of situations are based on

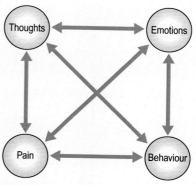

Fig. 8.1 Thoughts, emotions, behaviour and bodily sensations influence one another

many factors. Some of these, accompanied by examples relating to pain include:

- Past experiences (e.g. having coped well with a previous experience of pain)
- Family beliefs (e.g. must remain stoical in the face of illness)
- Past observations (e.g. seeing someone with the same condition who is coping well)
- Messages and stories told by influential people (e.g. a doctor telling someone that they will end up in a wheelchair)
- Memories (e.g. a parent with a disabling condition who did not cope well)
- Current and past mood (e.g. depression, anxiety).

Cognitive behavioural theory does not deny the reality of peoples' pain and distress. It recognizes that people have a pain condition but that their beliefs and thoughts about their pain and situation influence their response to their pain and their level of distress. It is essential that the reader and the patient understand that the model is not suggesting that pain is caused by psychological factors and if only someone thought differently then all their troubles would be over.

As the diagrammatic form of the cognitive model suggests, the influence between thoughts, feeling, behaviour and the body is not linear but cyclical. One can influence another which can influence another and another and so the cycle continues. If these influences are unhelpful, over time the detrimental impact of the pain can become wide ranging. Figure 8.2 outlines a typical situation that can occur over a few months or years.

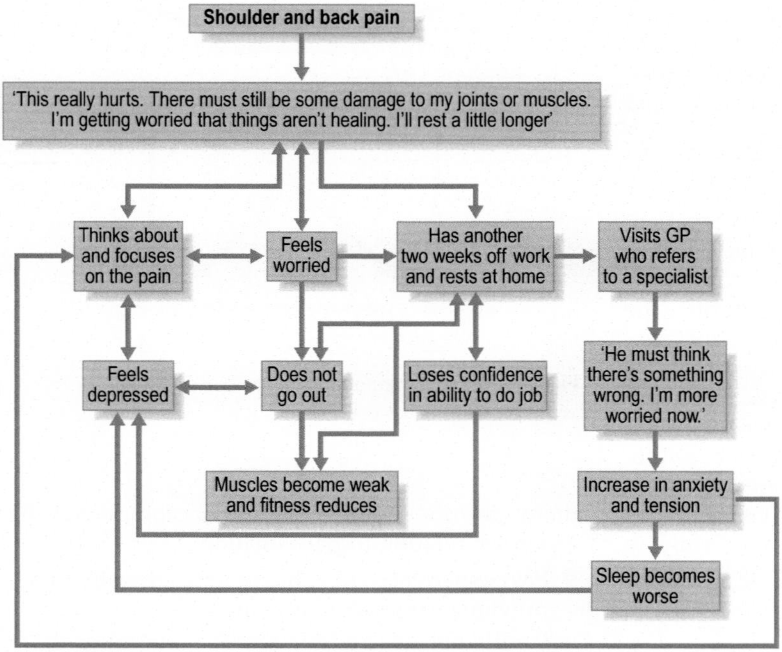

Fig. 8.2 A typical situation that can occur over a few months or years

Cognitive behavioural interventions aim to help people recognize their unhelpful cognitive and behavioural responses to pain, re-evaluate them and replace them with more helpful alternatives that will reduce distress and disability. This brief description does not do justice to the intricacies of this intervention and the skills required in its implementation. The application of this model requires the therapist to undergo appropriate training and to be supervised in their clinical practice.

Over 40 published randomized controlled trials have assessed the efficacy of cognitive behavioural interventions for chronic pain (Morley 2004). These trials suggest that when compared with waiting list controls, cognitive behavioural interventions are more effective in restoring function, improving mood and reducing disability and unhelpful pain-related behaviours (Morley et al 1999). Compared with a range of heterogeneous interventions (such as those provided by pain clinics, physiotherapy, occupational therapy and educational packages) cognitive behavioural interventions produce significantly greater changes in the pain experience (intensity, unpleasantness and sensation), improved cognitive strategies to manage pain and reduced behavioural expression of pain (Morley et al 1999). McCracken and Turk (2002) support

these findings and add that cognitive behavioural interventions lead to an overall decrease in health care costs and an increased chance of returning to work.

The outcome literature suggests that cognitive behavioural interventions help to make a significant impact on improving the physical and psychological function of people with FM (Thieme et al 2006, van Koulil et al 2007, 2008). Clinical outcome measures suggest that people with JHS make significant gains in a pain management programme for people with JHS across a range of physical and psychological measures (Daniel et al 2006). However, to the author's knowledge there are no studies published on cognitive behavioural interventions for JHS. This may be for the following reasons:

- Those with JHS may be treated in a group of people with many conditions that are associated with chronic pain and therefore are reported as part of a chronic pain cohort in the literature.
- It is known that JHS is under-recognized and neglected in clinical practice (Grahame & Hakim 2008) as are the psychosocial sequelae (Grahame 2001). It is therefore likely that the need for cognitive behavioural interventions for JHS is overlooked.

AIMS AND CONTENT OF COGNITIVE BEHAVIOURAL INTERVENTIONS

The wide-ranging effects of chronic pain are reflected in the aims of cognitive behavioural interventions. The overall aim is to help people develop skills to help them manage their pain and reduce the psychological and physical impact on their lives. The specific aims of cognitive behavioural pain management are listed below and then described in more detail in the text. When reading about the intervention it is important to remember than each element of the intervention does not exist in isolation, rather each works in association with the others to:

- Improve understanding of chronic pain
- Reduce pain-related distress
- Improve communication with others, in particular about chronic pain
- Return to valued and enjoyable activities
- Improve physical functioning and reduce disability
- Improve sleep
- Develop ways to manage increases in pain.

Clinical experience suggests that it is helpful if patients and clinicians do not view a reduction in pain as a main aim of these interventions. The research in the effectiveness of cognitive behavioural interventions for chronic pain suggests that a reduction in pain is reported. This may be due to a reduction in the number of days during which the pain increases rather than a reduction in the normal baseline level of pain. If patients focus on pain reduction as their primary aim some may have difficulty focusing on developing self-management skills.

Although cognitive behavioural interventions for chronic pain can be provided by one psychological therapist, those patients whose pain is having a greater physical and psychological impact on their lives may gain more benefit from a multidisciplinary team intervention. The British Pain Society (2007) suggests that the core team should consist of:

- A medically qualified person such as a consultant in pain management or another medical specialist, for example a GP, neurologist, or rheumatologist
- A chartered clinical psychologist or BABCP-registered cognitive behavioural therapist
- A state-registered physiotherapist.

Other members that can provide valuable input are:

- An occupational therapist
- A nurse
- A pharmacist
- An assistant psychologist.

It is essential that all the team members have appropriate training in the application of their professional skills to chronic pain and are supervised in their work.

Cognitive behavioural interventions for chronic pain are typically delivered in a group format known as pain management programmes (PMPs). This approach works well because the team provides consistent and reinforced messages and because group members can gain a great deal from meeting people with the same condition. A debate exists about whether PMPs should be provided for diagnostic groups rather than chronic pain per se (Turk & Okifuji 2001, Daniel 2005, Daniel et al 2006). Whilst the overriding principles and techniques are the same for all chronic pain regardless of the cause, when the pain is related to a specific condition or syndrome that is associated with other difficulties then groups for specific diagnoses may be beneficial because these difficulties could be addressed to some extent within the group context. In addition it has been recognized that those who feel different from the other group members are more likely to leave the group before the end of the intervention (Coughlan et al 1995). The author's clinical observations suggest that having one or two people with JHS in a group of people with chronic pain not associated with JHS can lead to group disharmony and the people with JHS feeling dissatisfied with the intervention and misunderstood by the team. Conversely, being in a group specifically for people with JHS can provide a containing and supportive environment for the group to develop self-management techniques.

Improving understanding of chronic pain

Many of the difficulties experienced following the onset of pain are the secondary physical and psychological effects. These arise partly due to a misunderstanding about chronic pain. Many people respond to chronic pain as though it were acute. Acute pain is pain that lasts for less than 3 months and is generally associated with damage.

If we believe that our pain is acute, our response is often rest to allow healing to take place, medication to reduce the pain, and protecting the painful areas by restricting movement. Although not always the case, we tend not to worry about acute pain because although it may be unpleasant we believe that any damage will heal and the pain will resolve. However, these responses in the presence of chronic pain can cause more difficulties. In chronic pain the relationship between pain and damage is less clear. Very often there is no damage even if the initial pain began following an injury. It is because of the need to respond differently to acute and chronic pain that education is an important element of cognitive behavioural interventions. Learning about the differences between the physiology of acute and chronic pain helps people to understand chronic pain and the need to change their responses to it.

People who have JHS are more susceptible to injury, dislocation and subluxation (see Chapter 2). Therefore it can be hard, but necessary, for people with JHS to understand the differences between pain that is a result of injury and their long-term chronic pain and to know how to respond to both.

Reducing pain-related distress

Due to the association between thoughts, feelings, behaviour and bodily symptoms it is common for people with chronic pain to experience a range of distressing emotions and those with JHS and FM are no exception (Gurely-Green 2001, Gupta et al 2007, Verbunt 2008). Although research papers allude to JHS being associated with distress, to the author's knowledge there are no published data on the prevalence of specific psychological difficulties in this population. However, the data collected in a PMP specifically for people with JHS suggest that their distress is similar to those with chronic pain that is not associated with JHS. The types of distress that are commonly reported by people with chronic pain are:

- Low mood or depression due to losses associated with long-term pain
- Frustration because the pain is a barrier to achieving goals
- Anxiety about the nature and cause of the pain
- Fear about the pain increasing, the future and losing independence
- Guilt due to feeling a burden on other people.

The cognitive behavioural pain literature recognizes that people's beliefs and thoughts about themselves and their pain can contribute to this distress and reinforce unhelpful behaviours which can increase distress further (Crombez et al 1999, Lamé et al 2005). For example, the belief that having chronic pain takes away everything worthwhile may result in low mood which in turn may result in a reluctance to engage in life outside the home, which has the consequence of lowering activity level which in itself results in many unhelpful effects. Common unhelpful meanings and beliefs about chronic pain that can increase distress and unhelpful behaviours include:

- My pain means that something inside me is damaged
- An increase in my pain means I have done something I shouldn't have
- An increase in my pain means that the damage has become worse
- My pain means that I'll never live a happy life
- My pain means that I'll never fulfil any of my dreams
- Having pain means that I won't have a meaningful future
- I'll never be able to cope with chronic pain.

Although these thoughts are understandable, they are not helpful and are not necessarily fact. Cognitive behavioural interventions help people to understand the link between thoughts, emotions, behaviour and pain. They are encouraged to become aware of their unhelpful thoughts, particularly in relation to the meaning of the pain and ongoing damage. They learn that thoughts are our own interpretations of a situation and that they tend not to be fact. These interpretations are influenced by normal but often unhelpful biases in the processing of information. Patients are encouraged to consider any biases that may be resulting in an unhelpful interpretation of the situation. These biases include:

- Hypervigilance to physical symptoms
- Selective memory towards negative information
- Filtering out or negating evidence that supports a more helpful viewpoint
- Viewing situations with an 'all or nothing' perspective. For example, 'Unless I get back to the sport I used to do and at the level I achieved, then there's no point in trying to return to anything'

- Predicting the future. For example, 'I know my pain will just become worse and I won't be able to cope with it'
- Processing information with a 'catastrophic' bias (see below).

Catastrophizing

Pain research suggests that catastrophizing in the presence of chronic pain can be particularly unhelpful (Vlaeyen et al 1995). Catastrophizing has been defined as 'an exaggerated negative mental set brought to bear during actual or anticipated pain experience' (Sullivan et al 2001). The fear-avoidance model aids our understanding of the role of catastrophizing and fear in the presence of pain (Vlaeyen et al 1995). The model proposes that catastrophic interpretations about pain are thought to be the salient feature associated with hypervigilance and fear of increased pain and/or damage/injury (Crombez et al 2004). This leads to avoidance of activity and increased fear (Crombez et al 1999, 2005) and in the long-term disuse, disability and mood changes (van den Hout et al 2001, Buer & Linton 2002, Sullivan et al 2002). Fear-avoidance beliefs predict disability in daily or occupational activity, treatment outcome and return to work (Pfingsten et al 2000). There is evidence that the same association between catastrophizing, fear and avoidance of activity exists in people with FM (Turk et al 2004, Edwards et al 2006).

Once they are aware of their unhelpful thoughts and thought patterns patients learn how to re-evaluate or 'challenge' the content of these thoughts and to seek more helpful thoughts. Table 8.1 gives two examples of unhelpful thoughts, their influence on emotions and possible challenges to these thoughts.

Gathering evidence that supports the helpful thought will increase the strength of belief in that thought. Cognitive behavioural interventions use 'behavioural experiments' to encourage people to engage in activities that will provide them with experiences that do not fit with their unhelpful thoughts (Bennett-Levy et al 2004). This strategy has been researched in chronic pain and has been found to significantly reduce unhelpful thoughts about pain and injury and associated fear (de Jong et al 2005).

Improve communication with others, particularly about chronic pain

It may appear out of context to talk about communication in a chapter about cognitive behavioural interventions for chronic pain. However, as already stated, we live in systems and the relationships within these systems require communication if they are to flourish. People with chronic pain often talk about their anger and frustration with people around them. They believe that people do not understand their pain and its effects and receive the message that their pain is not real. These emotions are also directed at healthcare providers (HCPs). Patients have often visited many HCPs over the years in the search for a diagnosis and a cure. Unfortunately many people find that a diagnosis is not given or they are given many conflicting diagnoses. Many undergo unsuccessful treatments which can result in disappointment and some feel disbelieved and labelled by HCPs. JHS and FM are no exception (Gawthrop et al 2007, Simmonds & Keer 2007, Merskey 2008) and reports of delays in being diagnosed are common (Gurley-Green 2001, Gawthrop et al 2007,

Table 8.1	Two examples of unhelpful thoughts, their influence on emotions and possible challenges to these thoughts		
UNHELPFUL THOUGHT	**EMOTION(S)**	**MORE HELPFUL THOUGHT CHALLENGE**	
'This pain is ruining my whole life. I can't do anything worthwhile'	Worry Depressed	'It can be hard having this pain all the time but there are times when I smile and feel happy and times when I achieve things. I can still manage my job. Even though I can't dance like I used to, maybe I can return to it in some form, even if just for pleasure'	
'I can't get it out of my head that I'll get worse and worse and I won't be able to cope any more with my pain'	Angry Despondent Worried	'OK, I really have to think this through. I have become less fit and can't do what I used to. However, now I understand my pain a bit better I can begin to set goals and build up my fitness and strength gradually even though I have pain. I must remember that the physiotherapist told me that there isn't a clear relationship between pain and damage and that it's safe to exercise. No one can predict the future but what I do know is that I can do things to prevent me from becoming worse'	

Grahame & Hakim 2008). The anger and frustration that results from these situations can impede communication.

Education about the nature of chronic pain and the difficulties in diagnosis and cure can increase people's understanding about why they have been through such difficult experiences. However, the patients' experiences are very real and the team needs to openly acknowledge this and spend time listening to their distress to prevent them from believing that the team is yet another set of HCPs that is not taking their condition, experiences and distress seriously. This then allows the group to address issues around communication such as:

- Developing a clear and concise explanation about their condition and pain that they can use when talking to other people
- Developing the confidence to ask questions and ask for clarification of information at appointments with HCPs
- Strategies to deal with emotions and events that may be impeding communication
- Recognizing that excellent communication skills will not always result in the other person listening or engaging in communication
- Skills in assertive communication.

Return to valued and enjoyable activities

People with chronic pain often report that over time their activity level decreases. The less essential activities such as going out socially are often the ones to stop first because people put their effort into maintaining the more essential ones such as a job, childcare and home maintenance. Gradually activity in other areas of life can begin to cease as does a sense of achievement and enjoyment. Goal setting is an important aspect of cognitive behavioural interventions for chronic pain if people are to re-engage in meaningful activities. It helps people to focus on an aim, to do something each day, and to engage in something that will provide a sense of achievement and self worth.

People can find it hard to set goals, especially if they have been living from day-to-day just managing their pain or if they have had the experience of the pain blocking them from reaching their goals which can result in a deep sense of disappointment and despondency. The acronym 'SMART' can help people to set goals.

S	Specific: Define the goal, decide on a specific activity, e.g. Swim twice a week
M	Measurable: Add an element of measurement in the goal so that you know when you've achieved it, e.g. Build up to swimming two lengths
A	Achievable: Reflect on the goal to ensure it is achievable in terms of finance, time demands etc.
R	Relevant: Ensure the goal is relevant to your lifestyle, what you want to do or what you enjoy
T	Time frame: Set a time for when you aim to achieve the goal by, e.g. 2 months.

Although long-term goals, for example planning to complete something in 2 years time can be valuable, it is important to also set goals that will be achieved in a shorter time frame. This will help to maintain motivation because the end point can be kept in sight.

To enable someone with pain to work towards the goal, once the goal is set it is important to identify its components, particularly the ones that are blocking the person from achieving the goal. For example, a goal of returning to swimming two lengths in 2 months' time is not just about being in the pool, swimming and getting out of the pool. The components involved and the ones that are blocking achieving the goal are listed in Table 8.2.

Once the difficulties have been identified, with the help of the therapist the patient decides what they will work on in order to achieve their goal. Table 8.3 continues with the example of swimming.

The next stage is to begin to work on these components but in a way that does not result in overactivity and increased pain. How to achieve this is described in the next section.

Improve physical functioning and reduce disability

As a result of having chronic pain many people change the way that they approach activity. Many, but not all, use pain as a guide to the amount of activity they do. On what they may call a 'good' or 'better' day they engage in more activity. They tend to push until their pain increases and use this as a sign to stop. The response to this increase in pain is often a decrease in activity. When the pain returns to its usual level, their activity level increases until the pain also increases, following

Table 8.2	An example of breaking down a goal into its components		
COMPONENT	**CAN I DO IT NOW?**	**WHAT DO I FIND HARD?**	
Packing a bag at home	Yes	——	
Getting to the swimming pool (carrying a bag)	No	Sitting down for the 15 minute bus journey is hard and I can't carry bags	
Buying a ticket	Yes	——	
Getting changed	Yes	——	
Walking to the edge of the pool	Not sure	I'm worried about the slippery floor and hurting myself	
Getting into the pool (maybe steps, maybe graduated walk)	Yes	——	
Swimming	Not 2 lengths	I think I can only do half a width at the moment	
Getting out of the pool	Yes	——	
Having a shower and hair wash	Yes	—	
Getting dry	Yes	——	
Getting dressed	Yes	——	
Drying hair	No	I can't lift my hands above my head and hold a hair dryer	
Getting back home (carrying a bag)	No	Sitting down for the 15 minute bus journey is hard and I can't carry bags and I will be tired by then	

Table 8.3	An example of identifying areas of a goal to work on
WHAT DO I FIND HARD?	**WHAT DO I NEED TO WORK ON?**
Sitting down for the 15 minute bus journey is hard and I can't carry bags	Sitting Shoulder flexibility Shoulder and arm strength Carrying bags
I'm worried about the slippery floor and hurting myself	Confidence with walking on uneven surfaces Confidence with walking on wet surfaces
I think I can only do half a width at the moment. My whole body aches afterwards	Body flexibility, especially shoulder Build up my swimming gradually
I can't lift my hands above my head and hold a hair dryer	Arm strength Shoulder flexibility
Sitting down for the 15 minute bus journey is hard and I can't carry bags and I will be tired by then	Sitting Shoulder flexibility Shoulder and arm strength Carrying bags

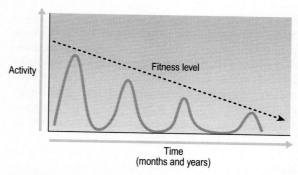

Fig. 8.3 The over–under activity cycle, activity cycling or the boom and bust cycle

which their activity reduces and so on. This pattern is called the over–under activity cycle, activity cycling or the boom and bust cycle (Fig. 8.3). The length of each cycle varies from person to person; it may run over the course of a day, a few days, a few weeks or sometimes months.

Patients state that the advantages to this cycle are that tasks are completed and a sense of achievement is gained. Over time however these are outweighed by the disadvantages. When people are asked about the disadvantages to this pattern they list some or all of the following:

- Pushing leads to an increase in pain
- Mood plummets as the pain increases and activity decreases
- They feel very frustrated when the pain prevents them from continuing with a task
- They are often angry with themselves for causing an increase in pain
- People often feel isolated when their mood and activity level decreases
- They are unable to plan because they cannot predict the intensity of their pain during the next few days or weeks.

It is important that patients know that another disadvantage of this cycle is that, over time, levels of fitness and flexibility decrease, the periods of activity become less and the periods of rest become longer. When this happens people experience life as closing in on them; they see fewer people; do fewer enjoyable activities; stop work and so on.

When addressing activity level and patterns, cognitive behavioural pain management helps people to:

- Understand the disadvantages of the over–under activity cycle
- Stop the pain from guiding their activity level but to use time instead
- Develop a less erratic pattern and maintain a similar level of activity whether it is a good or a bad day
- Gradually build up their level of activity and fitness.

Pacing

The above points are achieved by 'pacing' activity. The aim of pacing is to break the over–under activity cycle and maintain a relatively even level of activity regardless of pain level (Birkholtz et al 2004). The principle behind this is that chronic pain is not serving a useful purpose and so should not be used as a guide for activity level. However, this does not mean that people should push through the pain. Despite there being a lack of research evidence for the efficacy of pacing (Gill & Brown 2009), a lack of consensus as to what constitutes pacing (Birkholtz et al 2004) and some suggestions that it may actually encourage avoidance of activity (McCracken & Samuel 2007) it is a strategy that is widely used in the clinical context and many patients report finding it helpful. For the purposes of this chapter a common pacing technique will be described.

Pacing involves doing small amounts of regular activity that is guided by time rather than pain. People often say that they are pacing but are actually using pain level as a cue to stop activity. The aim of pacing is to stop doing something before the pain increases and to maintain an even level of activity day by day thus breaking out of the over–under activity cycle. When activity is discussed in the context of pacing, it is done in the broadest sense. Any 'activity' can be paced.

To work out how much activity is manageable without increasing the pain the following steps are followed.

Step one: Initially people set a goal and decide on the components that are blocking them from reaching that goal. For the purposes of describing pacing, the example of swimming (above) will be used: to be swimming two lengths twice a week in 2 months' time.

The components that are currently difficult are:

- Sitting
- Swimming
- Carrying
- Body flexibility, especially shoulder
- Shoulder strength
- Arm strength
- Confidence with walking on uneven surfaces
- Confidence with walking on wet surfaces.

Step two: The 'tolerances' for the activities that make up the difficult components are calculated. In this example the components are sitting, carrying and swimming. A tolerance is the length of time that someone can do something for without increasing their pain for more than 2 hours. Two hours is used as a guide because it is normal for the body to feel symptoms after carrying out an activity that has not been done for a while.

The person needs to time themselves three times at different times of the day and on different days. In the example of sitting, someone might time themselves once in the morning and see how long they can sit for without increasing their pain. This may be 6 minutes. Then they might time themselves in the afternoon. This may be 4 minutes. Then they might time themselves the next day at lunchtime. This may be 5 minutes. They then take an average of these three times ($6 + 4 + 5 = 15 \div 3 = 5$ minutes). And then reduce this average by 20% (or one fifth). This is because it is better to start at an achievable level. In this example the sitting tolerance would be 4 minutes so ideally after sitting for 4 minutes this person needs to change position or do something else such as stretching before returning to sitting. In this example, sitting for longer than 4 minutes increases the risk of overdoing the activity and contributing to an increase in pain. Timers that make an audible sound or vibrate can help people to remember to change position or stop an activity.

When chronic pain is accompanied by other symptoms such as fatigue, it may be helpful if the patient considers these symptoms in addition to the pain when they are setting their tolerance levels. The cognitive behavioural principles outlined in this chapter have been shown to be effective in chronic fatigue (Quarmby et al 2006).

Step three: The tolerance level (for example 4 minutes) is gradually increased (Figure 8.4). When someone is comfortable and confident with

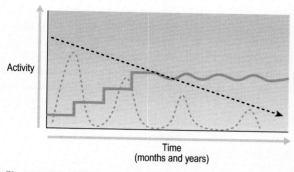

Fig. 8.4 Step 3: the tolerance level is gradually increased

their initial tolerance they increase it. Although it is the patient who decides when and how much they increase their tolerance by, they are encouraged not to increase it by any more than 10%. This is to prevent them from over-doing the activity. Again, when the person is comfortable and confident with this level, the tolerance is increased and so on until they reach a level that is not increasing the pain and is enabling them to achieve a goal (such as sitting on a bus).

When pacing is applied to an activity such as carrying, two variables need to be considered, (i) the time something is carried and (ii) the weight carried. The therapist and patient decide how to do this depending on the goal. For example, if the goal was to carry shopping bags, they may start with a bag in each hand with a light weight in both. If the goal were to go walking with a rucksack, the initial tolerance could be walking with the rucksack on their back with a small weight in (for example a small bottle of water).

PACING EXERCISE AND STRETCH

In cognitive behavioural pain management there is no physiotherapy 'hands on' treatment. Instead the emphasis is on pacing exercise and stretch. Again the term 'exercise' is used broadly and it certainly does not mean that everyone is encouraged to go to a gym. It is important that the exercises relate to the person's goals (Simmonds & Keer 2007). In the swimming goal above, the person has decided that they need to increase their arm and shoulder strength and overall flexibility. The physiotherapist will suggest what exercises the patient could do and the patient, not the physiotherapist, uses the principles of setting a tolerance (described above) to decide, for example, the weight used (if there

is weight involved) or the number of repetitions done.

The same principles can be applied to stretch. The physiotherapist teaches the patients the principles of stretch and the patients learn about the importance of stretch, even for hypermobile joints. They are encouraged to stretch slowly and gently and not to bounce into the stretch but to hold it steadily without pushing too far and maintaining a steady and gentle breathing pattern. Patients are encouraged to hold a stretch for five to ten normal breaths.

SLEEP DISORDER

Sleep problems are common in people with pain, including those with JHS (Hakim & Grahame 2004, Adib et al 2005) and FM (Bigatti et al 2008). Problems range from finding it hard to initiate sleep, waking through the night and not being able to return to sleep after waking. Lack of or disturbed sleep can result in people feeling mentally and physically slowed, irritable and/or low in mood and being less able to enjoy things. The link between heightened arousal, poor sleep, and pain amplification is discussed in Chapter 5.

The focus of the sleep aspect of cognitive behavioural pain management is not necessarily about helping people to find a comfortable position. Although this may be helpful for some, many patients have spent many years trying to do this themselves. The focus is on sleep hygiene principles. These are discussed below.

Expectations of sleep

It is important that patients know what a 'normal' nights sleep is. Many believe that others go to sleep, stay asleep for about 7 to 8 hours and then wake up refreshed.

This is not a normal sleep pattern. If people expect to sleep in this way they will become disappointed and more frustrated. A normal sleep pattern is divided up into cycles that are partly characterized by the depth of sleep. One sleep cycle has five stages in it and people tend to go through four to five sleep cycles a night. When sleep is plotted on a graph it looks much more like a roller coaster than a U shape (Fig. 8.5).

Patients report that knowing it is normal to come into a light sleep during the night and to sometimes wake up helps them to feel less

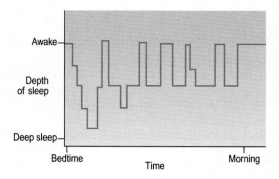

Fig. 8.5 Sleep plotted on a graph

frustrated and worried when this does happen, are less likely to blame the pain for waking them (although undoubtedly this also happens) and consequently find it easier to return to sleep.

Many people believe that they should have 7–8 hours a night. Although this is recorded in sleep studies, this is an average and is not something that we all must achieve. Rather than focusing on the number of hours of sleep, a helpful guide is whether the amount of sleep achieved is enabling someone to do what they would like to and have to do the following day.

Bedtime routine

Although people recognize the need for children to have a bedtime routine, this tends to be forgotten during our adult years. Patients are encouraged to have a relaxing bedtime routine to help prepare mentally and physically for sleep.

Time to go to bed and get up

Having a regular time to get up each morning will aid sleep. It can be tempting to stay in bed after a disturbed night's sleep but this will not be helpful as it may encourage people to go to bed later that evening.

It is important to go to bed when feeling tired. This will mean that the person is less likely to lay awake in bed unable to sleep and associate the bed and bedroom with restlessness and frustration.

When sleep difficulties become entrenched the boundaries between night and day can become blurred. Some people find themselves sleeping for many hours during the day and not going to bed until early in the morning. There are disadvantages to this, for example not being able to interact with other people and not being able to carry out a

daytime job. If people decide to change this pattern they need to do so gradually. For example, if they normally go to bed at 4 o'clock in the morning and get up at 1 o'clock in the afternoon, the following day they should go to bed 15 minutes earlier and get up 15 minutes earlier and when they are used to this repeat it and continue to do so until they have reached their goal.

Daytime sleeping

Fatigue is associated with JHS and FM which can make it hard for people not to sleep during the day. Some find that they do this without disrupting their night-time sleep. However, if people do sleep during the day and have problems sleeping at night they are encouraged not to sleep during the day but to instead go for a walk or do some exercise even though this may feel counterintuitive.

Stimulants

People need to know what stimulants are and what they do. Some are unaware that caffeine is in certain food and drinks. They are encouraged to avoid these foods 4–6 hours before bedtime and during the night.

Nicotine in cigarettes is a stimulant and something that people should also avoid if they are having problems sleeping.

Alcohol

Some people use alcohol to relax and initiate sleep. Although this may be successful, alcohol is associated with other sleep difficulties. It disrupts the sleep pattern making sleep less refreshing and it can result in earlier waking.

Exercise and stretch

Aerobic exercise during the day will help people to sleep at night. However, because exercise stimulates people it should not be done close to bedtime. Gentle stretching prior to bedtime or during the night might aid sleep.

The bedroom environment

When sleep problems are long-standing, the bedroom can become associated with frustration and worry, making it harder to sleep. To build up a helpful association between the bedroom and sleep patients are encouraged to remove items from the bedroom that are associated with behaviours other than sleep, for example televisions, computers, telephones and desks. If someone's home situation demands that they work in the bedroom it will be helpful to delineate an area that can be separated from the rest of the room and is used solely for work.

Thoughts, feelings and sleeplessness

Sleep difficulties are often associated with unhelpful thoughts that are associated with worry, anxiety and frustration and of course these make it even harder to sleep. Examples of these thoughts are:

- 'I must get to sleep in the next few minutes otherwise I just won't be able to cope with tomorrow'
- 'I'll know that I'll never be able to get sleep'.

As described earlier, cognitive behavioural interventions address the association between thoughts, emotions and behaviour. Sleep is no exception. Patients are encouraged to become aware of any thoughts that are preventing sleep and to re-evaluate and challenge them.

Strategies to deal with worries can help to reduce night-time worrying. Some examples are:

- Write down worries at least 2 hours before bedtime. Then should someone wake at night they can remind themselves that they have already given these worries time and that they can address them the next day.
- Keep a pad of paper by the bed. Should someone wake up with a new worry, they write it down and tell themselves that they will give it time tomorrow but now it is time to sleep.
- Imagery can help some people 'push' away their worries. For example, imagine putting worries in boxes that are hanging from a pulley system and then pushing them away. Or place worries in a boat that drifts away.

Lying awake in bed

Some people spend hours laying awake in bed in the hope that they will get to sleep. Unfortunately this will not aid sleep and will increase the likelihood that the bed will be associated with sleeplessness. Rather than lying awake they should get up after about 15–20 minutes, go to another room and engage in something that will not stimulate their mind, until they feel sleepy and then return to bed. Stretches may help at this time.

Clock watching

Looking at the clock during the night may prevent people from sleeping. Knowing the time may result in irritation that there are many sleepless hours until the morning or that there are not enough hours to catch up on sleep. Putting the clock in a drawer or turning it to face away will help reduce the temptation to 'clock watch'.

DEVELOPING WAYS TO MANAGE INCREASES IN PAIN

Despite practising pain management skills, there will be times when people's pain increases. This is often called a 'flare-up' and is the nature of chronic pain. Cognitive behavioural pain management helps people to apply pain management techniques during a flare-up.

Many people respond to flare-ups with rest as they believe that this will reduce their pain. Although this may help in the short term, in the long term it can cause more physical and psychological problems. Other people respond to flare-ups by pushing themselves because they are determined not to let the pain beat them. Unfortunately this only serves to further increase their pain. Cognitive behavioural pain management helps people to understand the disadvantages of these responses and encourages them to consider, apply and evaluate alternative strategies during these times. People are encouraged to use the pain management strategies listed:

- Challenging thoughts and feelings
- Pacing
- Planning and prioritizing
- Stretches and exercise
- Relaxation.

Challenging thoughts and feelings

Common thoughts during a flare-up include:

- 'This is terrible, it'll never end'
- 'I can't do anything today. I'll have to cancel all my plans'
- 'I must have done more damage to myself'.

Table 8.4	Common thoughts during a flare–up	
THOUGHT	EMOTION	RESPONSE
'This is terrible, it'll never end'	Depressed	Go to bed all day
'I can't do anything today. I'll have to cancel all my plans'	Frustrated	Cancel meeting with friend. Spend the day on your own not doing anything enjoyable
'I must have done more damage to myself'	Worry	Panic. Think about the pain all day and monitor if your pain gets worse.

Thoughts such as these will have an unhelpful effect on emotions and how people respond to a flare-up (Table 8.4).

Developing skills to challenging these thoughts (as described above) will help to reduce people's distress during these times and therefore be more able to manage the flare-up effectively.

Pacing

It can be very tempting to retreat to bed for long periods of time during a flare-up. However, this can result in:

- The pain-controlling activity level which increases the likelihood of someone returning to the over–under activity cycle
- Joint stiffness and loss of fitness
- Being unable to engage in meaningful activities and therefore not gaining a sense of achievement or enjoyment.

During a flare-up the patients are encouraged to maintain a gentle paced level of activity and not to reduce their tolerance levels. This follows the principle that the person and time rather than the pain is guiding activity levels. If a flare-up lasts for longer than 2 days then tolerance levels can be cut down by around 50% or less and a plan made to gradually increase these tolerances back to the level before they were reduced within about 7 days.

Planning and prioritizing

Flare-ups in pain can stop people from engaging in any planned activity. Cognitive behavioural pain management encourages people to continue with some planned activity despite the pain. This does not mean pushing too far but dovetailing pain management strategies with these activities. People

need to prioritize their plans for the day and to re-schedule some things, but not everything, and possibly changing plans slightly to make the day more manageable.

Stretches

Some people feel confident about stretching during times of increased pain. Others are more reluctant due to fear of injury or increased pain. Patients learn that stretching can be helpful during times of increased pain. Whilst recognizing that it can be hard to stretch, on these days the team encourage people to stretch using the principles of gently, slowly, little and often. They are also told that the range they are able to stretch may be less during a flare-up and are encouraged to stretch just as far as is comfortable without causing more pain.

OTHER ISSUES TO CONSIDER THAT RELATE TO JHS

The author's clinical experience suggests that there are issues that are more apparent in some people with JHS or are specific to JHS and not discussed in the cognitive behavioural literature.

The search for a diagnosis

Many people with JHS feel angry and frustrated about the time they have spent searching for a diagnosis and acknowledgement of their problems. They are frustrated and disappointed to find that a diagnosis does not lead to a cure. If not addressed, this may induce helplessness and serve as a barrier to developing self-management strategies.

Relationships with healthcare providers

Many people with JHS believe that all healthcare providers do not understand JHS. This has implications for their views on the PMP team and for their future contact with healthcare providers.

Hereditary nature of JHS

The majority of people with JHS who attend cognitive behavioural pain management are young women who have or are considering having children. They voice concerns about the hereditary nature of JHS. Some delay the decision to have children. Many of those with children are hypervigilant to their children's complaints of pain. They strive to receive a diagnosis of JHS early in their child's life in the hope that they will receive the treatment and support that they never received. Many parents with children with JHS believe that their children should 'be careful' and avoid certain activities for fear of injury and increased pain. This may have a long-term impact on the child because:

- Modelling from a parent is a known mechanism by which fear and avoidance are acquired early in life.
- Fear of pain/injury and avoidance of activity play significant roles in the detrimental physical and psychological impact of persistent pain.

The clinical team need to ensure that these issues are addressed in the context of cognitive behavioural pain management of the patient's distress.

SUMMARY

People with chronic pain can suffer physical and psychological secondary effects. Unfortunately these effects can be neglected by the healthcare system, particularly in people with joint hyper-mobility syndrome.

Using a dualistic model to understand chronic pain is unhelpful for the patient and interventions. Recent neurophysiological studies suggest that biological, psychological and social factors play a role in pain perception and pain reports in all people.

Psychosocial factors can increase the detrimental psychological and physical experience of the pain. This impact can be addressed by cognitive behavioural pain management interventions.

Cognitive behavioural interventions for chronic pain are carried out by a team of skilled clinicians. They support the patient in developing physical and psychological strategies to help them self-manage the pain and reduce its impact on their life.

Each strategy learnt as part of the cognitive behavioural intervention should not be used in isolation but alongside the other strategies if the pain is to be addressed holistically.

There is very little published research that addresses cognitive behavioural interventions for JHS despite it being a condition that has a wide-ranging physical and psychological impact.

References

Adib N, Davies K, Grahame R, et al: Joint hypermobility syndrome in childhood. A not so benign multisystem disorder? *Rheumatology* 44:744–750, 2005.

Beck AT: *Cognitive Therapy and the Emotional Disorders*, New York, 1976, International Universities Press.

Bennett-Levy J, Butler G, Fennell M, et al: *Oxford Guide to Behavioural Experiments in Cognitive Therapy (Cognitive Behaviour Therapy: Science & Practice)*, Oxford, 2004, Oxford University Press.

Bigatti SM, Hernandez AM, Cronan TA, et al: Sleep disturbances in fibromyalgia syndrome: relationship to pain and depression, *Arthritis Rheum* 15:961–967, 2008.

Birkholtz M, Aylwin L, Harman RM: Activity pacing in chronic pain management: one aim, but which method? part one: introduction and literature review, *Br J Occup Ther* 67:447–452, 2004.

Buer N, Linton SJ: Fear-avoidance beliefs and catastrophizing: occurrence and risk factor in back pain and ADL in the general population, *Pain* 99:485–491, 2002.

Carr DB, Loeser D, Morris DB: Narrative, Pain, and Suffering in *Progress in Pain Research and Mangement*, vol 34, Seattle, USA, IASP Press, 2005.

Coghill RC, McHaffie JG, Yen Y: Neural correlates of interindividual differences in the subjective experience of pain, *Proc Natl Acad Sci U S A* 100:8538–8542, 2003.

Coughlan GM, Ridout KL, Williams AC de C, et al: Attrition from a pain management programme, *Br J Clin Psychol* 34:471–479, 1995.

Crombez G, Vlaeyen JWS, Heuts PHTG, et al: Pain-related fear is more disabling than pain itself; evidence on the role of pain-related fear in chronic back pain disability, *Pain* 80:329–339, 1999.

Crombez G, Eccleston C, van den Broeck A, et al: Hypervigilance to Pain in Fibromyalgia: The Mediating Role of Pain Intensity and Catastrophic Thinking About Pain, *Clin J Pain* 20:98–102, 2004.

Crombez G, Van Damme S, Eccleston C: Hypervigilance to pain: an experimental and clinical analysis, *Pain* 116:4–7, 2005.

Daniel HC: *Do we need different pain management programmes for different diagnoses? Oral presentation at The British Pain Society's 10th National Pain Management Programme Conference*, 2005.

Daniel HC, Williams AC de C, Croucher S, et al: *Joint

hypermobility syndrome: the pain management programme puzzle, *Poster presentation at The British Pain Society Annual Scientific Meeting*: Harrogate; 2006.

de Jong JR, Vlaeyen JWS, Onghena P, et al: Fear of movement/(re)injury in chronic low back pain, *Clin J Pain* 21:9–17, 2005.

Dworkin RH, Corbin AE, Young JP Jr, et al: Pregabalin for the treatment of postherpetic neuralgia: A randomized, placebo-controlled trial, *Neurology* 60:1274–1283, 2003.

Edwards RR, Bingham CO 3rd, Bathon J, et al: Catastrophizing and pain in arthritis, fibromyalgia, and other rheumatic diseases, *Arthritis Rheum* 15:325–332, 2006.

Engel GL: The need for a new medical model: A challenge for biomedicine, *Science* 196:129–136, 1977.

Frank AW: *The Wounded Storyteller: Body, Illness and Ethics*, Chicago, 1997, Chicago University Press.

Gawthrop F, Mould R, Sperritt A, et al: Ehlers-Danlos Syndrome, *Br Med J* 335:448–450, 2007.

Gill JR, Brown CA: A structured review of the evidence for pacing as a chronic pain intervention, *Eur J Pain* 13:214–216, 2009.

Grahame R: Time to take hypermobility seriously (in adults and children), *Rheumatology* 40:485–491, 2001.

Grahame R, Hakim A: Hypermobility, *Curr Opin Rheumatol* 20:106–110, 2008.

Gupta A, Silman AJ, Ray D, et al: The role of psychosocial factors in predicting the onset of chronic widespread pain: results from a prospective population-based study, *Rheumatology* 46:666–671, 2007.

Gurley-Green S: Living with the hypermobility syndrome, *Rheumatology* 40:487–489, 2001.

Hakim A, Grahame R: Non-musculoskeletal symptoms in joint hypermobility syndrome. Indirect evidence for autonomic

dysfunction, *Rheumatology* 43:1194–1195, 2004.

Hutton JM: Issues to consider in cognitive-behavioural therapy for irritable bowel syndrome, *Eur J Gastroenterol Hepatol* 20:249–251, 2008.

Lamé IE, Peters ML, Vlaeyen JWS, et al: Quality of life in chronic pain is more associated with beliefs about pain, than with pain intensity, *Eur J Pain* 9:15–24, 2005.

Linton SJ: A review of psychological risk factors in back and neck pain, *Spine* 25:1148–1156, 2000.

Main C, Williams AC de C: ABC of psychological medicine, *Br Med J* 325:534–537, 2002.

McCracken LM, Turk DC: Behavioral and cognitive–behavioral treatment for chronic pain, outcome, predictors of outcome, and treatment process, *Spine* 27:2564–2573, 2002.

McCracken LM, Samuel VM: The role of avoidance, pacing, and other activity patterns in chronic pain, *Pain* 130:119–125, 2007.

Melzack R: Pain and the neuromatrix in the brain, *J Dent Educ* 65:1378–1382, 2001.

Merskey H: Social influences on the concept of fibromyalgia, *CNS Spectr* 13:18–21, 2008.

Moorey S, Greer S: *Cognitive Behaviour Therapy for People with Cancer*, Oxford, 2002, Oxford University Press.

Morley S, Eccleston C, Williams A: Systematic review and meta-analysis of randomized controlled trials of cognitive behaviour therapy and behaviour therapy for chronic pain in adults, excluding headache, *Pain* 80:1–13, 1999.

Morley S: Process and change in cognitive behaviour therapy for chronic pain, *Pain* 109:205–206, 2004.

Morris DB: *The Culture of Pain*, Chicago, 1993, University of California Press.

National Institute for Health and Clinical Excellence, *Cognitive*

behavioural therapy for the management of common mental health problems, 2007, http://www.nice.org.uk/ [accessed 26th November 2008].

Pfingsten M, Kroner-Herwig B, Leibing E, et al: Validation of the German version of the Fear-Avoidance Beliefs Questionnaire (FABQ), *Eur J Pain* 4:259–266, 2000.

Quarmby L, Rimes KA, Deale A, et al: Cognitive-behaviour therapy for chronic fatigue syndrome: comparison of outcomes within and outside the confines of a randomised controlled trial, *Behav Res Ther* 45:1085–1094, 2006.

Sharpe M, Williams AC de C: Treating patients with somatoform pain disorder and hypochondriasis. In Turk DC, Gatchel RJ, editors: *Psychological Approaches to Pain Management: A Practitioner's Handbook*, New York, 2002, Guilford Press, pp 515–533.

Simmonds JV, Keer RJ: Hypermobility and the hypermobility syndrome, *Man Ther* 12:298–309, 2007.

Sullivan MJ, Thorn B, Haythornthwaite J, et al: Theoretical perspectives on the relation between catastrophizing and pain, *Clin J Pain* 17:52–64, 2001.

Sullivan MJ, Rodgers WM, Wilson PM, et al: An experimental investigation of the relation between catastrophizing and activity intolerance, *Pain* 100:47–53, 2002.

The British Pain Society, *Recommended guidelines for pain management programmes for adults*, 2007, http://www.britishpainsociety.org/.

The International Association for the Study of Pain, *How prevalent is chronic pain? Pain Clinical Updates*, 2003, http://www.iasp-pain.org/ [accessed 24th October 2008].

Thieme K, Flor H, Turk DC: Psychological pain treatment in fibromyalgia syndrome: efficacy of operant behavioural and cognitive behavioural treatments, *Arthritis Res Ther* 8: R121, 2006.

Turk DC, Okifuji A: Matching treatment to assessment of patients with chronic pain. In Turk DC, Melzack R, editors: *Handbook of Pain Assessment*, New York, 2001, Guilford Press, pp 400–413.

Turk DC, Monarch ES: Biopsychosocial perspective on chronic pain. In Gatchel RJ, Turk DC, editors: *Psychological Approaches to Pain Management: A Practitioner's Handbook*, New York, 2002, Guilford Press, pp 3–29.

Turk DC, Robinson JP, Burwinkle T: Prevalence of fear of pain and activity in patients with fibromyalgia syndrome, *J Pain* 5:483–490, 2004.

van den Hout JH, Vlaeyen JW, Houben RM, et al: The effects of failure feedback and pain-related fear on pain report, pain tolerance, and pain avoidance in chronic low back pain patients, *Pain* 92:247–257, 2001.

van Koulil S, Effting M, Kraaimaat FW, et al: Cognitive-behavioural therapies and exercise programmes for patients with fibromyalgia: state of the art and future directions, *Ann Rheum Dis* 66:571–581, 2007.

van Koulil S, van Lankveld W, Kraaimaat FW, et al: Tailored cognitive-behavioral therapy for fibromyalgia: two case studies, *Patient Educ Couns* 71:308–314, 2008.

Verbunt JA, Pernot DH, Smeets RJ: Disability and quality of life in patients with fibromyalgia, *Health Qual Life Outcomes* 22:6–8, 2008.

Vlaeyen JWS, Kole-Snijders AMJ, Boeren RGB, et al: Fear of movement/(re)injury in chronic low back pain and its relation to behavioral performance, *Pain* 62:363–372, 1995.

Waddell G: *The Back Pain Revolution*, ed 2, Edinburgh, 2004, Churchill Livingstone.

Wall P: *The Science of Suffering (Maps of The Mind)*, ed 2, London, 2000, Phoenix Publishing.

Chapter 9

Physiotherapy and occupational therapy in the hypermobile adult

Rosemary Keer

Katherine Butler

INTRODUCTION

Joint hypermobility syndrome (JHS) is under-recognized, poorly understood and, sadly, often poorly managed (Beighton 1999). The syndrome does not necessarily cause problems and for many individuals it can be an asset, amply illustrated in the world of music, dance and sport. For others it can be a liability, producing significant problems which are often ignored by the medical profession (Phipps 2003, HMSA 2006). Early recognition and appropriate management can decrease suffering, reduce the need for unnecessary tests and invasive procedures, help to avoid surgery, reduce chronic pain and fear (Cherpel & Marks 1999) and prevent the destructive spiral into depression and physical deconditioning. It is the aim of this chapter to discuss the presentation of the syndrome to aid recognition and diagnosis by primary care practitioners and to explore assessment and management strategies to decrease suffering and disability, increase function and enable the hypermobile individual to effectively self-manage the condition.

PRESENTATION

ASSESSMENT

Pain is the most common complaint, often being widely distributed, involving several joints and areas of the body, and varying in duration from acute (15 days) to as long as 45 years (El-Shahaly & El-Sherif 1991). A typical presentation is illustrated in Keer & Grahame (2003), and Simmonds

& Keer (2007). The onset frequently occurs in childhood or adolescence, particularly in girls between the ages of 13–19 years, with 75% of hypermobile adolescents developing symptoms by the age of 15 (Kirk et al 1967) (Chapters 2, 10 and 11). Anecdotally, onset is also often associated with trauma, pregnancy, childbirth, a change in physical activity, such as a marked decrease contributing to deconditioning, or an unresolved joint problem which leads to compensatory strategies producing other joint problems. In addition, the patient will often report past episodes of medical or therapy intervention which were unhelpful and may even have exacerbated their symptoms. Exploring their history in this respect not only helps to identify potential generalized hypermobility, but will also give valuable information regarding what has not helped in the past, so that mistakes are not repeated.

It is unusual for pain to be the only symptom, so asking for details about other symptoms can give clues to tissues or systems which may be potential causes of the problem and may require examination (Table 9.1). Stiffness is a very common complaint and may seem at odds with the range of movement on testing. This is a subjective feeling of stiffness and although the range of movement may appear normal it may not be normal for that particular patient. Asking 'have you ever been able to touch the floor with your palms flat' (Oliver 2000) can be a useful indicator of previous hypermobility, a factor that is acknowledged in both the 5-point questionnaire (Hakim & Grahame 2003) and the Brighton Criteria (Grahame et al 2000) (Chapter 1). The reports of stiffness may also be a reflection of decreasing flexibility with

© 2010 Elsevier Ltd.
DOI: 10.1016/B978-0-7020-3005-5.00013-6

Table 9.1	Common symptoms reported and possible tissue or system at fault	
SYMPTOM REPORTED	**SYSTEM TO BE EXAMINED**
Stiffness	Muscle system (muscular tension)
'Feeling like a 90 year old'	Joints Hormonal
Audible clicking, popping, clunking, sensations of subluxation, vulnerability, instability or frank dislocation	Motor control Stability system
Sensations of parasthesiae, tingling, numbness, deadness	Neural system
Tiredness, fatigue, faintness, feeling unwell, flu-like symptoms	Autonomic nervous system Physical deconditioning

age, or due to injury or muscle stiffness/spasm. Paraesthesiaes are frequently non-dermatomal and there may be an increased disposition to development of a neuropathy (Francis et al 1987, March et al 1988).

Aggravating factors to determine the Severity, Irritability & Nature (SIN) (Maitland 1986) are not clear cut. Latency is frequently a problem, with symptoms developing several hours or even a day later, making it very difficult to identify the aggravating activity. This makes it difficult to judge the response to a physical examination and treatment. Careful questioning about the individual's response to physical activity will help, although caution is advised with regard to the amount and vigour of testing, particularly initially.

Hypermobile individuals frequently dislike static postures and report difficulty with standing still, such as when queuing, shopping or attending exhibitions, and sitting for prolonged periods of time. Hypermobility of the spine was found to increase the prevalence of back pain in industrial workers working in standing/sitting postures (Larsson et al 1995) and hypermobility of the spine and knees produced symptoms in musicians due to sustained standing postures (Larsson et al 1993).

In addition, hypermobile individuals dislike repetitive activities, being more likely to develop musculoskeletal lesions (Acasuso-Diaz et al 1993) and reporting an increased frequency of previous episodes and more recurrent episodes of overuse soft tissue lesions such as bursitis, tendonitis and fasciitis at a single site (Hudson et al 1995, 1998)

as well as fibromyalgia (Goldman 1991, Acasuso-Diaz & Collantes-Estevez 1998) (Chapter 5). It is often the case that pain or injury has occurred with minimal provocation during everyday activities, such that the patient cannot say what has brought the pain on. This can be very frustrating for the therapist and patient alike, but it is worth viewing this as a valuable piece of the jigsaw, leading to more accurate recognition and diagnosis of generalized hypermobility.

Certain aspects of the patient's history can be valuable in providing clues to hypermobility. Back and knee pain are reported most commonly as a source of pain in childhood (Biro et al 1983) (Chapter 11). Individuals who no longer demonstrate hypermobility due to age, injury or stiffness secondary to pain, may be able to confirm that they were more flexible when younger, or that there is a family history of increased flexibility. Studies have shown that 27–65% of patients with symptomatic hypermobility seen in clinic had relatives with hypermobility (Finsterbush & Pogrund 1982, Biro et al 1983, Bridges et al 1992). There may also be evidence of involvement of other connective tissue, because patients report that they bruise easily (Al-Rawi et al 1985, Kaplinsky et al 1998) and there is frequently a history of varicose veins, hernia, or prolapses (Wynne-Davies 1971, Al-Rawi et al 1985, El-Shahaly & El-Sherif 1991).

Hypermobile individuals frequently recount a long history of soft tissue injuries, strains and sprains (Acasuso-Diaz et al 1993), which can be suggestive of vulnerable tissues or areas of vulnerability due to increased tissue laxity, poor control and muscular weakness. Dislocations and subluxations are more common (Finsterbush & Pogrund 1982). This should prompt a holistic assessment looking at the functioning of the whole body, to identify reasons why a particular area is causing a problem. How well the individual recovered from previous injury/problems will have a bearing on subsequent treatment, expectations and prognosis, particularly as there is anecdotal evidence of poor healing and a slower recovery in this patient group (Russek 2000).

In addition, questions relating to gender, age, ethnicity, weight, details of work or daily activities, leisure and exercise or sport activities will help to give a full picture of the impact of JHS on the individual. It is also important to ask special questions regarding general health and medical history in terms of surgery or illnesses, related or not, such as fatigue, chronic fatigue syndrome and fibromyalgia, as well as details of medication, so that the physical examination can be tailored to the individual's presentation without risking a flare-up. Discussing medication may also highlight the possibility of JHS as a diagnosis, because there is often a poor response to non-steroidal anti-inflammatory drugs (NSAIDs), and local anaesthetics have been reported as less effective in EDS type III patients (Arendt-Neilson 1990, Hakim et al 2005).

EXAMINATION

Observation of the patient's mannerisms and postures during history-taking may give an indication of hypermobility. Contact of the hand to the face may reveal hyperextension of the digits, constantly changing position or fidgeting and/or sitting in an unusual posture (legs wound round each other, slumped to the side or resting on the lateral border of the feet) are familiar sightings (Fig. 9.1).

Skin is a very important feature and helps to confirm a diagnosis of hypermobility. To the touch it is silky, soft, extensible and thin. Elasticity can be tested by picking up a section from the back of the hand between the thumb and first finger (Chapter 2). Wounds may show poor healing with a thinner or papery scar. There may be stretch marks (striae atrophicae) not associated with weight loss or pregnancy, which appear during the growth phase in certain areas such as across the lumbar spine and pelvis, around the hips, thighs and shoulders.

The Beighton scale (Beighton et al 1973) gives an indication of hypermobility in certain joints (JHM), and while it is quick and easy to use in the clinic, it is limited in its application as only a few joints are tested. Other scales are discussed in more detail in Chapter 1. A diagnosis of JHS can be confirmed using the Brighton Criteria (Grahame et al 2000) which assesses the effect of weaker connective tissue on the body as a whole, but its use is primarily as a research tool. In an out-patient setting, making a diagnosis of JHS will depend on a thorough history and physical examination of the whole body.

It may be appropriate or indeed necessary to refer a patient, whom one suspects of being hypermobile, to a rheumatologist for a definitive diagnosis or further investigations when:

- the patient's symptoms do not fit the examination findings (except with regard to the range of movement as mentioned below)
- a clear diagnosis regarding the nature of the connective tissue disease is required and it is necessary to exclude other pathology

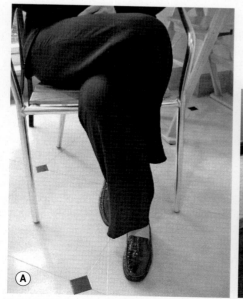
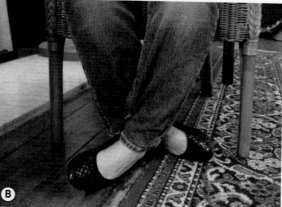

Fig. 9.1 Typical sitting posture: (a) legs wound round each other, (b) resting on the lateral border of the feet

- a complex presentation involving many body areas and systems requires access to other health care professionals
- further investigations are required to provide more information regarding pathology, such as in the spine or peripheral joints to identify degeneration or instability (Grahame 2003).

Pain is also thought to arise because the connective tissue (ligament, tendon, muscle, capsule) in hypermobile individuals is more lax and less resilient and suggests a predisposition to the effects of trauma (acute and chronic) from overuse and misuse. Microtrauma occurs more frequently and with less provocation (Acasuso-Diaz et al 1993, Hudson et al 1998), meaning that even everyday activities can be the cause of tissue trauma and pain. For some, there is the added problem of subluxation, dislocation or instability which can produce, or be the result of, poor movement control. The hypermobile individual has an increased susceptibility to instability due to increased extensibility in the connective tissue restraints (capsule, ligament, muscle, tendon), affecting the passive control system, decreased muscle tone and strength, affecting the active control system, and deficient proprioceptive acuity (Mallik et al 1994, Hall et al 1995), affecting the neural and feedback control system, which is further outlined in Panjabi's model of stability (1992) (Chapter 12.8).

Poor movement control has the potential to lead to further joint problems, setting off a chain reaction or 'domino' effect whereby a problem in one joint can develop into widespread pain affecting many joints over a period of time. Increased healing time may lead to more well-developed compensatory strategies which affect other areas, progressing onto chronic pain and physical deconditioning (Fig. 9.2).

It is helpful to think in terms of compensatory relative flexibility, a concept proposed by Sahrmann (2002). This states that movement occurs more readily at a joint with less stiffness than at a joint with relatively more stiffness. For example, hamstring muscle tension or stiffness either as a result of habitually sitting for long periods, or as a result of injury, will inhibit movement at the hip into flexion during forward bending, potentially leading to overflexion in the spine. It is common to see decreased hip flexion and increased spinal flexion in hypermobile individuals and this may be contributing to low-grade irritation and

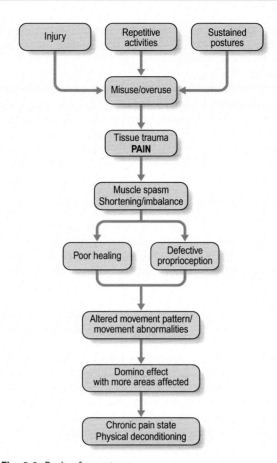

Fig. 9.2 Basis of symptoms

strain to lumbar spine tissues, producing pain. Figure 9.3a is an example of this and is in contrast to Figure 9.3b which shows well-balanced full range flexion in a hypermobile individual.

There is evidence of neurophysiological defects such as pain enhancement and autonomic dysfunction (Gazit et al 2003) (Chapter 6.1), which will have the effect of increasing disability, leading to less activity and a vicious spiral of chronic pain and physical deconditioning (Rose 1985). Psychological distress is common, with concerns and difficulties occurring around work, home life and raising children, as well as fear of pain, serious illness or permanent disability. Individuals have often had to withstand years of having their complaints dismissed, being misunderstood or not being believed by the medical profession at large (Phipps 2003). This has, understandably in some cases, led to anger, confusion and depression.

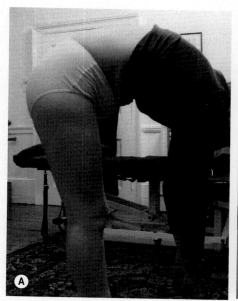
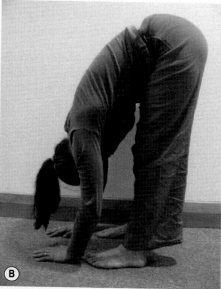

Fig. 9.3 Compensatory relative flexibility: (a) forward flexion with decreased hip flexion relative to spinal flexion, (b) forward flexion with balanced movement throughout the spine and hips

The physical examination starts with observation. The patient, undressed to their underclothes and standing in their normal stance, is assessed from all four directions (front, back and each side) and compared with what is considered the ideal skeletal alignment. This is a standard based on sound scientific principles which involves minimal stress and strain on the body tissues and allows maximal efficiency (Kendall et al 1993). Details of a thorough postural examination are given in Kendall et al (1993) and should include postural alignment, symmetry and weight distribution from head to toe.

Hypermobile individuals show a tendency to rest at the end of joint range and have poor postural alignment. Even if they are initially able to stand or sit in a good position, it is difficult to sustain the position for long periods. It is easier for their bodies to take the path of least resistance and settle into a position which requires decreased muscle work, resting on tension in their soft tissues. Familiar postures are slumped sitting, standing with hyperextended knees and hips (Fig. 9.4) and hanging on the hip. This leads to stress and strain in the collagenous tissues. If these postures are sustained, fluid is forced out and tissue nutrition is adversely affected. The tissue undergoes creep, which leads to deformation,

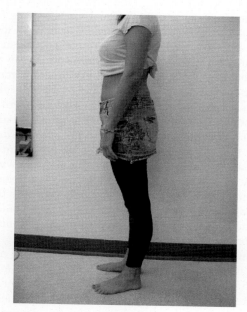

Fig. 9.4 Standing with hyperextending knees

stretching and weakening over time. There is also a weakening of surrounding muscles through disuse and changes in how and where load is transferred through the kinetic chain. Hyperextension at the knee provides a good illustration (Kendall et al 1993), with the patella displaced caudally and contact of the femoral condyles on the tibial plateau shifted more anteriorly. This has the potential to weaken and damage tissue, disrupt nutrition of joint tissue and produce pain. There are also effects along the kinetic chain at a distance from the knee, with the ankle joint held in plantarflexion, producing changes in the calf muscles, and also into the hip and lumbar spine.

ACTIVE MOVEMENT

Hypermobile individuals tend to look and move well, even if they have pain. Thus during active range of movement testing their reports of symptoms (subjective) are often at odds with the physical examination (objective). It is possible to see how misunderstandings may arise; the person who complains of widespread debilitating pain affecting several joints can, when asked, bend forward to touch their toes. This tends to go against medical wisdom and may lead to the individual being dismissed or considered a hypochondriac. The explanation may be that although the movement looks to be full range, it may not be 'normal' or full range for that particular person. Additionally, it may be that some areas are moving into hypermobile range (such as lumbar spine) and masking reduced range in an adjacent area (such as the hip joint). It is important to assess the quality of movement and critically appraise where, when and how much movement is occurring throughout the body or kinetic chain, while keeping the biomechanics in mind. Hypermobility may be masked when range of movement is decreased due to fear, pain or stiffness following injury or inactivity or in the case of an older person who may have lost their normal degree of flexibility with age. Clinical reasoning will lead to examination of other areas (skin, other joints, historical flexibility) for confirmation of hypermobility.

It is helpful to examine the effect of moving one area in the context of the whole body. This may mean examining ease and range of movement in all areas of the spine as well as some peripheral joints, if symptomatic. For instance, full flexion at the shoulders may only be possible with lumbar spine extension, because latissimus dorsi is shortened or overactive (Sahrmann 2002), producing an area of relative stiffness. This has the potential to lead to overuse injuries at the shoulder through repetition of an overhead activity, particularly relevant in the sports person. It would therefore be necessary to assess the shoulder and whole spine. For the less active, it may be as simple as increased pronation in the midfoot as a result of stiffness at the ankle into dorsiflexion, either through talocrural stiffness (from injury) and/or soft tissue shortness/tightness in the calves or higher in the kinetic chain. Poor movement patterns may also be due to muscle deconditioning and weakness. A case highlighted in Simmonds and Keer (2008) involved an individual lifting with poor muscle control around the wrist which led to the wrist being pushed into ulnar deviation under load, causing strain to the ligament and tendon on the radial side. Close questioning and detailed examination of everyday habitual activities can highlight significant problems, which can be easily rectified once identified.

Functional activities, assessed as relevant to the individual, need to be examined. These include walking (over a set distance), climbing stairs, sitting to standing, bending, mini squat to full squat, one-leg stand, heel raise and any specific activity known to cause problems. In addition to pain, it is also helpful to look for even weight bearing, balance, co-ordination, symmetry and load transfer (Lee & Lee 2007). Pain is not always reproduced on testing unless the problem area is in the acute stage. This appears to be due to the tendency for pain to be aggravated by sustained postures or repeated activities. If repeating an activity or sustaining a posture does not reproduce pain, the examination must rely on an analysis of the quality and patterns of movement throughout the kinetic chain. Forward spinal bend is useful for assessing the relative contribution of lumbar, thoracic and hip joints into flexion as well as highlighting segmental hinging or translation. Mini squat is helpful in assessing lower limb alignment during a functional activity. One-leg stand assesses the ability to transfer load effectively through the pelvis and hip. Heel raise can be helpful in assessing control around the foot and ankle.

Hypermobiles frequently use a 'bracing' pattern with breath holding in an attempt to improve stability and produce more force. As the global muscles of the trunk are used, the ribs can become fixed so that chest expansion, and therefore efficient respiration, is affected. The individual either breathes apically or into the abdomen, with the risk of increasing abdominal pressure downwards which can have a deleterious effect on the pelvic floor. It is useful to assess the breathing pattern at rest and with activity.

Many hypermobiles suffer from feelings of instability and 'giving way', subluxations and dislocations, and due to the lax connective tissue, joints may become unstable through injury. Treatment is therefore focused on control of movement and it is important to assess the local postural muscles associated with trunk stability, such as transversus abdominus, deep multifidus and the pelvic floor muscles in terms of timing, atrophy, loss of tonic function, loss of co-ordination and asymmetry. There is also support for the use of real time ultrasound imaging to assess performance of the deep stability muscles, which can be particularly useful for identifying 'cues' which the patient can use to activate the correct muscle (Fig. 9.5).

Examination continues with detailed inspection of individual structures that have been identified as possible contributors to the patient's symptoms.

1. Articular movement testing, both passive and accessory movement, to identify hypermobility, hypomobility and symptom reproduction.

2. Muscle testing, assessing strength, tone, length, timing and tenderness of trigger points.

3. Neural testing, both in terms of function (sensation, reflexes and power) and mobility (Butler 2000). This may involve testing straight leg raise (SLR), upper limb tension tests (ULTTs), slump and thoracic slump, particularly if involvement of the autonomic nervous system is suspected.

4. Specific tests to identify pathology such as impingement (hip and shoulder) and active straight leg raise (ASLR).

PROPRIOCEPTION

It is known that proprioceptive acuity is diminished in individuals with JHS (Mallik et al 1994, Hall et al 1995) and this can have a significant effect on the way an individual moves. The research shows that both joint position sense and threshold to detection of movement are impaired such that they have less awareness of approaching the end of joint range (Chapter 6.4). The reason for this impairment is not known but may be related to increased laxity and elasticity in the tissues, which may explain why the application of tape has been found to enhance proprioception in those with a deficit (Callaghan et al 2002, 2008) and also why supportive, tight garments have been reported as helpful in improving proprioceptive feedback (Simmonds & Keer 2007).

In the laboratory, threshold to detection of passive movement has been found to be more reliable than joint position sense (Juul-Kristensen et al 2008), but detection is affected by the position in range of movement when testing (Ageberg et al 2007). In addition, the effect of pain and injury should be taken into consideration as Juul-Kristensen et al (2008) found that proprioception was poorer in elbows with epicondylitis than in the controls' elbows.

It can be difficult to measure proprioception accurately in the clinic and tests are generally linked to function. The ability to stand on two legs with eyes closed, or on one leg with eyes open and closed as in the Romberg test, will reveal exaggerated swaying and/or loss of balance once the eyes are closed. As in the study above, pain

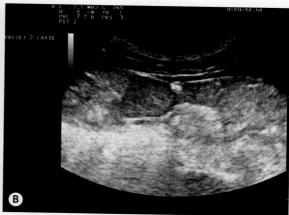

Fig. 9.5 Real-time ultrasound scans of transversus abdominus (TrA): (a) TrA at rest (b) TrA contracting, note slight thickening and sliding of third layer

may contribute to the increased sway observed due to poor stability/control around the ankle, knee, hip and/or sacro-iliac joint. Standing on one leg and observing the strategies employed in order to remain balanced can highlight poor load transference through the lower limb, but particularly through the pelvis and hip. Hip hitch, or a pseudo-Trendelenburg, is frequently observed.

MANAGEMENT

A management plan is formulated following discussion between the patient and the therapist. It is based on the findings of the assessment in terms of what is causing the problem and where treatment should be directed, and an in-depth discussion with the patient about their expectations. Many patients are hoping for a miracle cure, others want to help themselves but have received conflicting advice, while others are fearful of getting worse and 'ending up in a wheelchair'. Recent research has shown greater benefit and cost-effectiveness in treatment for musculoskeletal disorders when patients, who expressed a preference, received their preferred treatment, compared to those who expressed no preference (Preference Collaborative Review Group 2008). In addition, a qualitative study (Cooper et al 2008) exploring perceptions of physiotherapy in a group of chronic low back pain patients highlighted the importance that patients place on communication. It underpinned the other key themes which included individual care, good explanation regarding diagnosis and treatment and involvement in decision making and treatment time. Amanda Sperritt (Gawthrop et al 2007) echoes these findings in an article in the *BMJ* about her experiences of EDS. She comments that 'the most helpful professionals treat me as a partner in the management of the condition' and states that listening and support from the therapist help 'to make life that bit easier'. Amanda also reports that physiotherapy was valuable because it allowed her to play an active part in her treatment, as well as teaching her to use her muscles to protect her joints. It is only by listening to the patient's story that a prioritized problem list and achievable and appropriate goals, which are the key to successful client care, can be agreed (Simmonds & Keer 2007). Gaining a clear understanding of the patient's problem through a comprehensive assessment helps to ensure appropriate and effective intervention.

However, there are reports of physical therapy being unhelpful or even exacerbating symptoms. There may be several reasons for this and most are underpinned by a failure to recognize that the patient has JHS and, as such, has more lax, less resilient connective tissue (Acasuso-Diaz et al 1993). Extra care should be taken with manual therapy. Recovery and healing is slower than in the non-hypermobile, so if this factor is not appreciated there is a temptation to progress more quickly or with more vigour in order to produce a change.

Functional restoration is the main aim of treatment since this enables the individual to self-manage the condition. It is made up of different components.

1. Restoration of a normal range of movement for that particular individual, even if it is hypermobile (Keer et al 2003, Maillard & Murray 2003).
2. Restoration of efficient and effective movement patterns throughout full range of movement, including the hypermobile range. This will include correcting and preventing movement dysfunction and regaining joint stability.
3. Education, reassurance, advice and problem-solving (Rose 1985, Russek 1999).
4. Improving general fitness (Simmonds & Keer 2007) (Chapter 13).

Three patterns of presentation have been proposed (Finsterbush & Pogrund 1982), which require different therapeutic approaches.

1. Episodes of *acute* musculoskeletal pain, dislocation and subluxation, initially respond well to the usual therapeutic modalities of electrotherapy, support, ice, movement and advice.
2. Recurrent episodes or a series of episodes of pain at different sites with some physical deconditioning characterize the *intermediate* stage and require therapeutic modalities which are adapted and modified to provide functional restoration.
3. *Chronic*, long-standing, severe and unremitting pain with profound physical deconditioning may require a multidisciplinary pain management programme using cognitive behavioural skills (Harding 2003) (Chapter 8).

It is important to try to give treatment that has meaning for the patient. This may be a treatment modality or exercise which instantly takes the pain away, or addresses an area of particular concern. This gives the patient a sense of control or more comfort and as such promotes improved movement patterns and muscle recruitment but also has the power to motivate compliance to exercises or advice.

Acute symptom strategies

In the acute stages the primary aim is relief of pain. To this end the usual therapeutic modalities listed above are utilized. Rest is usually recommended for up to five days while the inflammatory stage takes place (Mattacola & Dwyer 2002), with movement to prevent the deconditioning effects of immobilization thereafter. Supporting the injured part can be very important because it allows movement of the body without strain to the injured tissue. Support can vary from a tight garment to a specific splint or brace. If the skin can tolerate it, tape is extremely useful as it moves more readily with the body. Support can help rest an area and put less stress on the body as a whole, but also, more importantly, it can allow pain-free movement. This has the real potential to prevent development of chronic pain by helping to reduce afferent stimulation of peripheral nociceptors. Vierck (2006) suggests that if tissue injury healing (particularly injury to deep tissues) and pain do not settle within 3 months there is a risk of developing chronic widespread pain and fibromyalgia.

'Injury' in a hypermobile individual may be a small everyday incident, such as picking up a bag, which provokes instantaneous pain (Simmonds & Keer 2007) or a sustained posture with joints at the end of their range of movement. In both these cases, if hypermobile connective tissue is not recognized it may be hard to analyse what caused the problem and easy to dismiss the patient's complaints. Inflammation is not necessarily a dominant feature.

There is an increased risk of deconditioning (Rose 1985) and an increased healing time (Russek 2000) in the hypermobile individual, so, while being mindful of the normal healing times, it is wise to be cautious and proceed slowly. Pacing of activities and specific exercises which do not provoke pain are important to prevent an exacerbation. Care should be taken during the proliferative stage up to 21 days after injury and it may be necessary to continue using support. During the remodelling stage controlled stress needs to be applied to produce a robust repair, but again care is needed in this patient group with particular attention to a gradual controlled progression of stress.

Taping has several uses. It can provide support for injured tissue, such as a medial ligament strain at the knee and reduce pain (Macgregor et al 2005, Aminaka and Gribble 2008). There is also evidence that it can facilitate better muscle activation and patterning. Macgregor et al (2005) found that patella tape which produced a lateral stretch across the patella increased VMO activity in people with patellofemoral pain. Christou (2004) found similar effects with both medial tape and placebo tape and suggested the mechanism is via cutaneous stimulation. Interestingly, they also found that tape had the opposite effect in healthy individuals. There is evidence for tape enhancing proprioception, but only in those whose proprioception is poor (Callaghan et al 2002, 2008). Individuals with normal proprioception were either shown to have no effect or a worsening of joint position sense when tape was applied to the knee. This was true whether the subject had a healthy knee (Callaghan 2002) or suffered from patellofemoral pain syndrome (Callaghan 2008). There is also evidence of patella taping having a beneficial effect on dynamic postural control in patients with patellofemoral pain syndrome compared to healthy individuals (Aminaka & Gribble 2008).

Intermediate symptom strategies

This group may have progressed from the acute stage without good healing or resolution and find themselves with a 'domino effect', whereby one initial injury sets off a chain reaction. This may be the result of resting too much and becoming deconditioned, or through developing poor compensation strategies, or being encouraged to push through the pain and irritating more tissues. At this stage it is very important to assess the whole person and all areas of symptoms in order to be able to identify what is continuing to 'drive' the problem and thereby apply appropriate treatment.

The treatment is now based on rehabilitation and functional restoration with the aim of returning the individual back to their former self. Once pain is under control, treatment is concerned with restoring a full range of movement and ensuring good motor control throughout the movement, even if it is hypermobile. Manual therapy is often used at this stage to restore normal movement and can be applied to the affected tissue(s) as indicated by the assessment.

1. Joints. Gentle, rhythmic, large-amplitude oscillations (Maitland 1986) have been found anecdotally to be most effective at reducing pain and improving joint range. However, high-velocity thrust techniques (HVT) are generally thought to be contraindicated, particularly in the cervical spine, although they can be successfully applied to a stiff thoracic spine in skilled hands.

2. Neural tissue. Restriction to normal neural mobility can be treated effectively with gentle mobilizing techniques as described by Butler (2000). Sustained end of range mobilization is not recommended in the hypermobile individual and overzealous 'stretching' can result in muscle spasm and guarding.

3. Muscle and fascia. Myofascial release, a massage therapy aimed at releasing tension in muscles and fascia (Gordon & Gueth 2006) uses long, stretching, gentle sustained pressure. It is thought to improve relaxation and circulation, and decrease pain, anxiety and lactic acid build up. It can be a useful technique to release muscles that have developed an overactive and dominant pattern, but for best effect is used with patient participation and awareness (Lee & Lee 2007). This helps to highlight to the patient where they may be overworking their muscles and how to release them in the future. It may be necessary to 'switch off' and relax an overactive muscle before an inhibited or 'switched off' muscle can be voluntarily contracted.

Re-educating good movement patterns and motor control often starts with an appreciation and practice in attaining and maintaining good postural alignment, firstly in static postures and progressing onto dynamic postures and specific tasks. Maintaining a good standing and sitting posture for more than a few seconds can be challenging in the beginning for some hypermobiles, because their postural muscles are unused to holding joints (the knee, pelvis and spine in particular) in a more neutral position, so their endurance capabilities need to be built up slowly and gradually.

It is usually necessary to begin this process in non-weightbearing positions to decrease the load through the joint(s). Effective and efficient joint control begins with gaining control of the pelvis and

trunk before moving to the peripheral joints. Assessment will have identified which of the deep stability muscles (transversus abdominus, pelvic floor multifidus) need facilitation to recruit effectively both in isolation and in a co-ordinated fashion. Activation is then practised while maintaining a neutral pelvic/lumbar spine position as well as a relaxed breathing pattern to prevent a 'bracing' or co-contraction rigidity strategy. This is often started in lying (supine, prone and side lying) and progressed to sitting and standing. The emphasis is on a low-level (20–30% of maximal voluntary contraction (Richardson et al 2004)) isometric hold repeated several times with relaxation in between.

The ability to maintain good control during weight-bearing is challenged by standing, initially on both legs, and progressed to one leg. All the time attention is paid to ensuring good joint alignment and relaxed but accurate and balanced muscle activation. Once control with static postures is being achieved, movement can be added in the form of knee bends or practising weight transference in stride stand in preparation for gait training. In addition, proprioception and balance can be challenged by introducing an unstable base, in the form of a gym ball, balance board (Fig. 9.6) or foam roller.

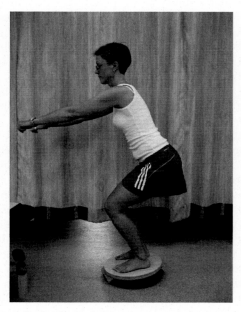

Fig. 9.6 Challenging balance and proprioception through knee bending on a balance board

There has been little research into effective treatment for symptoms as a result of JHS, although there is now evidence in the medical literature that low back pain, function and recurrence can be significantly improved through re-educating spinal stability strategies (Hides et al 1996, O'Sullivan 2000, Richardson et al 2004) and it seems logical that these recommendations can effectively be applied to the hypermobile population. Furthermore it seems that it is not only weakness of the stability muscles that is the problem but also delayed activation which allows unprotected displacement of the trunk to occur with movement of the limbs (Hodges & Richardson 1996, 1998). Specific, low-threshold training of transversus abdominus (TrA) (O'Sullivan 1997) and multifidus (Hides et al 1996) has been shown to be effective in treating chronic low back pain and preventing recurrences, and more recently Tsao and Hodges (2007) have shown this specific training can correct the timing delay in a relatively short period of time. However, there is conflicting evidence on the effectiveness of specific stabilization exercises in chronic back pain, with some considering them no better than other active physiotherapeutic interventions (May & Johnson 2008). Clinical experience provides anecdotal evidence of the ineffectiveness and harm of non-specific exercises, so the decision of what form of exercises to use will depend on clinical reasoning.

For peripheral joints there is evidence that utilizing close chained exercises in the lower limbs over an 8-week period is effective in reducing pain, improving proprioception, muscle strength and quality of life in JHS (Ferrell et al 2004). A study by Kerr et al (2000) showed similar findings in children with JHS. Gaining control of knee extension or hyperextension is vitally important for hypermobile individuals. Not only does it relieve pressure on the knees and prevent ligament damage, it also has a beneficial effect on the rest of the kinetic chain. Exercises can be started in a non-weightbearing position, but close chained to improve proprioceptive feedback. Knee flexion and extension without allowing the knee to fall into a 'lock' position can be practised by bending and straightening the knees through contact with the heels on a gym ball (Fig. 9.7). This can be advanced by performing controlled knee bends in standing on both legs and then on a single leg and progressed further by using an unstable base such as a foam pad or balance board. Exercising is always cognitive with attention on maintaining good alignment through the leg, effective pelvic control, relaxed breathing and low effort.

Similar principles can be applied in the upper limb with low load, close chained exercises being used to improve shoulder and elbow control. These often start by learning how to achieve a good shoulder position, or 'setting' the scapula (Mottram 1997). This is progressed to maintaining good scapula control during movement, such as moving a ball on a work surface and then into

Fig. 9.7 Re-educating knee control using a gym ball

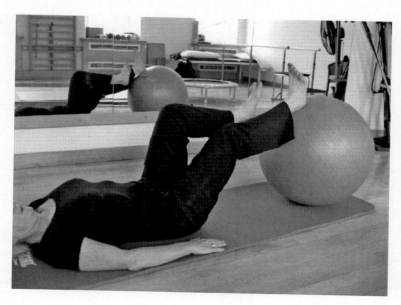

more range on a wall. Further progression can be achieved by increasing the resistance and moving into weightbearing in four-point kneeling.

Once good effective joint control has been established and exercising has begun to work on maintaining control throughout movement, attention progresses to improving the endurance and strength capabilities of the body in order to withstand high load activities without losing control. Muscle endurance training is thought to be important, because type I muscle fibres (slow twitch) atrophy at a faster rate than type II fibres (Harrelson 1998). The emphasis is therefore on increased repetitions and hold time. It is important to ensure that there is good relaxation between muscle contractions, to delay the onset of fatigue. In addition, eccentric muscle work appears to be particularly difficult for the hypermobile individual. Patients frequently use gravity to return the limb to the starting position rather than using slow controlled eccentric muscle activity. Right from the early stages of the rehabilitation programme control through the full range of movement should be emphasized and worked on.

In order to build strength in a muscle, the load is progressively increased in terms of force and speed. Resistance can be applied using free weights or exercise bands. There is some evidence that muscle hypertrophy (through strength training) can lead to increased muscle/joint stiffness (Ocarino et al 2008), which may be a useful additional mechanism to gain control of the hypermobile joint.

Ramsay and Riddoch (2001) found that ballet dancers were far superior to physiotherapy students in proprioceptive accuracy and suggested that rehabilitation should encourage repetition of movement with verbal and visual feedback to improve sensory motor performances. Biofeedback in the form of mirrors and photography (stills and video) can be used to increase awareness of posture and joint control, both in static positions and during performance of specific exercises and tasks. More specialized biofeedback, such as surface electromyographic (EMG) biofeedback, can help detect the presence of excessive muscular activity during the performance of a functional task (Polnauer & Marks 1964, Philipson et al 1990) (Chapter 12.1.). Video is particularly useful when assessing and treating musicians, because the patient can face a video monitor and play their instrument while postural cues are given by the therapist (Dommerholt & Norris 1997). The video

camera is placed at various angles, allowing the musician to see his or her posture from several perspectives and the session can be recorded for further study and review. This assessment technique can easily be utilized to review writing, sporting activities, or performance of daily living tasks.

Chronic symptom strategies

Individuals who fall into this group have often had symptoms for a long time, with severe deconditioning, kinesiophobia and psychological effects. They may have become dependent on using aids (collars, braces, sticks, crutches or even wheelchairs), be unable to work and claiming incapacity benefit or registered disabled. Like many chronic pain patients they will very often hold unhelpful beliefs about their pain and disability. But being hypermobile may add additional concerns regarding the weakness or vulnerability of their tissues, which increases the fear and belief that pain equates to damage. Understanding and then challenging these beliefs through interactive informative discussion and paced exercising and activity can encourage a more positive attitude and improve confidence.

Pacing is vital to those with hypermobility (Harding 2003) and fibromyalgia. Cycles of overactivity/underactivity are common and result in a flare-up of pain which requires a period of rest to recover. Repetition of this cycle leads to a downward spiral resulting in deconditioning and a confirmation (in the patient's mind) of weakness and inadequacy. Teaching pacing skills allows the patient to work at their own pace but within recognized guidelines (Harding 2003). The emphasis is on maximizing tissue health and endurance with a range of exercises and activities. Variety is key, with frequent changes between more active and more sedentary tasks, different postures (flexed, extended), smaller movements and larger movements, more intense and less intense muscle work as well as balancing flexibility with strength and endurance (Harding 2003). As has been seen with exercising in general, individuals with JHS need to increase activity levels more slowly to reduce the risk of flare-ups.

SPECIFIC EXERCISE

It is important that the exercises prescribed are specific and target the intended muscle, movement or task. The form of the exercise or movement is of paramount importance. Remedial exercise becomes as much cognitive as it is physical. For the patient to learn the skills necessary to gain effective control of movement it is necessary for them to engage with their body and develop greater body awareness. Education regarding anatomy, biomechanics and how this particular exercise will help their problem, along with imagery and biofeedback, are powerful tools. Mental practice of motor imagery (mental representation of movement without any body movement) has been shown to improve motor and task performance with the greatest improvement occurring when interventions combine physical and mental practice (Dickstein & Deutsch 2007). In addition, studies have shown that motor imagery can increase muscle strength (Zijdewind et al 2003, Sidaway & Trzaska 2005). This is thought to occur as a result of neural adaptations such as degree of motor unit activation, improved coordination and decreased co-contraction of antagonist muscles (Sidaway & Trzaska 2005). Although the effects of motor imagery in JHS have not been studied clinical experience suggests it is a valuable adjunct to treatment.

While exercising they can be taught techniques to check that their postural alignment remains good, that a certain muscle is not dominant, that a weaker or more inhibited muscle is working. This can be achieved through the use of video, mirrors, pressure biofeedback and the therapist's input. However, if the patient is ultimately to be able to make use of these skills to prevent and correct problems in the future, they have to develop the ability to correct themselves.

Generic exercises do not work without good instruction and practice, because invariably an individual will 'take the path of least resistance'. Patients usually take the easy option, or if they have been in pain, long-standing compensatory strategies may inhibit weaker, less dominant or 'forgotten' muscles. The inhibition of the vastus medialis obliquus (VMO) following knee surgery is well known to physiotherapists. Facilitation is needed to 'switch' the correct muscle on, as is ensuring the reduction of swelling and pain. It is important that an assessment highlights an individual's muscle imbalance and corrects it. It may be appropriate to use manual therapy to inhibit overactive muscles and facilitate underactive ones. This then forms the exercise and is practised in a simple easy way and gradually made more challenging. Although hypermobile individuals do not appear to suffer inflammation in the same way, the principles are similar. Without EMG devices (Chapter 12.1) it is often difficult to tell which muscle is working, but palpation (therapists or patient) and feel (patient feedback) can be used successfully, as well as being critical of the form the exercise is taking from the perspective of the whole body.

In the fibromyalgia literature it is thought that 'exercises that are too vigorous might trigger immune activation with release of pro-inflammatory cytokines provoking a sickness response' (Maier & Watkins 1998), which may be a factor in the exacerbation of symptoms that JHS individuals often report. Exercise should be pain free, although a distinction is made between training pain and an aggravation of symptoms. If an exercise is painful it is either not being performed correctly or is not 'right' for that patient at that particular moment in time. In the author's experience this is particularly true for individuals with fibromyalgia and JHS and time spent modifying an exercise until it is pain-free but still achieving its aim pays dividends in terms of patient confidence and progression.

For those individuals who do not achieve a good response with the treatment approach outlined above, a multi-disciplinary pain management programme (PMP) may be required. There is, however, some evidence to suggest that patients with chronic pain, either caused by hypermobility or in the presence of hypermobility, do not respond as well as expected in a PMP. Hakim & Ashton (2005), on analysing the characteristics of those who did poorly in a PMP, found hypermobility to be a common finding. This does not appear to be an isolated case and a programme modified to hypermobile individuals is going some way to address this problem (Chapter 8).

STRETCHING

Many hypermobiles like to stretch, but have been advised not to by health professionals for fear of damaging their tissues or joints through overstretching. An unpublished audit at Guy's Hospital in 1986 reported by Harding (2003) revealed that patients with joint hypermobility found stretching helpful. This came as a surprise to the audit's authors, but has been borne out repeatedly in clinical experience. Stiffness is a common complaint, with many hypermobiles saying they 'feel like a 90-year-old', but it is not clear what produces this feeling. We know that hypermobile joints, like non-hypermobile joints, stiffen through disuse in response to pain, but it is also possible that hypermobile individuals are more likely to use their global muscles for stability and are therefore subject to more increased muscle tension and spasm. Stretching can be a helpful antidote to this, but it is important that the hypermobile individual does not overstretch, which is potentially easy to do.

It becomes necessary to differentiate between stretching performed in order to regain and maintain muscle length, relieve muscle tension, or restore and maintain joint range, and stretching to increase an already hypermobile range of motion. It is good to stretch, but care is required. Educating an individual about how they can stretch safely without overstretching into their hypermobile or more vulnerable areas will help develop better body awareness, a skill which can be used in the future to ensure safe exercising.

EDUCATION AND ADVICE

The power of finally receiving a diagnosis after years of searching, suffering and frustration can not be overemphasized. Knowledge is empowering. It allows the patient to move from negative to more positive emotions and start to focus on ways of managing their condition, safe in the knowledge that it is not a life-threatening disorder, and that with the correct input they can make a significant change, not only to their own life, but also to the lives of family and friends.

Understanding the implications of the disorder is thought to help an individual cope more effectively with pain (Russek 1999). Education about the condition is one of the most important aspects of medical intervention and forms a major part of physiotherapy and occupational therapy input. It will generally consist of advice regarding joint care, lifestyle modifications, the judicious use of aids and supports, help with associated problems, exercise and fitness. As therapists we are usually able to give our patients more time, to listen to their individual anxieties or concerns. This helps to gain a full understanding of how the condition is impacting on their life and reassures the patient that someone is finally taking them seriously. Detailed discussion about their daily activities can identify specific problems, which, with a problem-solving approach, can be resolved, better managed and prevented from recurring.

JOINT CARE

Hypermobile individuals tend to rest at the end of their range of movements, particularly at the knees, hips and lumbar spine. Educating patients to avoid unhelpful postures such as 'W' sitting (Fig. 9.8), sitting with the leg tucked under the buttock, sitting cross-legged 'Indian style' and kneeling on plantarflexed feet or resting on the lateral borders of the feet (Fig. 9.1b) for prolonged periods will help to prevent soft tissue strain and subsequent symptoms. Further advice on joint care is given in Chapter 12.2.

Joint care for therapists

Work-related thumb pain is an occupational hazard for manual therapists around the world (Glover et al 2005, McMahon et al 2006, Campo et al 2008), and the presence of hypermobility may be a significant factor in its development (Fig. 9.9). The lifetime prevalence of thumb problems in Australian physiotherapists was 65% with a current prevalence of 41% in the observational study by McMahon et al (2006). Factors found to be significantly associated with thumb problems included thumb joint hypermobility or an inability to stabilize the joints of the thumb. Hypermobility of the carpometacarpal (CMC) joint (see Chapter 12.2) of the thumb and decreased thumb strength were significant factors

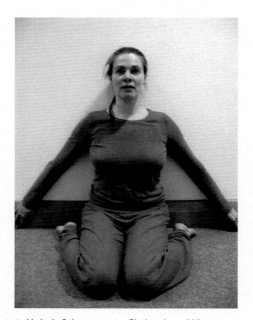

Fig. 9.8 Unhelpful postures. Sitting in a 'W'

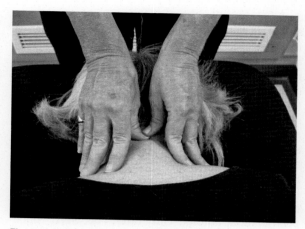

Fig. 9.9 Hypermobility in the thumb and fingers of a therapist while performing manual therapy techniques on the cervical spine

contributing to thumb pain in another study of Australian physiotherapists (Snodgrass et al 2003) and generalized joint hypermobility (considered with a score of 3/9 on the Beighton scale) was more prevalent (although not statistically significant) in the pain group compared to the non-pain group. Interestingly, although there was no difference between the prevalence of osteoarthritis (visible on radiographs) in the pain and non-pain groups, the prevalence of osteoarthritis in females in this study was higher than in a normal population (19% compared to 2% respectively). This suggests that female physiotherapists are more at risk of developing osteoarthritis at the CMC joint than the normal population and that hypermobility (both at the joint and in general) in addition to occupation may be a contributing factor.

The type and duration of therapy is also a contributing factor. Campo et al (2008) found that manual techniques of soft tissue work and joint mobilizations increased the risk of work-related musculoskeletal disorders in the wrist and hand by 14 and 8 times respectively in those Physical Therapists in the USA who treated ten or more patients a day. It is clearly important that therapists engaged in manual therapy are made aware of the risks and encouraged to take appropriate measures. These will include modifying techniques, using equipment (massage tools, mobilization wedge), reducing hours or patients and wearing protective splints (Chapter 12.2).

Other areas of the body have the potential to cause problems in an occupation as physically

active as physiotherapy. Patient transfers, patient repositioning and bent or twisted postures have been given as factors in the development of back pain (Campo et al 2008) and the hypermobile physiotherapist would be well advised to take extra care to avoid problems. As yet, hypermobility is not screened for in the student physiotherapy population, but should possibly be considered in order to highlight those at risk of problems from performing or having performed on them repeated mobilization/manipulation techniques during their under- or particularly post-graduate studies.

LIFESTYLE MODIFICATIONS

There can be specific areas of concern regarding work, home and family life. Helpful advice on activities of daily living is given in Keer et al (2003) and the issues of hypermobility and work-related musculoskeletal disorders are discussed in Mangharam (2003).

Computer use is ubiquitous, often ergonomically unsound, and frequently intense. Optimal ergonomic positioning while at the computer should be encouraged for all patients and keyboard short cuts should be used wherever possible in order to decrease mouse usage during a session at the computer.

Some general concepts that are readily accepted when using a computer keyboard and mouse are:
- keep wrists neutral
- do not rest wrists while typing
- move the whole arm while keying
- avoid stretching the fingers to reach keys that are far away
- keep fingers curved and relaxed
- use a light touch
- keep fingernails short (Stegink-Jansen et al 2000)
- avoid double clicking as much as possible when using the mouse
- position mouse within easy reach to avoid overstretching.

Specific advice regarding pregnancy is discussed in Chapter 12.6 and sport and performance in Chapter 13.

AIDS AND SUPPORTS

In general, the use of aids and supports is discouraged because it can encourage muscle weakness and dependency. However, there is a place for supporting an area during the recovery phase of an injury with a gradual decrease in use, as discussed above. Furthermore, if there is a risk of continued strain to a joint, despite attempts to improve stability and muscle strength, there is an argument for judicious use of an aid or support. This may involve wearing a collar for travelling, to help prevent a neck strain as a result of sudden stops or humps in the road, or wearing a support on the knee to be able to take part in a particular sport. Aids and supports can be particularly helpful in the hand to enable individuals to continue to work and these are described in more detail in Chapter 12.2.

ASSOCIATED PROBLEMS

There may be other areas in the body producing symptoms as a consequence of lax connective tissue. Flat feet are common and it may be sensible to enlist the help of a podiatrist to perform a gait analysis and possibly fit orthotics. Urogenital problems, such as prolapse and urinary incontinence, may require referral to a specialist physiotherapist for a pelvic examination and advice regarding pelvic floor exercises (Chapter 12.6). Many hypermobiles suffer symptoms of irritable bowel and in cases advice on diet and reduction in constipation-inducing medication can be sufficient while others benefit from more extensive investigations and treatment as described in Chapters 6.2 and 6.3. A poor response to local anaesthetics, if present (Arendt-Niesen et al 1990, Hakim et al 2005), can be distressing for some hypermobiles when attending the dentist or obstetrician and liaison and education with other health professionals can reduce anxiety. The tendency towards low blood pressure and (pre-) syncope may be relieved by an increase in lower limb muscle work and taking in a little more water and salt, but if these measures fail, further investigation and treatment of the autonomic nervous system may be required (Chapter 6.1).

GENERAL EXERCISE AND FITNESS

Once the patient has regained a good level of function and has control of their pain, attention can move to developing a fitness programme

and helping the patient return to their chosen activities and sport (Chapter 13). In general, unsupervised sessions in the gym are not advisable for the hypermobile patient, because they may over-do the exercises or do them incorrectly, or indeed exercises may take the patient into their hypermobile range and thus sessions with a trained therapist are advised initially. The therapist can teach, observe and correct the patient to ensure they can perform the exercises/tasks in an accurate and controlled way. We only retain a little of what we are taught and this lends weight to the argument of a review with the patient to check performance at a later date. Some unexpected adaptations can often be seen once patients have been left to exercise on their own. Exercising in the gym is not for everyone, so discussion with the patient may identify sports, activities or other exercise which will enable maintenance of fitness. Particularly good suggestions include Pilates, Alexander Technique and Tai Chi where the emphasis is on slow, controlled movement. Yoga is not contraindicated but care should be taken to avoid overstretching. Good instruction and supervision in the initial stages is essential. It is helpful to find an activity which is enjoyable and achievable so the patient is motivated to develop a life-long habit of exercise (Keer 2003). This subject is discussed in more detail in Chapter 13.

SUMMARY

Generalized joint hypermobility and JHS are frequently overlooked in musculoskeletal conditions, but they are not difficult to identify when looked for and should be a consideration in all musculoskeletal pain presentations. JHS requires a holistic approach in terms of assessment and management, which may involve a multidisciplinary team.

An individualized, modified, therapeutic programme is recommended, based on functional restoration with the emphasis on movement control, joint stability and self-management. Early, accurate diagnosis and effective intervention will help to prevent the downward spiral into chronic pain and deconditioning and thereby reduce suffering.

References

Acasuso-Diaz M, Collantes-Estevez E, Sanchez Guijo P: Joint hyperlaxity and musculoskeletal lesions: study of a population of homogenous age, sex and physical exertion, *Br J Rheumatol* 32:120–122, 1993.

Acasuso-Diaz M, Collantes-Estevez E: Joint hypermobility in patients with fibromyalgia, *Arthritis Care Res* 11:39–42, 1998.

Ageberg E, Flenhagen J, Ljung J: Test-retest reliability of knee kinaesthesia in healthy adults, *Bio Med Central Musculoskeletal Disorders* 8:57, 2007.

Al-Rawi ZS, Al-Aszawi AJ, Al-Chalabi T: Joint mobility among university students in Iraq, *Br J Rheumatol* 4:326–331, 1985.

Aminaka N, Gribble PA: Patellar taping, patellofemoral pain syndrome, lower extremity kinematics and dynamic postural control, *Journal of Athletic Training* 43:21–28, 2008.

Arendt-Nielsen L, Kaaland P, Bjerring P, et al: Insufficient effect of local analgesics in Ehlers-Danlos type III patients (connective tissue disorder), *Acta Anaesthesiol Scand* 34:358–361, 1990.

Beighton PH, Solomon L, Soskolne CL: Articular mobility in an African population, *Annals of Rheumatology Disease* 32:413–418, 1973.

Beighton P, Grahame R, Bird H: *Hypermobility of Joints*, ed 3, London, 1999, Springer Verlag.

Biro F, Gewanter HL, Baum J: The hypermobility syndrome, *Pediatrics* 72:701–706, 1983.

Bridges AJ, Smith E, Reid J: Joint hypermobility in adults referred to rheumatology clinics, *Ann Rheum Dis* 51:793–796, 1992.

Butler DS: *The Sensitive Nervous System*, Adelaide, Australia, 2000, Neuro Orthopaedic Institute (NOI) Publications.

Callaghan MJ, Selfe J, Bagley PJ, et al: The effects of patellar taping on knee joint proprioception, *Journal of Athletic Training* 37(1):19–24, 2002.

Callaghan MJ, Selfe J, Mc Henry A, et al: Effects of patellar taping on knee joint proprioception in patients with patellofemoral pain syndrome, *Man Ther* 13(3):192–199, 2008.

Campo M, Weiser S, Koenig KL, et al: Work-Related Musculoskeletal Disorders in Physical Therapists: A Prospective Cohort Study With 1-Year Follow-up, *Phys Ther* 88(5):608–619, 2008.

Cherpel A, Marks R: The benign joint hypermobility syndrome, *New Zealand Journal of Physiotherapy* 27:9–22, 1999.

Christou EA: Patellar taping increases vastus medialis oblique activity in the presence of patellofemoral pain, *J Electromyogr Kinesiol* 14(4):495–504, 2004.

Cooper K, Smith BH, Hancock E: Patient-centredness in physiotherapy from the perspective of the chronic low back pain patient, *Physiotherapy* 94:244–252, 2008.

Dickstein R, Deutsch JE: Motor imagery in physical therapy practice, *Phys Ther* 87(7):942–953, 2007.

Dommerholt J, Norris RN: Physical therapy management of the instrumental musician, *Orthopaedic Physical Therapy Clinics of North America* 6:185, 1997.

El-Shahaly HA, El-Sherif AK: Is the benign hypermobility syndrome benign? *Clin Rheumatol* 10:302–307, 1991.

Ferrell WR, Tennant N, Sturrock RD, et al: Amelioration of symptoms by enhancement of proprioception in patients with joint hypermobility syndrome, *Arthritis & Rheumatism* 50:3323–3328, 2004.

Finsterbush A, Pogrund H: The hypermobility syndrome. Musculoskeletal complaints in 100 consecutive cases of generalised joint hypermobility, *Clin Orthop* 168:124–127, 1982.

Francis H, March L, Terenty T, et al: Benign joint hypermobility with neuropathy: documentation and mechanism of tarsal tunnel syndrome, *J Rheumatol* 14(3):577–581, 1987.

Gawthrop F, Mould R, Sperritt A, et al: A patient's journey: Ehlers-Danlos syndrome, *Br Med J* 335:448–450, 2007.

Gazit Y, Nahir AM, Grahame R, et al: Dysautonomia in the hypermobility syndrome, *Am J Med* 115:33–40, 2003.

Glover W, McGregor A, Sullivan C, et al: Work-related musculoskeletal disorders affecting members of the Chartered Society of Physiotherapy, *Physiotherapy* 91:138–147, 2005.

Goldman JA: Hypermobility and deconditioning: Important links to Fibromyalgia/Fibrositis, *South Med J* 84:1192–1196, 1991.

Gordon C, Gueth JN: Fibromyalgia Syndrome: Fact, Fiction, and Future Remedies, *Critical Reviews in Physical and Rehabilitation Medicine* 18(4):343–369, 2006.

Grahame R, Bird HA, Child A, et al: The revised (Brighton 1998) criteria for the diagnosis of benign joint hypermobility syndrome (BJHS), *J Rheumatol* 27:1777–1779, 2000.

Grahame R: Hypermobility and the heritable disorders of connective tissue. In Keer R, Grahame R, editors: *Hypermobility Syndrome: Recognition and Management for Physiotherapists*, Edinburgh, 2003, Butterworth Heinemann, pp 23–24.

Hakim A, Grahame R: A simple questionnaire to detect

hypermobility: an adjunct to the assessment of patients with diffuse musculoskeletal pain, *Int J Clin Pract* 57:163–166, 2003.

Hakim AJ, Ashton S: Undiagnosed, Joint Hypermobility Syndrome patients have poorer outcome than peers following chronic back pain rehabilitation, *Rheumatology* 44(3 Suppl 1):255, 2005.

Hakim AJ, Norris P, Hopper C, et al: Local Anaesthetic Failure; Does Joint Hypermobility Provide The Answer? *J R Soc Med* 298(2):84, 2005.

Hall MG, Ferrell WR, Sturrock RD, et al: The effect of the hypermobility syndrome on knee joint proprioception, *Br J Rheumatol* 34:121–125, 1995.

Harding V: Joint Hypermobility and chronic pain: possible linking mechanisms and management highlighted by a cognitive-behavioural approach. In Keer, Grahame, editors: *Hypermobility Syndrome: Recognition and Management for physiotherapists*, Edinburgh, 2003, Butterworth Heinemann, pp 147–161.

Harrelson GL: Physiological factors of rehabilitation. In Andrews JR, Harrelson GL, Wilk KE, editors: *Physical Rehabilitation of the Injured Athlete*, ed 2, London, 1998, WB Saunders, pp 13–37.

Hides JA, Richardson CA, Jull GA: Multifidus muscle recovery is not automatic after resolution of acute, first-episode low back pain, *Spine* 21:2763–2769, 1996.

HMSA Newsletter, Autumn 2006, p 6 & 9.

Hodges PW, Richardson CA: Inefficient muscular stabilization of the lumbar spine associated with low back pain. A motor control evaluation of transverses abdominus, *Spine* 21:2640–2650, 1996.

Hodges PW, Richardson CA: Delayed postural contraction of transversus abdominis in low back pain associated with

movement of the lower limb, *J Spinal Disord* 11:46–56, 1998.

Hudson N, Starr MR, Esdaile JM, et al: Diagnostic associations with hypermobility in rheumatology patients, *Br J Rheumatol* 34:1157–1161, 1995.

Hudson N, Fitzcharles M-A, Cohen M, et al: The association of soft tissue rheumatism and hypermobility, *Br J Rheumatol* 37:382–386, 1998.

Juul-Kristensen B, Lund H, Hansen K, et al: Poorer elbow proprioception in patients with lateral epicondylitis than in healthy controls: a cross sectional study, *J Shoulder Elbow Surg* 17:72S–81S, 2008.

Juul-Kristensen B, Lund H, Hansen K, et al: Test-retest reliability of joint position sense and kinaesthetic sense in the elbow of healthy subjects, *Physiother Theory Pract* 24:65–72, 2008.

Kaplinsky C, Kenet G, Seligsohn U, et al: Association between hyperflexibility of the thumb and an unexplained bleeding tendency: is it a rule of thumb? *Br J Haematol* 101:260–263, 1998.

Keer R, Edwards-Fowler A, Mansi E: Management of the hypermobile adult. In Keer R, Grahame R, editors: *Hypermobility Syndrome: Recognition and Management for Physiotherapists*, Edinburgh, 2003, Butterworth Heinemann, p 89.

Kendall FP, McCreary EK, Provance PG: *Muscles Testing and Function*, ed 4, Baltimore, 1993, Williams & Wilkins.

Kerr A, Macmillan C, Uttley W, et al: Physiotherapy for children with hypermobility syndrome, *Physiotherapy* 86:313–316, 2000.

Kirk JA, Ansell BM, Bywaters EGL: The hypermobility syndrome. Muscular complaints associated with generalized joint hypermobility, *Ann Rheum Dis* 26:419–425, 1967.

Larsson LG, Baum J, Mudholker GS, et al: Benefits and disadvantages of joint hypermobility among musicians, *N Engl J Med* 329:1079–1082, 1993.

Larsson LG, Mudholker GS, Baum J, et al: Benefits and liabilities of hypermobility in the back pain disorders of industrial workers, *J Intern Med* 5:461–467, 1995.

Lee D, Lee LJ: *Course notes 10 day series: The lumbopelvic hip course*, 2007, Twickenham, UK.

Macgregor K, Gerlach S, Mellor R, et al: Cutaneous stimulation from patellar tape causes a differential increase in vasti muscle activity in people with patellofemoral pain, *Journal of Orthopaedic Research* 23(2):351–358, 2005.

Maier SF, Watkins LR: Cytokines for psychologicals: implications of bidirectional immune-to-brain communication for understanding behaviour, mood, and cognition, *Psychol Rev* 105:83–107, 1998.

Maillard S, Murray K: Hypermobility Syndrome in children. In Keer R, Grahame R, editors: *Hypermobility Syndrome: Recognition and Management for Physiotherapists*, Edinburgh, 2003, Butterworth Heinemann, p 42.

Maitland GD: *Vertebral Manipulation*, ed 5, London, 1986, Butterworth Scientific.

Mallik AK, Ferrell WR, McDonald AG, et al: Impaired proprioceptive acuity at the proximal interphalangeal joint in patients with the hypermobility syndrome, *Br J Rheumatol* 33:631–637, 1994.

Mangharam J: Joint hypermobility and work-related musculoskeletal disorders (WRMSD). In Keer R, Grahame R, editors: *Hypermobility Syndrome: Recognition and Management for Physiotherapists*, Edinburgh, 2003, Butterworth Heinemann, pp 127–146.

March LM, Francis H, Webb J: Benign joint hypermobility with neuropathies: documentation and mechanism of median, sciatic, and common peroneal nerve compression, *Clin Rheumatol* 7(1):35–40, 1988.

Mattacola CG, Dwyer MK: Rehabilitation of the ankle after acute sprain or chronic instability, *Journal of Athletic Training* 37:413–429, 2002.

May S, Johnson R: Stabilisation exercises for low back pain: a systematic review, *Physiotherapy* 94:179–189, 2008.

McMahon M, Stiller K, Trott P: The prevalence of thumb problems in Australian physiotherapists is high: an observational study, *Australian Journal of Physiotherapy* 52:287–292, 2006.

Mottram SL: Dynamic stability of the scapula, *Man Ther* 2:123–131, 1997.

Ocarino JM, Fonseca ST, Silva PL, et al: Alterations of stiffness and resting position of the elbow joint following flexors resistance training, *Man Ther* 13:411–418, 2008.

Oliver J: Hypermobility: Recognition and Management, *In Touch* 94:9–12, 2000.

O'Sullivan PB, Phyty GD, Twomey LT, et al: Evaluation of specific stabilizing exercise in the treatment of chronic low back pain with radiologic diagnosis of spondylolysis or spondylolisthesis, *Spine* 22:2959–2967, 1997.

O'Sullivan PB: Lumbar segmental 'instability': clinical presentation and specific stabilizing exercise management, *Man Ther* 5:2–12, 2000.

Panjabi MM: The stabilizing system of the spine. Part1. Function, dysfunction, adaptation and enhancement, *J Spinal Disord* 5:383–389, 1992.

Philipson L, Sorbye R, Larsson P, et al: Muscular load levels in performing musicians as monitored by electromyography, *Medical Problems of Performing Artists* 5:79–82, 1990.

Phipps C: I still don't think anybody believes me, *The Guardian* 14th Oct, 2003.

Polnauer FF, Marks M: *Senso-motor study and its application to violin playing*, Urbana, Ill, 1964, American String Teachers Association.

Preference Collaborative Review Group: Patients' preferences within randomized trials: systemic review and patient level meta-analysis, *Br Med J* 337:a1864, 2008.

Ramsay J, Riddoch J: Position-matching in the upper limb: professional ballet dancers perform with outstanding accuracy, *Clin Rehabil* 15:324–330, 2001.

Richardson C, Hodges PW, Hides J: *Therapeutic Exercise for lumbopelvic stabilization*, ed 2, Edinburgh, 2004, Churchill Livingstone.

Rose BS: The hypermobility syndrome. Loose-limbed and liable, *New Zealand Journal of Physiotherapy* 13:18–19, 1985.

Russek LN: Hypermobility syndrome, *Phys Ther* 79:591–599, 1999.

Russek LN: Examination and treatment of a patient with hypermobility syndrome, *Phys Ther* 80:386–398, 2000.

Sahrmann SA: *Diagnosis and Treatment of Movement Impairment Syndromes*, St Louis, 2002, Mosby Inc.

Sidaway B, Trzaska (Robinson) A: Can mental practice increase ankle dorsiflexor torque? *Phys Ther* 85(10):1053–1060, 2005.

Simmonds JV, Keer R: Hypermobility and the hypermobility syndrome, *Man Ther* 12:298–309, 2007.

Simmonds JV, Keer R: Hypermobility and the hypermobility syndrome Part 2: Assessment and management of hypermobility syndrome: illustrated via case studies, *Man Ther* 13(2):e1–e11, 2008.

Snodgrass SJ, Rivett DA, Chiarelli P, et al: Factors related to thumb pain in physiotherapists, *Aust J Physiother* 49:243–250, 2003.

Stegink-Jansen CW, Patterson R, Viegas SF: Effects of fingernail length on finger and hand performance, *J Hand Ther* 13(3):211–217, 2000.

Tsao H, Hodges PW: Immediate changes in feedforward postural adjustments following voluntary motor training, *Exp Brain Res* 181:537–546, 2007.

Vierck CJ: Mechanisms underlying development of spatial distributed chronic pain (fibromyalgia), *Pain* 124:242–263, 2006.

Wynne-Davies R: Familial joint laxity, *Proc R Soc Med* 64:689–690, 1971.

Zijdewind I, Toering ST, Bessem B, et al: Effects of motor training on torque production of ankle plantar flexor muscles, *Muscle Nerve* 28(2):168–173, 2003.

Chapter 10

Physiotherapy and occupational therapy in the hypermobile adolescent

Alison Middleditch

INTRODUCTION

During adolescence the physical, physiological and psychological changes that occur have an impact on the diagnosis and management of joint hypermobility syndrome (JHS). Joint laxity is usually greatest at birth, decreases during childhood, and continues to reduce during adolescence and adult life. The tightness or relative laxity of a ligament is an important factor in governing the available joint range of an individual. Other factors, such as the shape of the joint surfaces, muscle length and the mobility of the neural structures also affect range of movement. These factors continue to change throughout the adolescent growth period and affect the extent of range of movement in both those with JHS and those with 'normal tissues'.

An adolescent may be unaware that their joints are hypermobile (JHM) but may believe they are 'double-jointed' and use their excessive range to do contortionist or 'party tricks'.

PREVALENCE

Studies on the prevalence of JHS in children must be viewed with caution because of the variability of diagnostic criteria used. The reported prevalence of JHM in children varies from 6.7% of British school children (Carter & Wilkinson 1964) to 39.6% of Caucasian Brazilian school children (Forleo et al 1993) (Chapter 11). There have been no studies that have specifically investigated the incidence of JHS in adolescents (Table 10.1).

GROWTH

During adolescence, the rapid rate of growth affecting both the bony and soft tissue elements can be a contributory factor in the development of symptoms in individuals with JHM or JHS. It is essential to have a thorough understanding of normal growth and developmental characteristics to provide a basis for realistic expectations when dealing with adolescents.

Growth rates

In early childhood both girls and boys grow at a similar rate in height and weight. The most rapid rate of growth occurs just before birth and it then remains relatively steady until adolescence. The rate of growth is disproportionate throughout the body: until the teenage years the rate of growth is greater in the limbs than the spine, but during adolescence the rate of growth is greater in the trunk. The peak height velocity (adolescent growth spurt) occurs approximately two years after the onset of puberty (Porter 1989). The onset of puberty is approximately 10.5 years of age in girls and 12.5 years in boys. There is a change of body shape and proportion in various body parts during this growth period. On average girls add between 6–11 cm and boys 7–12 cm to their height during this period. Most girls have reached 99% of their adult height by the time they are 15 whereas boys reach adult stature between 18 and 21 years old. Although peak height velocity occurs earlier in girls, boys eventually surpass girls to attain a larger adult stature. By the age of 18, the average boy is 12 cm taller and 10 kg heavier than the average 18-year-old girl (Riddoch 1991).

DOI: 10.1016/B978-0-7020-3005-5.00014-8

Table 10.1 Prevalence of joint hypermobility in different populations of adolescents					
POPULATION	CRITERIA USED	AGE	NO. OF SUBJECTS	TOTAL % HYPERMOBILE	REFERENCE
US adolescent athletes	Beighton 5/9	15.5 average	264	12.9%	Decoster et al 1997
Dutch school children	Beighton 5/9	12–17	658	13.4%	Rikken-Bultman et al 1997
Icelandic school children	Beighton 4/9	12	267	26.7%	Qvindesland & Jonsson 1999
Turkish high school children	Beighton 4/9	13–19	861	11.7%	Seçkin et al 2005

When treating an adolescent it is useful to monitor whether the individual is going through a rapid growth phase. Some adolescents will grow steadily throughout their teenage years whereas others will have periods of rapid growth spurts. It is essential to measure standing height and sitting height separately to give an indication of the relative rate of growth of the limbs and spine. Measurement of sitting height (stem height) is considered to be a measurement of spinal height.

Co-ordination

There is a perceived 'adolescent awkwardness' that accompanies the growth spurt and manifests in poor co-ordination and balance. There is some evidence (Beunen & Malina 1988) that this clumsiness affects one-third of teenage boys, lasts up to 6 months and is probably a result of the disproportionate rate of growth between the trunk and legs.

Flexibility

In adolescence there is often a reduction in flexibility in both those with JHM and those with normal tissues. It has been thought that during the growth spurt, the growth of the bony elements often outstrips that of the soft tissue elements (Thein 1996) and there is a subsequent decrease in strength and flexibility. It is this stage in development that tissues can become overstressed in a cumulative overload, and many adolescents find that their joints are less lax and movements are stiffer. Until the muscles catch up with the increase in bone length they are under a degree of tension that is felt as increased muscle tightness and this may be one of the causes of growing pains in adolescents. In addition, the lumbar fascia may not be able to keep pace with the bony growth spurt during adolescence which can result in increased tension and tethering in the thoracolumbar fascia giving rise to an increased lumbar lordosis. Typical postural changes at this time include:

- tight thoracolumbar fascia
- tight hamstrings
- increased lordosis
- decreased abdominal strength
- a compensatory thoracic kyphosis.

Some adolescents with JHM will not notice any increase in stiffness, but others will notice a reduction in joint laxity in a range that nevertheless remains hypermobile. As changes occur in the muscles and more sarcomeres (the contractile unit of muscle) are laid down, flexibility may improve again. However, a study of 600 high-school children did not find any correlation between growth and decreased flexibility during the peripubescent period (Feldman et al 1999).

Weight

Weight increases steadily throughout childhood and adolescence. Peak weight velocity follows peak height velocity and is closer to age in boys than girls. In boys the difference between peak height velocity and peak weight velocity ranges from 0.2 to 0.4 years whereas the ratio for girls is 0.3 to 0.9 years (Malina et al 2004). A study measuring pre- and post-puberty weight change showed that boys increase in weight by an average of 113% and girls by an average of 67% (Buckler 1990). This increase in mass (body weight) substantially increases the ground reaction forces to which the joints are subjected, and the more fragile tissues of a child with JHS become vulnerable if joint stability is further compromised by poor muscle control.

Increase in muscle mass and strength are proportional to weight gain during adolescence (Thein 1996). A boy's muscle mass will double between the ages of 11 and 17 years, and peak height and muscle growth occur simultaneously. A girl's muscle mass doubles between 9–15 years of age, and the fastest growth is approximately 6 months after peak height velocity. In both sexes increases in muscle strength closely follow increases in muscle mass, which occur approximately 9–12 months after peak height and weight gain (Porter 1989).

Bone

Bone maturation is the process whereby the tissue undergoes changes from the embryonic rudiment of bone to the adult form (Roche 1986). Before puberty chronological age correlates well with bone age but during adolescence bone age is more closely related to adult maturity levels, so that bone age is related to the timing of puberty and growth in height in an individual (Roche 1986). Hence, two adolescents of the same chronological age can have different levels of bone maturation owing to differences in timing of onset of puberty. This can be particularly relevant in teenagers who are playing contact sports (Chapter 13) in teams where the selection criterion is based on age rather than skeletal maturity.

The increase in height and decrease in muscle strength and coordination that occurs during adolescence is compounded further by dramatically changing hormone levels. Furthermore, changes in body shape and size also challenge the self-image of the teenager and this must be considered when treating an adolescent with JHS.

CLINICAL PRESENTATION

The presence of JHM in adolescents, as in other age groups, does not equate to having JHS so that hypermobile individuals do not necessarily develop problems and may even consider the increased flexibility to be an asset (Grahame 2003). Symptoms may arise as a result of hypermobility at any age and JHS is seen more frequently in girls. JHS is a common cause of referral for musculoskeletal symptoms in children and adolescents (Murray & Woo 2001) and one study reported three-quarters of hypermobile subjects had developed symptoms before the age of 15 (Kirk et al 1967). JHS is under-diagnosed and adolescents with the condition are often dismissed as having growing pains or emotional problems (Chapter 2).

Pain

Although pain is usually the predominant symptom, the adolescent may present with a variety of different problems. Pain may be widespread, or confined to just one joint. Common symptoms described by hypermobile adolescents include joint and muscle aches which are often worse at night, frequent and excessive joint noises (clicking, popping, clunks), a history of subluxation or dislocation (particularly of the patella, shoulder or temporomandibular joint), non-specific low back pain, joint effusions and repetitive strain injury (RSI). They may also complain of a feeling of weakness or vulnerability as if a joint is going to lock or 'go out of place'. Other symptoms include paraesthesia, chest pain, fainting and light-headedness. Headaches are also a familiar feature of JHS in adolescents. Symptoms may be worse after periods of prolonged inactivity, such as a long journey, or following vigorous or unusual activity. At a time when the adolescent body is going through rapid physiological and psychological change the onset of symptoms can be particularly worrying to the teenager.

Function and posture

There are a number of functional activities that adolescents with JHS may find problematic. They often have difficulty sitting still for any length of time, probably owing to their inability to find a comfortable, stable position, and have a tendency to fidget. In the classroom this may result in the child being labelled as inattentive or hyperactive. Adolescents have particular difficulty sitting on high stools in science laboratories because they are unsupported without an adequate back support. The problem can be compounded further if the stool does not have a foot rest that would allow transference of body weight through the legs. The inability to place the feet on a foot rest or the ground also compromises the stability of the trunk.

In common with adults, some adolescents with JHS report that prolonged standing brings on symptoms of low back, knee and foot pain. Standing in queues and school assemblies can be a particular problem. An upright relaxed balanced posture requires good muscle tone and conditioning.

Adolescents with JHS tend to shift their weight frequently from foot to foot, often locking one knee into hyperextension and pushing the hip into extension. In this position, the individual hangs on the hip ligaments rather than using the pelvic postural muscles for support. This creates an accumulative overload of the joints and soft tissues, often giving rise to symptoms.

Another common problem is pain in the forearm, wrist and fingers when writing or using the computer for a sustained period. This can lead to symptoms of repetitive strain injury and can be particularly difficult when writing at speed and under stress in exam conditions.

Co-ordination

Adolescents with JHS may also report that they are clumsy, have poor co-ordination, bruise easily and may fall more frequently than children with 'normal tissues'.

Fatigue

Adolescents with JHS may complain of an overwhelming fatigue. In a matched case-control study comparing Beighton joint hypermobility scores (Chapter 1) in 58 consecutive children with chronic fatigue syndrome (CFS) with 58 healthy controls (Barron et al 2002), it was found that there was a higher incidence of JHM in those with CFS than in the control group. Nijs et al (2006) also found that generalized JHM is more common in patients with CFS than in healthy controls (Chapter 6.1).

A study has shown an association between JHM and malnutrition. A cross-sectional field study of 829 children of the lower urban socio-economic strata in Mumbai, aged 3–11 years, found that moderate and severe malnutrition were associated with JHM and that moderately and severely malnourished hypermobile children were more likely to have musculoskeletal symptoms as compared to their non-hypermobile counterparts (Hasija et al 2008).

COMMON PROBLEMS IN THE HYPERMOBILE ADOLESCENT

Adolescents with JHS may present with pain in a single joint or pain at multiple sites. Problem areas include the back, knees, feet, shoulders and temporomandibular joint.

SPINAL PROBLEMS

Lumbar spine

Hypermobile subjects are particularly susceptible to low back pain, and the incidence of lumbar disc prolapse, pars interarticularis defects and even spondylolisthesis occurs with increased frequency in hypermobile individuals (Chapter 12.8).

Non-specific low back pain is a common problem in hypermobile adolescents and occurs in the absence of demonstrable radiological change, neurological signs or identifiable back pathology. Studies have shown that there is a relationship between joint laxity and low back pain (Chabot 1962, Hirsch et al 1969, Howes & Isdale 1971, Gedalia et al 1985).

Adolescents with non-specific low back pain and JHS frequently have poor static and dynamic control of the deep trunk and pelvic stabilizing muscles thus compromising their ability to perform normal functional activities. This control is frequently inadequate in static postures and is compromised further during daily functional activities, particularly those that are performed at speed or include a change in direction of motion.

Scoliosis

It is reported that there is a link between adolescent idiopathic scoliosis (AIS) and JHM. A study of a group of 109 Chinese girls with AIS found them to have more joint flexibility than a control group (Binns 1988). Another study set out to compare the influence of physical and sporting activities on AIS (Perrin 2006). It was found that girls with AIS had a higher level of joint laxity than a control group, regardless of whether they were practising gymnasts. The researchers concluded that girls with high joint laxity may be more prone to developing AIS.

Cervical spine

A history of recurrent episodes of acute torticollis is a common finding in adolescent JHS (Chapter 12.7a). This is a painful unilateral condition that develops after minor trauma or an acute respiratory infection (Staheli 2007). It can also manifest on rising in the morning, particularly in teenagers who sleep prone with their head rotated and extended. A sudden uncontrolled movement of the head can cause the neck to become 'locked or stuck'. Poor control of the deep neck and shoulder girdle stabilizing muscles is a contributing factor, and it has been proposed that overstretching of the neck may cause partial subluxation of the facets, or straining of the muscles and ligaments. A case report in which magnetic resonance imaging (MRI) was performed on a 15-year-old male adolescent within a few hours of onset of an acute torticollis showed there was a signal intensity compatible with a fluid collection at C2–3, and that the lesion was probably linked to a sudden disruption of the disc collagen fibres, thereby causing excessive lateral pressure, pushing C2 to the left; MRI 3 weeks later was unremarkable (Maigne et al 2003).

A study of 564 pre-adolescent children with musculoskeletal pain showed that at 4-year follow-up, neck pain was the most persistent/ recurrent musculoskeletal pain and that age, headache, JHM and having combined musculoskeletal pain were found to be independent predictors of pain in adolescence (El-Metwally et al 2004).

Persistent headaches are a feature of JHS in adolescence. Cervical spine JHM has been found to be a possible predisposing factor for new daily persistent headache (Rozen et al 2006).

PERIPHERAL JOINT PROBLEMS

The shoulder

Instability of the shoulder can vary from a vague sense of loss of shoulder function and control to a frank instability due to a traumatic dislocation. Atraumatic instability is a common finding in adolescents with JHS that can become symptomatic during the teenage years; it is seen more frequently in young women than young men. The individual may have had repeated episodes of recurrent transient subtle subluxations which eventually progress to atraumatic dislocations. Some hypermobile adolescents are able to dislocate or sublux their shoulders voluntarily and may do this as a 'party trick' and may present as a unilateral or bilateral problem.

The extensible shoulder joint capsule of an adolescent with JHS may allow humeroscapular positions outside the range of balanced stability, and poor neuromuscular control may fail to position the scapula to balance the net humeral joint reaction force. An excessively compliant capsule with relatively weak rotator cuff muscles and poor proprioception will also reduce the stability of the joint. This type of instability is often most prevalent in mid-range positions and simple activities of daily living such as putting on a coat or reaching for an object can cause the shoulder to sublux. See Chapter 12.1 for more detail on shoulder pathology in JHS.

The hip

In hypermobile adolescents a snapping or clicking hip is a common phenomenon. The click may or may not be associated with pain and symptoms (Sanders & Nemeth 1996). The adolescent may complain that it feels as though their hip 'goes out of joint' and they may have intermittent difficulty in fully weight-bearing through the hip. Clicking of the hip has also been associated with excessive femoral head translation (in an anterior or posterior direction) that results from poor control of the muscles that stabilize the hip and pelvis (Sahrmann 2002). In particular, these individuals tend to have particularly weak gluteal muscles and iliopsoas. Hip problems associated with JHM are discussed in further detail in Chapter 12.3.

Knee joint

Patellofemoral pain is multifactorial and can be structural or non-structural. Over-pronation of the foot and hyperextension of the knee are common clinical findings in JHM and make the individual more susceptible to anterior knee pain. The balance of the soft tissues around the patella is influenced by these biomechanical defects and consequently tracking of the patella during knee movements may be altered. Patellofemoral instability is more common in females and those with generalized hypermobility. The hypermobile adolescent may present with a history of recurrent subluxation or dislocation of the patella and exhibit apprehension when the patella is passively moved laterally.

Another cause of knee pain in hypermobile adolescents is hyperextension of the knee that results in nipping or trapping of the pain-sensitive infrapatella fat pad in the knee. See Chapter 12.4 for more detail on pathology in the knee joint.

Foot and ankle joint

Pain and cramps in the muscles of the feet and legs may be the first problems reported by the hypermobile adolescent. A stable foot is essential for normal gait and function and in hypermobility excessive ligamentous laxity and poor muscle control can result in over-pronation of the foot. As the subtalar joint pronates it can cause excessive internal rotation of the tibia and femur, thereby causing abnormal function in the lower limb and pelvis. An unstable foot can compromise the individual's ability to stabilize other joints of the lower limb and pelvis. JHM of the foot has been linked to different clinical foot disorders such as hyperkeratosis on the toes and plantar surfaces of the feet, metatarsalgia, plantarfasciitis, hallux abductovarus, hallux limitus, muscle fatigue and strains in the lower leg (Root et al 1977). See Chapter 12.5 for further discussion on the foot.

Recurrent inversion injuries of the ankle are also associated with JHM. A study of 200 Australian junior netball players showed that those players with JHM sustained more injuries than those who had normal flexibility. The most common injuries were in the ankle (42%), knee (27%) and fingers (15%) (Smith et al 2005).

FUNCTIONAL ASSESSMENT OF THE HYPERMOBILE ADOLESCENT

SUBJECTIVE ASSESSMENT

Assessment of the hypermobile adolescent must take into account not only their physical problems but also their stage of development and maturity. It is essential to take a full history. This may be the first time the adolescent has developed a problem or they may have a history of recurrent problems in different soft tissues and joints. It is important that other conditions are excluded as a source of symptoms. It is also useful to explore whether there is a family history of JHM or lax joints.

The physical changes that occur during adolescence are accompanied by emotional and psychological development, which can make it a confusing and difficult time for a teenager. The onset of unexplained or ongoing pain and symptoms can be frightening and add to emotional distress. Teenagers under 16 years of age should be accompanied by a parent or guardian and it is important to build a good basis for communication with the teenager and their parents from the start. Adolescents with JHS may have seen a number of different doctors and healthcare professionals who have been unable to make a definitive diagnosis; both the adolescent and their parents may have become increasingly frustrated and believe that no-one is taking the problem seriously.

It is essential to understand the impact of the patient's problems on their school, social and home life. Some adolescents with JHS have poor attendance records at school due to recurrent episodes of pain and they can become withdrawn from interacting with their peer group. Those who have experienced pain over a prolonged period may have decreased their activity levels to such a point that they do not do any active exercise, whereas other hypermobile adolescents may take part in a range of different sporting activities both outside and inside school.

The overwhelming fatigue experienced by some hypermobile adolescents can present in a number of different ways and the therapist must be aware of these. Common features of fatigue include:

● Constantly feeling tired and having no energy
● Unable to concentrate at school, when watching television or reading a book
● A lack of interest in anything
● Impatience with friends and family
● Poor appetite.

Adolescents can suffer from a number of different problems that they do not associate with their musculoskeletal problems and these can include urinary and faecal incontinence, bruising, clumsiness, pre-syncope, chest tightness and fatigue. Orthostatic hypotension was found in 78% of patients with JHS who fulfilled the 1998 Brighton Criteria (Gazit et al 2003); adolescents with JHS commonly complain of fainting and giddiness (Chapter 6.1).

OBJECTIVE ASSESSMENT

The five-point hypermobility questionnaire (Hakim & Grahame 2003) (Chapter 1) is a simple and useful tool in aiding assessment as to the likelihood of JHM being present. It has been shown to have a sensitivity of 85% and a specificity of 90%.

A full physical assessment must be carried out and this will include an analysis of posture, normal physiological and functional movements and observation of the functional activities that are painful or difficult.

Maximal exercise capacity is significantly reduced in adolescents with symptomatic hypermobility

(Engelbert et al 2006) and it is therefore important to include a form of fitness testing such as the '6-minute walk test' (Boardman et al 2000). Wittink et al (2000) compared three fitness tests (treadmill, upper extremity ergometer, and bicycle ergometer tests) on individuals with chronic low back pain and found that the best method of aerobic fitness testing was a treadmill test.

The extent of the JHM must be identified when assessing the range of motion at all joints. This is not just a quantitative measure, but also includes the quality of movement during physiological and functional activities. When assessing adolescents who are going through a growth phase it must be remembered that they may have had a recent and sometimes dramatic reduction in range of motion. This is seen often in trunk flexion when the hamstrings of the adolescent become relatively tight and for the first time a teenager with JHS may find that they can no longer bend forward to put their hands flat on the floor.

Muscle strength testing is essential and muscles should be tested both specifically and as part of their normal functional activities. It is important that hypermobile individuals have good muscle control throughout their normal hypermobile range; hence, muscle control and stability should be assessed throughout the hypermobile range.

Balance and proprioception are often compromised in adolescents with JHS and an assessment should include the ability to balance on one leg. In single-leg standing, the control of the foot can be observed, as well as whether the adolescent stands in significant hyperextension in an attempt to stabilize the knee. At the pelvis it should be noted if there is a positive Trendelenburg sign. The proprioceptive element (Chapter 6.4) can be more specifically addressed by asking the patient to close their eyes when performing a single-leg balance test. The single-leg balance test can be made more dynamic by assessing the patient's ability and muscle control when performing a single-leg squat. In the active hypermobile adolescent who is playing sport, it is essential to assess the ability to cope with the increasing dynamic demands of hopping and jumping. Functional assessment in weight-bearing should also include step-up and step-down on a stair and repeated sitting to standing from a chair.

A common feature of JHM is pain in the fingers, wrists and forearms, particularly in relation to writing and using the computer. The therapist should observe the hand and forearm position and the position adopted when writing and using a keyboard. If the adolescent is complaining of pain when playing a musical instrument it can be helpful if it is possible to observe the patient whilst performing on their musical instrument (Chapter 12.2). If the adolescent has pain or difficulty with a particular skill or functional activity then the therapist should observe the patient doing the activity.

Observing the gait pattern is an essential component in the assessment of JHS. The excessive laxity, weak muscles, altered proprioception and poor stamina can have an effect on the efficiency of the patient's gait. A number of abnormalities are common in adolescents with JHS and these may include over-pronation of the feet, hyperextension of the knee, adduction and internal rotation at the hip and a positive Trendelenburg gait.

It is important to know if the patient is going through a period of growth at the time of treatment. The patient's standing and sitting height (to give an idea of spine height) should be measured at the initial assessment and then at monthly intervals. If the teenager is going through a rapid growth phase it may be necessary to modify certain exercises and to reassess expectations in terms of rate of improvement.

Finally, it may be necessary to assess the patient's shoes to see if they are providing adequate support and control and also to discuss how they carry their books and other equipment to school.

MANAGEMENT OF THE HYPERMOBILE ADOLESCENT

Management of the hypermobile adolescent can be challenging but also rewarding. The principles of rehabilitation should be applied to the management programme. Identification of realistic short- and long-term goals is essential. These goals may be musculoskeletal but should also include lifestyle issues such as exercise and sport participation, school attendance and social activities.

The aims of a rehabilitation programme for adolescents with JHS are:

- Pain control
- Improving proprioception, co-ordination and kinaesthetic sense
- Reconditioning muscles to improve control, stability and endurance

- Restoring the individual's natural joint range
- Improving general fitness
- Restoring normal function
- Coping with fatigue
- Teaching self management.

PAIN CONTROL

In general, pain control improves as the patient's general fitness, kinaesthetic sense and muscle condition improve. These factors can take a little while to retrain and in the short term modalities such as heat, ice, soft tissue manipulation, transcutaneous electrical nerve stimulation (TENS), acupuncture and joint mobilizations may provide some temporary respite from pain. If there has been an acute injury, splinting may be used to reduce pain, but splints should be withdrawn as quickly as possible so that muscles do not become increasingly deconditioned and the patient does not become reliant on the splints. Taping may also help to ease pain, although hypermobile individuals often have particularly sensitive skin and they may not be able to tolerate taping, even if a hypoallergenic tape is used.

IMPROVING PROPRIOCEPTION, CO-ORDINATION AND KINAESTHETIC SENSE

Proprioception and kinaesthetic sense should be emphasized at all stages in the rehabilitation programme and there are many ways in which they can be incorporated into an exercise regimen. Proprioception will be enhanced in weight-bearing positions and weight-bearing should be used as much as possible when planning exercise prescription (Fig. 10.1). The use of mirrors and biofeedback machines can help in giving vital information to the patient about their posture and movement patterns.

There are many pieces of simple equipment that can make proprioceptive training fun and relevant. These include, balance and rocker boards, sit-fit cushions (Fig. 9.7), rolls, and the Swiss ball (Fig. 10.2a, b). In addition equipment such as a dance mat and a Wii Fit™ are fun and popular with the adolescents. Exercises should be performed in a pain-free range initially and as close to a functional pattern as possible.

RECONDITIONING MUSCLES

A muscle-conditioning programme will need to address stability, strength and endurance and devising a muscle-reconditioning programme for the hypermobile adolescent must take into account the patient's specific functional difficulties and the muscle work required for the teenager's sporting or leisure activities.

For a muscle to increase strength it must be made to work at a higher level than it is accustomed to – this is termed the overload principle. If the overload principle is not used, a muscle will be able to maintain

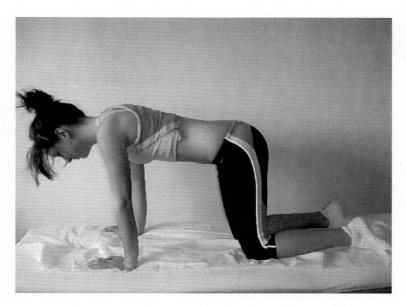

Fig. 10.1 Four-point kneeling is an effective weight-bearing position to enhance proprioception

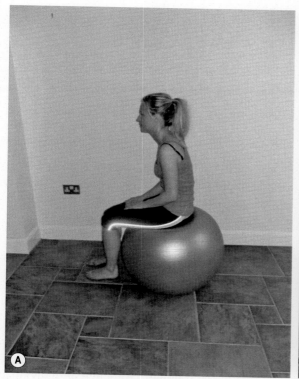 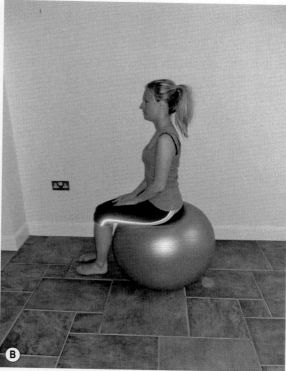

Fig. 10.2 Re-educating good sitting posture on the Swiss ball: (a) slouched posture, (b) good posture

strength as long as training is continued against a resistance to which the muscle is accustomed, but no added strength gains will be made. To effectively increase muscle strength, resistance training requires a consistent, increasing effort against a progressively increasing weight (Prentice 1989).

In rehabilitation, progressive overload is limited by the healing process and if the adolescent is recovering from an acute injury, it is essential not to overstress the healing tissues. At all stages of rehabilitation, exercises are chosen on the basis that they do not underload or overload the healing tissue. An exercise that overloads the tissues may delay healing whereas insufficient loading may leave the tissue weakened and unable to withstand applied loads (Porterfield & DeRosa 1991). In the hypermobile teenager it is especially important to implement a careful and graded programme that promotes tissue healing and at the same time promotes increases in muscle strength. Signs of excessive overload following exercise are:

- Increased pain for more than 12 hours after exercise
- Pain increases at an earlier stage than in previous training sessions
- Increased swelling, warmth and redness in the area of the injury
- Decreased ability to use the part.

Hypermobile adolescents often have a fear of doing exercise in case their symptoms are aggravated and it should be explained that it is normal to experience some reconditioning discomfort but if an exercise causes moderate levels of pain it should be modified or discontinued.

The type of activity or exercise chosen is based on the specific adaptations to imposed demands principle (SAID). The SAID principle states that soft tissues remodel according to the stress imposed on them and that exercise is specific to the posture, mode, movement, exercise type, environment and intensity used (Hall et al 2005). Hence, exercises should be devised that are specific to the skills required and work toward regaining normal function.

Low load stretching techniques are useful in helping the hypermobile adolescent to maintain their range, particularly when the individual is going through a growth spurt. Hypermobile adolescents should be discouraged from doing excessive and vigorous stretching. Low-load long-duration stretches are safer and more effective than high-load short-duration stretches. Stretches should be performed to the point where the individual feels a light tension and they should never be performed into pain or severe discomfort. Preheating the tissues has been shown to enhance the effectiveness of the stretch (Cosgray et al 2004). Commonly the muscle groups that become tight in adolescent individuals with JHM are the hamstrings, iliopsoas, calf muscles and the lumbar erector spinae. Stretches should be performed at least once a day but during a growth spurt the adolescent may need to increase the frequency of stretching.

Exercise takes time to work and strength gains appear to be slower in individuals with JHM (Simmonds & Keer 2007). It is helpful to set realistic goals for exercise programmes so that the teenager does not become despondent at what can seem like a slow rate of improvement in muscle strength.

IMPROVING NATURAL JOINT RANGE

It is a misconception that reducing hypermobile range improves symptoms. It is essential that the adolescent retains the range of movement that is normal to them; this is individual and there are no criteria for the range of motion that is 'normal' for a hypermobile individual. Range of movement may improve with general and specific exercises, but in some cases manual treatment can be effective in restoring range. The therapist must use extra care when using manual techniques on the fragile connective tissue of a hypermobile individual whilst they are going through the adolescent growth phase. In particular it is inadvisable to use high-velocity thrusts (HVT/Grade V manipulations) on hypermobile adolescents. Vigorous techniques can cause a flare-up of the symptoms and if too much vigour is used, tissue damage could occur; however, the judicious use of manual mobilizing techniques can be very helpful in restoring joint range. In some instances the patient may have one or two stiff joints (particularly in the thoracic spine) that are adjacent to the patient's normal hypermobile joints. Joints that have become stiff in a hypermobile adolescent often respond well to manual mobilization, but great care must be taken not to over stress the adjacent hypermobile tissues. If manual techniques have been used to gain joint range of motion, it is essential that the patient is taught how to maintain their range themselves.

IMPROVING GENERAL FITNESS

As stability and strength improve, treatment should also focus on addressing general fitness (Chapter 13). Cardiovascular fitness may have decreased due to higher levels of inactivity and the exercise programme should incorporate cardiovascular reconditioning along with the musculoskeletal and neurological elements of rehabilitation. Activities such as a graded walking programme, stationary bicycle, deep-water running and swimming can all be used to good effect. As the adolescent gains strength and confidence they may wish to progress to other activities such as dancing (ballroom or Latin American), tap dancing, cycling and sport.

COPING WITH FATIGUE

It is important for the adolescent, their family and schoolteachers to understand that fatigue is a common part of the condition. Although an individual with severe fatigue will want to spend the day in bed resting or sleeping, this does not help the problem. It is important for the teenager to try to maintain a normal daily routine even though they are feeling very tired. Taking regular exercise at the right level is helpful; this is individual to each patient and the therapist should help to devise an appropriate programme. Exercise should be balanced with resting and incorporated into the programme. Early intervention has been shown to be effective in the long term in adolescents with chronic fatigue (Gill et al 2004); treatment included exercise, continuing with school, trying to not let it take over the teenager's life and to try to keep going and work through it.

Some adolescents find relaxation techniques helpful in managing their fatigue. This could include relaxation classes, yoga, learning breathing control or using one of the many relaxation tapes available.

It is also useful to discuss diet, stressing the importance of a good balanced diet to provide energy and reduce the fatigue.

Cognitive behavioural therapy (Chapter 8) can be helpful in addressing many of the aspects of hypermobility and there is evidence that it can help to achieve a successful outcome with chronic fatigue (Stulemeijer 2004).

RESTORE NORMAL FUNCTION

The ultimate aim of any rehabilitation programme is to restore normal function and as the adolescent gains in stability, strength and confidence there is often an easy transition to improvements in normal function. However, if the patient is having specific problems with certain tasks, for example, using the computer to do their homework, it is necessary to evaluate the task specifically. In the example of computer use, the problem may be affected by one or a combination of factors such as an unsupportive chair, poor seat and desk height, inadequate forearm support, spending too long in a sedentary position without taking a break, inappropriate computer equipment, muscle fatigue in the neck, shoulder girdle and upper limb muscles. Even when a work position is optimal, sustained positions can cause discomfort, so that over a period of time soft tissue adaptations can occur. Advice on regular breaks and stretching exercises to maintain range of movement are essential.

Assessment of writing position and hand function is useful. The patient may require a specific exercise programme to improve co-ordination and endurance of the wrist and hand muscles. There is a variety of equipment such as therapeutic putty and resistance bands that can be used to recondition the muscles of the hand and thumb (Chapter 12.2).

Items such as writing slopes, copyholders, pens with a thick grip and ergonomic keyboards can all assist in aiding normal function. The use of a good back pack to carry schoolwork and other items will reduce the stresses on the spine and upper limbs.

The characteristic flat foot seen in many adolescents with JHS can be addressed by the use of orthotics. There is little scientific evidence as to how orthoses have their effect but studies suggest that they assist in altering foot biomechanics (Genova & Gross 2000, Woodburn et al 2003), increase muscle facilitation (Hertel et al 2005) and improve posture and balance (Meyer et al 2008). It is also thought that they enhance proprioception, which is particularly helpful for the adolescent with JHS.

Dynamic functional activities such as going up and down stairs often pose a problem and the adolescent may avoid doing them. Observing any abnormal movement patterns in using the stairs and then implementing a retraining programme

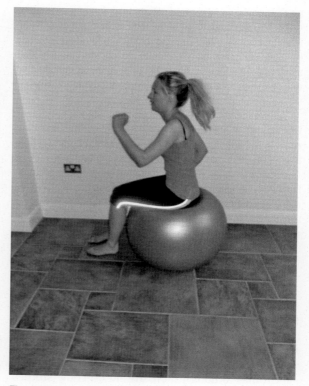

Fig. 10.3 Maintaining good posture while exercising on a Swiss ball

to incorporate an efficient movement pattern and muscle reconditioning can assist in returning the adolescent to normal activities.

Throughout the rehabilitation programme it is important to teach the teenager how to achieve a good balanced and relaxed posture in different functional positions. Postural exercise can be incorporated into muscle-reconditioning exercises and fitness training and the adolescent should be encouraged to work at maintaining a balanced posture at all times (Fig. 10.3).

TEACHING SELF-MANAGEMENT

The more the adolescent understands about their condition, the greater control they will have over their problems. The development of fear/avoidance pain patterns needs to be identified and addressed (Chapter 8). If a movement or activity is painful the individual may avoid performing various actions because they fear they are doing irreversible damage to their body. As movement patterns alter, elements within the musculoskeletal system adapt so that there is greater dysfunction and pain is provoked more easily. In turn, the individual restricts their activities further and a cycle develops which becomes increasingly difficult to change. Additionally, muscles become deconditioned due to lack of use, general fitness declines and a chronic pain state develops.

Adolescents with JHS must have an understanding of the nature of their condition and be reassured that it is helpful to maintain as normal a lifestyle as possible; this is essential in the prevention of chronic pain. In some instances it may be necessary for the adolescent to modify certain aspects of their lifestyle, although as they get fitter and stronger they may be able to return to their normal activities. Setting goals within the context of balancing schoolwork and activities outside of home is important. It is not unusual for adolescents to be out at weekends with their friends, shopping, playing sport and socializing, and then find on Monday that they are in too much pain to be able to go to school. Following a few days rest, their symptoms improve ready for the next weekend for the cycle to start again. Pacing activities is a well-established tool in the management of pain syndromes although there are no outcome studies on the effect of pacing for chronic pain (Gill & Brown 2008). The adolescent agrees a level of activity and specific tasks that they do on a daily basis, regardless of whether it is a good or bad day.

Designing a pacing programme will require the agreement of the teenager with help and support from parents, school and anyone else involved in the rehabilitation process. It is important that pacing does not become part of a passive coping strategy and as soon as the adolescent can start to manage their activity level, goals should be set to pace up, so that the individual increases agreed levels of activity and tasks.

During adolescence, the effect of lifestyle choices will affect both current and future health. The hypermobile adolescent needs to be encouraged to make healthy choices to optimize their general health and feeling of well-being and there is evidence that school, peer and parental support influence these choices (He et al 2004). The benefits of a healthy diet, good sleeping patterns and exercise should be discussed and encouraged and the risks of smoking, drugs and alcohol highlighted. It may be necessary to refer the teenager to other healthcare professionals for specific advice on any of these topics.

SPORT AND EXERCISE

There is mixed opinion as to whether individuals with JHM or JHS should participate in competitive sport. Ligamentous laxity has been linked with an increased risk of injury in athletes (Grana & Moretz 1978, Inklaar 1994, Stewart & Budgen 2006), but a study of North American lacrosse players found no significant difference in the overall injury rates between JHM and non-JHM players (Decoster et al 1999). More specifically in adolescents, a study of 200 Australian junior netball players concluded that young netball players with JHM are more likely to develop injuries (Smith et al 2005). Conversely, a study of 264 teenage athletes showed that the overall prevalence of JHM in an athletic population was similar to that of a non-athletic population and the authors question whether it is warranted to deprive youths with JHM from the benefits of regular or strenuous exercise (Decoster et al 1999).

In the authors' and editors' opinion JHM should not preclude taking part in sport, and hypermobile adolescents must be encouraged to take regular exercise or play sport. The benefits of physical activity include improving cardiovascular fitness, improvements in muscle strength and control, coordination and a feeling of wellbeing. There is no one particular form of exercise that is superior to any other for those with JHM, but it is important that it is an activity or form of exercise that the teenager enjoys and feels comfortable doing. Swimming is an excellent form of exercise, but it is also advisable to include an activity into any programme that is weight-bearing, to increase bone loading and improve proprioception. It is more effective to do a number of different forms of exercise and vary the routine rather than stick to just one type of activity. Participating in team sports and playing with other adolescents has many benefits, but playing contact sports such as rugby, may be inadvisable for some hypermobile individuals. The hypermobile adolescent will need a training programme that includes muscle control work specific to the needs and demands of their particular sport. If sport or exercise is painful, the adolescent should be assessed to identify any specific training needs.

It is also important to liaise with the individual's PE teachers, sports coaches or trainers so that those involved with teaching or training the adolescent are aware of the condition and are aware of potential problems (Chapter 13).

SUMMARY

An adolescent with JHS may present with a variety of different problems. A proactive approach is important to ease symptoms and restore normal function. Physiotherapy and occupational therapy are a vital part of the management of a hypermobile adolescent and consideration should be given in particular to the following:

1. It is important to take into account the normal physical, physiological and psychological changes that are taking place during the teenage years and ensure that the rehabilitation programme takes into account the physiological effects on musculoskeletal structures of the adolescent growth spurt.

2. Exercise is a vital component of any management programme for hypermobile teenagers. A good exercise programme will incorporate activities to improve muscle strength, flexibility and co-ordination as well as improve overall fitness. There is no one type of exercise that is superior, but it should be a form of activity that the adolescent is interested in and wants to do.

3. The hypermobile adolescent should be encouraged to maintain a normal daily lifestyle including good school attendance and socializing with their friends and family.

References

Barron DF, Cohen BA, Geraghty MT, et al: Joint hypermobility is more common in children with chronic fatigue syndrome than in healthy controls, *J Paediatr* 141(3):421–425, 2002.

Beunen G, Malina RM: Growth and physical performance relative to timing of the adolescent growth spurt in *Exercise and Sport Sciences Review, American College of Sports Medicine Series*, vol 24, Baltimore, 1988, Williams and Wilkins, pp 503–540.

Binns MS: Joint Laxity in Idiopathic Adolescent Scoliosis, *J Bone Joint Surg Am* 70-B3:420–422, 1988.

Boardman DL, Dorey F, Thomas BJ: The accuracy of assessing total hip arthroplasty outcomes: a prospective correlation study of walking ability and 2 validated measurement devices, *J Arthroplasty* 15:200–204, 2000.

Buckler J: *A Longitudinal Study of Adolescent Growth*, New York, 1990, Springer Verlag, p 433.

Carter C, Wilkinson J: Persistent joint laxity and congenital dislocation of the hip, *Journal of Bone and Joint Surgery (British)* 46:40–45, 1964.

Chabot J: *Les Consultations Journalières en Rhumatologie*, Paris, 1962, Masson, p 65.

Cosgray NA, Lawrence SE, Mestrich JD, et al: Effect of Heat Modalities on Hamstring Length: A Comparison of Pneumatherm, Moist Heat Pack and a Control, *Journal of Orthopaedic Sports Medicine* 34(7):377–384, 2004.

Decoster LC, Cailas JC, Lindsay RH, et al: Prevalence and features of joint hypermobility among adolescent athletes, *Archives of Pediatric Adolescent Medicine* 151(10):989–992, 1997.

Decoster LC, Bernier JN, Lindsay RH, et al: Generalized Joint Hypermobility and Its Relationship to Injury Patterns among NCAA Lacrosse Players, *Journal of Athletic Training* 34:99–105, 1999.

El-Metwally A, Salminen JJ, Auvinen A, et al: Prognosis of non-specific musculoskeletal pain in preadolescents: A prospective 4-year follow-up study till adolescence, *Pain* 110(3):550–559, 2004.

Engelbert RHH, van Bergen M, Henneken T, et al: Exercise Tolerance in Children and Adolescents with Musculoskeletal Pain in Joint Hypermobility and Joint Hypomobility, *Pediatrics* 118(3):e690–e696, 2006.

Feldman D, Shrier I, Rossignol M, et al: Adolescent growth is not associated with change in flexibility, 9:24–29, 1999.

Forleo LH, March L, Terenty T, et al: Benign joint hypermobility with neuropathy: documentation and mechanism of tarsal tunnel syndrome, *J Rheumatol* 14:577–581, 1993.

Gazit Y, Nahir AM, Grahame R, et al: Dysautonomia in the joint hypermobility syndrome, *Am J Med* 115:33–40, 2003.

Gedalia A, Person AD, Brewer EJ, et al: Juvenile episodic arthralgia and hypermobility, *J Pediatr* 107:873–876, 1985.

Genova JM, Gross MT: Effect of foot orthotics on calcaneal eversion during standing and treadmill walking for subjects with abnormal pronation, *Journal of Orthopedic Sports Physical Therapy* 30:664–675, 2000.

Gill AC, Dosen A, Ziegler JB: Chronic Fatigue Syndrome in Adolescence: A Follow-up Study, *Archives of Paediatric and Adolescent Medicine* March 158:225–229, 2004.

Gill JR, Brown CA: A structured review of the evidence for pacing as a chronic pain intervention, *Eur J Pain* 13(2):214–216, 2008.

Grahame R: Hypermobility and hypermobility syndrome. In Keer R, Grahame R, editors: *Hypermobility syndrome – recognition and management for physiotherapists*, Edinburgh, 2003, Butterworth-Heinemann, pp 1–14.

Grana WA, Moretz JA: Ligamentous laxity in secondary school athletes, *J Am Med Assoc* 40:1975–1976, 1978.

Hakim A, Grahame R: A simple questionnaire to detect hypermobility: an adjunct to the assessment of patients with diffuse musculoskeletal pain, *Int J Clin Pract* 57(3):163–166, 2003.

Hall CM, Thein L, Brody L: *Therapeutic Exercise. Moving Toward Function*, Lippincott Williams and Wilkins, 2005, pp 212–213.

Hasija RP, Khubchandani RP, Shenoi S: Joint hypermobility in Indian children, *Clin Exp Rheumatol* 26(1):146–150, 2008.

He K, Kramer E, Houser RF, et al: Defining and understanding healthy lifestyle choices for adolescents, *J Adolesc Health* 35(1):26–33, 2004.

Hertel J, Sloss BR, Earle JE: Effect of foot orthotics on quadriceps gluteus medius electromyography activity during selected exercises, *Arch Phys Med* 86:26–30, 2005.

Hirsch C, Jonsson B, Lewin T: Low back pain in a Swedish female population, *Acta Orthopedica Scandinavica* 3:171–176, 1969.

Howes RG, Isdale IC: The loose back: an unrecognized syndrome, *Rheumatol Phys Med* 11:72–77, 1971.

Inklaar H: Soccer injuries. II: Aetiology and prevention, *Sports Med* 18:81–93, 1994.

Kirk JA, Ansell BM, Bywaters EG: The hypermobility syndrome.

Musculoskeletal complaints associated with generalized joint hypermobility, *Ann Rheum Dis* 26:419–425, 1967.

Maigne J-Y, Mutschler C, Doursounian L: Acute Torticollis in an Adolescent: Case Report and MRI Study, *Spine* 28(1):E13–E15, 2003.

Malina R, Bouchard C, Oded Bar-Or: *Growth Maturation and Physical Activity. Timing and sequence of changes during adolescence*, ed 2, USA, 2004, Human Kinetics, pp 307–333.

Meyer C, Cammarata E, Haumont T, et al: Arch support use for improving balance and reducing pain in older adults, *Appl Nurs Res* 21(3):153–158, 2008.

Murray KJ, Woo P: Benign joint hypermobility in childhood, *Rheumatology* 40:489–491, 2001.

Nijs J, Aerts A, De Meirleir K: Generalized joint hypermobility is more common in chronic fatigue syndrome than in healthy control subjects, *J Manipulative Physiol Ther* 29(1):32–39, 2006.

Perrin PP: Why do idiopathic scoliosis patients participate more in gymnastics? *Scand J Med Sci Sports* 16(4):231–236, 2006.

Porter RE: Normal development of movement and function: child and adolescent. In Scully RM, Barnes MR, editors: *Physical Therapy*, Philadelphia, 1989, JB Lippincott.

Porterfield JA, DeRosa C: *Mechanical low back pain*, Philadelphia, 1991, W B Saunders, p 13.

Prentice WE: Impaired Muscle Performance: Regaining Muscular Strength and Endurance. In Voight ML, Hoogenboom BJ, Prentice WE, editors: *Musculoskeletal Intervention Techniques for Therapeutic Exercise*, USA, 1989, McGraw-Hill Medical, pp 135–152.

Qvindesland A, Jonsson H: Articular hypermobility in Icelandic

12-year-olds, *Rheumatology (Oxford)* 38:1014–1016, 1999.

Riddoch C, Savage JM, Murphy N, et al: The long-term health implications of fitness and physical activity patterns, *Arch Dis Child* 66:1426–1433, 1991.

Rikken-Bultman DG, Wellink L, van Dogen PW: Hypermobility in two Dutch school populations, *Eur J Obstet Gynecol Reprod Biol* 73:189–192, 1997.

Roche AF: Bone growth and maturation. In Falkner F, Tanner JM, editors: *Human Growth: A Comprehensive Treatise*, vol 2, ed 2, New York, 1986, Plenum, pp 25–60.

Root ML, Orien WP, Weed JH: Normal and abnormal function of the foot, *Clin Biomech* II:110–125, 1977.

Rozen TD, Roth JM, Denenberg N: Cervical spine joint hypermobility: a possible predisposing factor for new daily persistent headache, *Cephalagia* 26(10):1182–1185, 2006.

Sanders B, Nemeth WC: Hip and thigh injuries. In Zachazewski JE, Magee D, Quillen WS, editors: *Athletic Injuries and Rehabilitation*, Philadelphia, 1996, Saunders, pp 599–622.

Sahrmann S: *Diagnosis and Treatment of Movement Impairment Syndromes*, St Louis, 2002, Mosby, p 146.

Seçkin U, Tur BS, Yilmaz O, et al: The prevalence of joint hypermobility among high school students, *Rheumatol Int* 25(4):260–263, 2005.

Simmonds JV, Keer R: Hypermobility and the hypermobility syndrome, *Man Ther* 12:289–309, 2007.

Smith R, Damodaran AK, Swaminathan S, et al: Hypermobility and sports injuries in junior netball players, *Br J Sports Med* 39:628–631, 2005.

Staheli LT: *Fundamentals of Pediatric Orthopedics*, ed 4, Philadelphia, 2007, Lippincott, Williams and Wilkins, p 266.

Stewart DR, Budgen SB: Does generalized ligamentous laxity increase seasonal incidence of injuries in male first division club rugby? *Br J Sports Med* 38:457–460, 2006.

Stulemeijer M: Chronic Fatigue Syndrome: Topic Overview, *British Medical Journal,* Online First, Dec 7, 2004.

Thein L: The child and adolescent athlete. In Zachazewski JE, Magee D, Quillen WS, editors: *Athletic Injuries and Rehabilitation,* Philadelphia, 1996, Saunders, pp 933–958.

Wittink H, Hoskins TH, Kulich R, et al: Aerobic Fitness Testing in Patients with Chronic Low Back Pain: Which Test is Best? *Spine* 25(13):1704–1710, 2000.

Woodburn J, Heliwell P, Barker S: Changes in 3D joint kinematics support the continuous use of orthoses in the management of painful rearfoot deformity in rheumatoid arthritis, *J Rheumatol* 30(11):2356–2364, 2003.

Chapter **11**

Physiotherapy and occupational therapy in the hypermobile child

Susan M Maillard

Julie Payne

INTRODUCTION

The main focus of this chapter will be joint hypermobility syndrome (JHS), also known as Ehlers-Danlos syndrome – hypermobility type, and the multidisciplinary management of this condition in children. There are many symptoms that can be attributed to this condition and the therapies can provide solutions to many of these.

The management of hypermobility syndrome can be complex, but the key to success is to ensure that all the muscles are working effectively, especially in controlling the joints into their hypermobile range. In order to prescribe an effective treatment programme, a thorough assessment is required. It is also important at this stage that the family has a clear understanding of the condition. The ultimate aim is for the child and family to manage the condition relatively independently of medical intervention.

For some children the pain associated with hypermobility becomes chronic and unremitting and in some cases may progress to specific pain syndromes, such as complex regional pain syndrome (CRPS). The modified assessment and management of these in relation to hypermobility are discussed in more detail.

CLINICAL PRESENTATION

Many children have hypermobile joints, however only a percentage of those will suffer from symptoms. JHS is diagnosed when hypermobility becomes symptomatic and all other causes of the symptoms are excluded. Laboratory tests may be necessary to rule out other more serious conditions which may have similar symptoms, such as juvenile idiopathic arthritis (JIA) and other inflammatory conditions, the other forms of Ehlers-Danlos syndrome and Marfan syndrome (Chapter 1). Findings of marked hyperelastic skin, herniae and lenticular abnormalities are not usually seen in JHS, but relatively easy bruising and poor wound healing may be seen, indicating some overlap with these defined genetic conditions (El-Shahaly & El-Sherif 1991).

Children may present to an orthopaedic physician, rheumatologist, paediatrician or physiotherapist with any of a wide range of traumatic or non-traumatic pain complaints and other associated symptoms (Table 11.1). These children typically lack the positive laboratory findings found in rheumatological conditions and rarely develop any positive changes in radiological investigations. Occasionally mild swelling or puffiness, and more rarely joint effusions, may occur at very hypermobile joints, but usually only lasts for hours or, very occasionally, days (Kirk et al 1967, Scharf & Nahir 1982, Russek 1999). The prevalence of symptoms is variable however, being more common in the lower limbs.

There have been many scoring systems devised for measuring or defining hypermobility (Chapter 1), with the Beighton 9-point scale being the most popular (Beighton et al 1973). One intrinsic difficulty associated with the Beighton scale is measuring ranges of passive movement; the observed range depends upon the force applied to the moving part, which may vary with the enthusiasm

DOI: 10.1016/B978-0-7020-3005-5.00015-X

Table 11.1   Common presenting symptoms in JHS in children

MAIN PRESENTING SYMPTOM	MAIN AREAS AFFECTED
Pain	Joints
	Muscles
	Headaches
	Abdominal
	After physical activity
	Night-time pain
Fatigue	
Muscle weakness	Grip
	Hip abductors
	Hip extensors
	Inner range quadriceps
	Plantar flexors (ankle)
Joint symptoms	Clicking joints
	Mild and temporary effusion
	Flat feet
	Subluxations
	Sprained joints (ankles)
	Chondromalacia patellae
Skin	Easy bruising
	Poor skin healing
	Skin stretchiness increased
	Papyraceous scars
	Stretch marks
Developmental changes	Congenital dislocated hip
	Delayed walking
	Reduced co-ordination
	Gastric reflux
	Hernia
Changes to gait	Poor heel/toe action
	Flexed knees
	Flexed internally rotated hips
	Positive Trendelenburg action
	Tiptoe walking

of the examiner and the pain threshold and co-operation of the child (Silverman et al 1975). In addition, the scale only samples a few joints and focuses more on the upper limbs. As symptoms are more common in the lower limbs in children it is good practice to assess all joints for hypermobility initially in order to establish the degree of hypermobility, i.e. global or localized, as this will guide the treatment programme.

The Beighton scale forms part of the Brighton Criteria, a set of classification criteria for diagnosing JHS (Grahame et al 2000), which although not yet fully validated in children, is showing good potential and becoming the most commonly used measure (Chapter 1).

There are other recognized conditions that are closely linked with hypermobility in children.

ANTERIOR KNEE PAIN

There is a significant association between anterior knee pain and generalized joint laxity and, in addition, it is recognized that hypermobility may be a contributing factor in the development of chondromalacia patellae. This can cause a variety of difficulties, including muscle wasting (particularly the quadriceps) and pain in the hips and ankles, and can lead to associated flat feet and backache (Al-Rawi & Nessan 1997).

GROWING PAINS

It is believed that 'growing pains' or 'benign paroxysmal nocturnal leg pain' are related to generalized hypermobility (Maillard & Murray 2003). The pain is thought to be due to periods of unaccustomed excessive activity (such as after an intensive PE lesson) in those predisposed by underlying hypermobility with associated muscle imbalances and inefficiencies. It is very common for children with JHS to suffer pain at the end of the day and during the night, especially after a physically active day and the pain is more likely due to muscle spasm resulting from overuse of weak muscles and not due to 'growing' at all.

MOTOR DEVELOPMENT DELAY AND DYSPRAXIA

In the very young child, hypermobility may be detected with evidence of delayed motor development and a degree of clumsiness (Moreira & Wilson 1992, Davidovitch et al 1994). There is said to be a higher incidence of both gross and fine motor delay in children that are hypermobile, even in the absence of an identified neurological deficit (Jaffe et al 1988, Tirosh et al 1991). However, the motor delay is usually self limiting if hypermobility is the only cause and will improve either spontaneously or with a motor development rehabilitation programme. A number of parents of hypermobile children do report ongoing clumsiness in their children well into later childhood and beyond.

This is a difficult area as there is a considerable overlap between dyspraxia and JHS. The most common shared symptoms are those of impaired co-ordination, balance and proprioception. Many children who have a diagnosis of dyspraxia are also found to be hypermobile. It may be sensible to consider the diagnosis of dyspraxia and JHS along the same spectrum of conditions (Kirby & Davies 2007, Sugden et al 2008).

CHRONIC PAIN SYNDROMES

Fibromyalgia, a syndrome of diffuse muscle and joint pain diagnosed by the presence of 11 or more out of 18 specific tender points, although most common in adults, has been reported to cause diffuse musculoskeletal pain and fatigue in children (Gedalia et al 2000). Hypermobility has been shown to be a significant feature of this syndrome too, with studies showing an incidence of hypermobility in patients diagnosed with fibromyalgia of between 14–81% (Gedalia et al 1993) (Chapter 5).

Other pain syndromes, such as CRPS, have also been linked with hypermobility and up to 80% of children with CRPS are also hypermobile (Mato et al 2008).

FATIGUE AND CHRONIC FATIGUE SYNDROME

Fatigue is also a very common feature in children with JHS and it can present in several ways. It can be global, affecting the whole body, or it can be specific, affecting specific muscle functions. Both need to be considered as a symptom (Chapter 6.1).

Children with JHS will often report difficulty in walking any distance due to tiredness and aching and they will also report that they need to get to bed early and will wake late and will often not feel rested after the night's sleep. This pattern is also common in children with chronic fatigue syndrome (CFS). However, in CFS the fatigue will dominate their life and prevent most normal activities. CFS, characterized by unexplained fatigue that lasts for at least 6 months together with a constellation of other symptoms (Dinos et al 2009), has been associated with joint hypermobility. Barron et al (2002) found joint hypermobility to be more common in children diagnosed with CFS

when compared to otherwise healthy children. However, a study on adolescents was less clear cut, finding higher skin extensibility in those diagnosed with CFS, but no difference in joint mobility, Beighton score or connective tissue abnormality when compared to a group of healthy adolescents (van de Putte et al 2005). In common with dyspraxia, it is the authors' opinion that JHS and CFS should be considered on the same spectrum of conditions, because it is often unclear where one condition starts and the other finishes (Acasuso-Diaz & Collantes-Estevez 1998, Gedalia et al 2000).

There is no evidence to suggest, however, that JHS is linked with more serious conditions of the cardiac system, bone, skin or eyes (Mishra et al 1996, Grahame et al 2000). Although the incidence of 'pulled elbows' has increased due to children participating in more physically demanding sports, and there are reports of a link between hypermobility and 'pulled elbows', a study by Hagroo et al (1995) found no evidence of an increased prevalence of hypermobility in children with pulled elbows.

PREVALENCE

The reports of the prevalence of hypermobility must be viewed cautiously because of the variability in the measurement criteria used. Joint hypermobility has been reported in 6.7–43% of children depending upon age, ethnicity and criteria for assessing hypermobility (Table 11.2). The prevalence is higher in females, being between 7.1–57% compared to 6.0–35% in boys (Gedalia et al 1985, Decoster et al 1997, Russek 1999, Kerr et al 2000, Vougiouka et al 2000). Given the high proportion of subjects documented as 'hypermobile' in some studies, it is clear that the different systems of assessment have major limitations in defining a cohort at significant risk of musculoskeletal problems in different populations. Hypermobility is also more prevalent among Asians than Africans and more prevalent in Africans than Caucasians and decreases with age (Kirk et al 1967, Cheng et al 1991, El-Shahaly & El-Sherif 1991, Birrell et al 1994, Acasuso-Diaz & Collantes-Estevez 1998, El Garf et al 1998, Hudson et al 1998, Russek 1999) such that far fewer adults are hypermobile compared to the number of hypermobile children.

Table 11.2   Prevalence of joint hypermobility in different populations of children

POPULATION	CRITERIA USED (CHAPTER 1)	REFERENCE	AGE	NO. OF SUBJECTS	TOTAL % HYPERMOBILE	NO. OF SUBJECTS F/M	% MALE HYPER-MOBILE	% FEMALE HYPER-MOBILE
British school children	Carter – Wilkinson 4/5	Carter & Wilkinson (Carter & Wilkinson 1964; Kerr et al 2000)	6–11	285	6.7	140/145	6.2	7.1
US school children	Modified Beighton*	Gedalia et al 1985	5–17	260	12.3	126/134	6.7	18.3
US adolescent athletes	Beighton 5/9	Decoster et al 1997	15.5 avg.	264	12.9	114/150	6.0	21.9
US music students	Beighton 3/9	Larsson et al 1987	14–68	660	19.1	300/360	6.9	33.7
Non-caucasian Brazilian school children	Carter – Wilkinson 5/9	Forleo et al 1993	5–17	416	31.7			
Brazilian school children	Carter – Wilkinson 5/9	Forleo et al 1993	5–17	1,005	36.3	560/445	33.7	38.4
Caucasian Brazilian school children	Carter – Wilkinson 5/9	Forleo et al 1993	5–17	589	39.6			
Greek school children	Beighton ** 3/5	Vougiouka et al 2000	5–14	2,432	8.8	1152/1280	7.1	10.8
Icelandic school children	Beighton 4/9	Qvindesland & Jonsson 1999	12		26.7		12.9	40.5
People in Singapore	Modified Beighton*	Seow et al 1999	15–39	306	17			
Dutch school children	Beighton 5/9	Rikken-Bultman et al 1997	4–13	252	15.5			
Dutch school children	Beighton 5/9	Rikken-Bultman et al 1997	12–17	658	13.4			
West African people	Beighton 4/9	Birrell et al 1994	6–66	204	43		35.0	57.0

*Criteria as in Beighton et al, except for hyperextension of fingers to be parallel to forearm (as in Carter and Wilkinson) rather than hyperextension of 5th MCP joint to 90 degrees.
**Scoring using the right limbs only and lumbar flexion.

ASSESSMENT

SUBJECTIVE EXAMINATION

It is important to take a full history of the presenting condition, to rule out any other under-lying conditions and to establish a clear picture of the nature and severity of the symptoms and when and where they occur. This will enable the treatment plan to be specific to the child's symptoms and in addition, if recorded accurately, it can also be used as an outcome measure. The main areas to focus the questioning upon are given below.

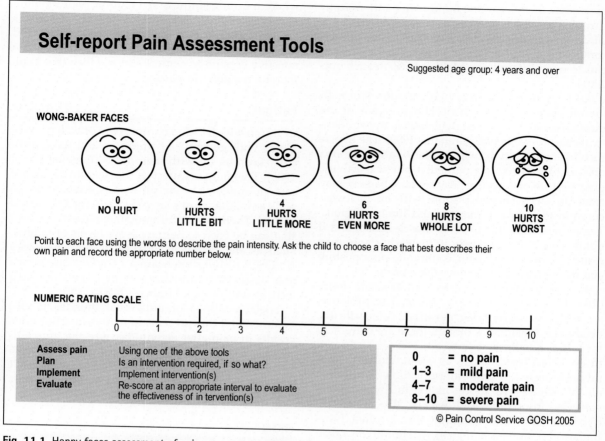

Fig. 11.1 Happy faces assessment of pain. *From Hockenberry MJ, Wilson D: Wong's Essentials of Pediatric Nursing, ed. 8, St. Louis, 2009, Mosby. Used with permission. Copyright Mosby.*

Pain

A body diagram can be used to record the pain distribution with a suitable measure of pain intensity, such as a Visual Analogue Scale (VAS), which is less subjective if the child is over 7 years old, or a 'Happy Face Scale' (e.g. Wong-Baker Faces, Wong et al 2001) (Fig. 11.1) or 'ouchometer' for younger children. Children with JHS will often present with painful joints and muscles that are worse in the evenings, after physical activities, and may wake them at night-time. The pain only occurs after an activity and not during it, which makes it difficult for the family to feel they can limit the activity to avoid the pain. It is worth spending time taking a good history of the pain, since this will help ensure that full understanding of the pain picture is established and it also reassures the family that they have been heard fully regarding their child's pain.

In JHS there is also the issue of the child developing a downward spiral of pain symptoms and this should be broken to avoid continuation of symptoms (Fig. 2.10). This idea should be explained to the family and from the assessment the relative proportion and timing of the rest periods and active periods should be defined. It is also important to ascertain when the episodes of pain occur, for example, always at weekends requiring the child to recover during the week instead of attending school because of the pain. This should be discussed as it will ensure the 'pacing programme' and returning to normal activity is appropriate.

Previous experiences of pain the child has had or personally observed before should be noted, because this may have an impact upon their coping mechanisms. A child's coping mechanisms can be adversely affected by their observations of another member of the family who suffers from chronic pain (McGrath 1995). An assessment by a clinical psychologist often identifies factors which compound the underlying cause of pain in such children and families (Malleson & Beauchamp 2001).

Back pain in children may require thorough investigation and assessment. However one of the most common differential diagnoses is hypermobility (Scharf & Nahir 1982, Grahame 1999). The hypermobility may affect the whole spine or a specific area only and be related to a particular physical activity, poor posture or carrying heavy school bags. It may result in an 's'-shaped posture with an increased curve in the cervical, thoracic and lumbar regions. The pain is often due to acute muscle spasm and if not managed appropriately in the early stages may result in chronic back pain, continuing poor posture and the associated difficulties these bring.

Back pain tends to affect adolescents more often than young children. Acute disc prolapse, as well as early degenerative osteoarthritis, need to be considered, though these are extremely rare. If the pain is severe, other diagnoses need to be considered, such as spondylolysis, spondylolisthesis or pain amplification syndrome, all of which are more likely in hypermobile subjects. Idiopathic scoliosis is also linked to hypermobility, and although this is often functional, and not pathological, it should be taken seriously and monitored closely, with a comprehensive central core stability and strengthening programme prescribed (Chapter 10).

It is also important to ask about headaches and abdominal pain, because both are common in children with JHS. Headaches are usually due to muscle spasm in the neck, affecting the trapezius muscle, and producing a frontal headache, while abdominal pains are linked to cramps in the gut, which is commonly known as irritable bowel syndrome (IBS) (Chapter 6.2).

Stiffness and joint swelling

Children occasionally complain of stiffness in the mornings. However, this rarely lasts for long and is often more related to the degree of pain felt the previous day. It is important to recognize the difference between stiffness that develops after activity and that is not associated with joint swelling, which is typical of mechanical conditions such as JHS, compared to those rheumatic diseases where morning stiffness and chronic joint swelling are more typical. The former pattern is seen as an indication that the musculo-tendonous and ligamentous structures around the joints are not effective enough to control and stabilize that joint, thereby resulting in pain.

Fatigue

Children with JHS and chronic pain often have problems with generalized tiredness and have difficulty keeping up with their peers (Engelbert et al 2006). This may manifest as the need to sleep and rest more often or may present as a reluctance to walk any distance or play physically for any period of time. There are useful assessment questionnaires that can be used to help measure levels of fatigue, such as the Pediatric Quality of Life Inventory (PEDSQL) Multidimensional Fatigue Scale which was designed to measure fatigue in patients aged 2–18 years (Varni & Limbers 2008).

Specific fatigue of individual muscles is also common and this presents in many ways but often results in pain after activity because the muscle is neither strong nor fit enough to cope with the activity. Fatigue may also present as shaking of a muscle and common functional activities such as gait, may alter with time and effort as fatigue occurs.

SKIN

Stretchy skin can often be an indication of hypermobility (Chapter 1), and may be associated with easy bruising and poor skin healing. Stretch marks are also more common in adolescents with hypermobility and become apparent during the growth period. There is a group of children with JHS/EDS who have more stretchy skin than normal and who often have a 'doughy' feel to their muscles. These muscles are often significantly weaker and more difficult to strengthen. Once strengthened they also, unfortunately, lose strength quickly after completing a training programme unless exercise is continued.

CO-ORDINATION

Children with JHS are often clumsier and less co-ordinated than other children. They generally have poor balance and co-ordination and often fall over a lot and bump into different objects. This is thought in part to be due to reduced proprioceptive acuity in the joints, particularly at the extremes of the movements (Mallik et al 1994, Hall et al 1995) (Chapter 6.4). This may affect their ability to play sport effectively, to cut up food and manage other fine motor tasks such as buttons and zips.

Generally, spatial awareness is reduced in hypermobile joints, which has an impact upon the child's balance mechanisms. These factors are compounded by the muscles around the joints not being at their optimum strength or stamina; either because joint pain is inhibiting muscle action, or because the child (or child's parents) are fearful of exacerbating pain and hence restrict movement. The result is that the muscles become weaker and more unfit.

SCHOOL

Attending school is the biggest activity for children and so it is important to ask about the area the school covers, the number of stairs involved and whether there are lockers easily available. The bigger and more spread out the school is, the stronger and fitter the young person needs to be.

Often children with JHS have difficulties with writing, affecting both speed and neatness, and this will have an impact on their performance abilities (Chapter 12.2).

Sport should be a big part of any young person's life, but it is especially important for an individual with JHS. It is therefore important to find out what they are doing with regard to physical education (PE), how often, to what level and what difficulties, if any, they are encountering.

HOBBIES AND SPORT

The hobbies and sport that a child either enjoys or is interested in should influence the treatment programme and goals. Hypermobility can be considered an advantage for many sporting, dancing and music activities but the child needs to be able to control their joints effectively and to be strong enough to cope with the activity.

GENERAL DEVELOPMENT AND PAST MEDICAL HISTORY

As mentioned above, motor development may be delayed and this can include walking. Children most commonly start to walk between the ages of 12–18 months. However, hypermobile children often start to walk slightly later. They often don't crawl normally but prefer to bottom shuffle.

Occasionally there may also be a delay in speech development, but usually no delay in cognitive ability and understanding.

Young children with hypermobility may become tiptoe walkers as a way of producing more stability at the ankle and this can be managed well by following a strengthening programme and wearing supportive ankle boots.

Occasionally young people with JHS may also have functionally reduced immune systems which render them more liable to pick up colds and small infections. This is thought to be due to their generalized deconditioning and improving their physical fitness and strength helps to make them more resilient.

OBJECTIVE EXAMINATION
Joint range of movement

The degree of hypermobility in affected joints can be scored using one of the scales mentioned above, but a full assessment of range of movement of every joint is likely to be useful, especially in children with multiple joint symptoms. Some children may have generalized hypermobility of most joints, while others may have a peripheral form affecting mainly hands and lower limbs.

Muscle strength

In a child with hypermobility it is important to assess the strength of the muscles surrounding a hypermobile joint, as well as the stamina of the muscles in the limb and trunk and the general stamina of the child. It is important for good control and stability of the joints that the muscles surrounding the joints have full strength and normal endurance, especially into the hypermobile range. If this is not the case then arthralgia and muscle fatigue are likely to occur with prolonged activity. The risk of subluxation of joints, although rare, is increased when muscle strength and control are not optimum. Muscle strength can be measured using either the Oxford Scale, or the expanded 11-point scale (0–10) (Kendall et al 1993) or by using myometry.

Stamina and fitness

Children with JHS are usually generally unfit and have very poor stamina and improving these will be an important part of a treatment programme.

Stamina is often assessed subjectively, but the '6-minute walk test' (Nixon et al 1996, Garofano & Barst 1999, Boardman et al 2000, Hamilton & Haennel 2000, King et al 2000, Pankoff et al 2000) is a better objective measure. This test requires the subject to walk as fast and as far as they can in 6 minutes. If they are unable to manage 6 minutes then the distance covered and the time taken are recorded.

Posture and gait

As with any musculoskeletal assessment, it is important to observe the posture and gait of the child, and to watch for any abnormalities in this due to the hypermobility. The most common postural disturbances are:

- hyperlordosis of the lumbar spine and increased kyphosis of the thoracic spine
- hyperextension of the knees in the weight bearing position
- pronated/flat feet.

    The most common changes to gait are:
- poor heel–toe strike
- over-pronation at the ankle
- flexion at the knees
- flexion and internal rotation at the hips
- positive Trendelenburg sign.

Balance and proprioception

Diminished balance and poor proprioception are often an issue for children with JHS, as discussed previously, and these need to be assessed at the initial stage. Balance can be tested by asking a child to stand on one leg at a time and observing postural sway to give a simple measure, which can be progressed further by asking them to close their eyes at the same time. Removing the visual input will assess proprioception more specifically (see Chapter 6.4). A more specific assessment of proprioception and body awareness can be achieved by isolating and passively moving a joint and assessing spatial awareness without the visual input; that is, asking a child to identify the direction of movement of a joint while they have their eyes shut.

    Once the child is fully assessed and the specific difficulties identified an individualized rehabilitation programme is developed.

AIMS OF TREATMENT

It is a common misconception that the purpose of treatment is to reduce the range of mobility of the joints. Rather, the main purpose of a rehabilitation programme is to improve joint stability and control whilst maintaining the full hypermobile range of movement which is normal for each hypermobile child. Therefore the aims of treatment are to:

- increase the strength of the muscles, especially into the hypermobile range
- improve the stamina of the muscles
- improve the general fitness of the child
- re-educate the gait to avoid/correct any abnormalities in the biomechanics
- return to normal activities and functioning
- educate the child and family to enable them to continue to manage the condition with minimal reliance on medical input, external support or medication.

    Success in achieving these aims will help to ensure that the child has a stable joint or joints, protected by strong, fit muscles which will enable them to manage their symptoms independently. Often a combination of a small and specific rehabilitation programme with regular activity in sporting activities is a very effective approach to reducing the symptoms of JHS.

TREATMENT METHODS

PAIN RELIEF

It is important for the child and family to understand that the pain is due to the hypermobility and associated musculoskeletal insufficiencies and not to any other pathology such as JIA or other rheumatological conditions. It is then easier to understand why a rehabilitation programme is the treatment of choice. The family often need to be reassured that the pain will ease but only when the muscles are strong and fit and are protecting the joints more fully, and when the child is functioning normally both biomechanically and generally (i.e. walking correctly and attending school fully etc). It is often found that the pain is the last thing to improve and only does so slowly and this should be emphasized at the start of the programme. Children and parents are often counselled that rehabilitation is often prolonged, e.g. for a child that has had 18 months of pain and disability it may take this time again before they return to full pain-free independent function. It is difficult to quantify the degree of pain that is acceptable within the rehabilitation programme, however we expect the pain to be of a moderate to mild degree and should be expected on and off over the years and will often worsen if they become unfit. It is important for the children and family to realize the pain of hypermobility is not signifying damage or illness, but indicating poor control of the joints, and is therefore benign.

Other methods of pain relief may be of use, such as hot packs or cold packs on specific joints. Trancutaneous electrical nerve stimulation (TENS) machines may also have a role to play in this aspect, but must be seen only as a supportive treatment and not a solution, and that their use will not replace the rehabilitation programme. Relaxation and distraction techniques can be used to help the child or young person manage their pain. This is often useful at night-time if they have difficulty sleeping due to the pain and discomfort. It can also be used in many other situations, for example during a school break, to ensure that they are able to manage the rest of the day. Massage may also be a very effective way of easing any pain, especially if it is due to muscle spasm.

It is important that families understand that there is always a physical and a psychological component to managing pain, so a clinical psychologist may be useful to help teach the child and the family different pain-coping strategies rather than relying on medication.

JOINT STABILITY AND MUSCLE STRENGTH

The inherent stability of a joint is determined by the efficiency or integrity of the musculoskeletal system (muscle, tendon, capsule, ligament and articular surfaces) and the neural control systems (motor and sensory). As discussed previously, one hypothesis suggests that JHS may be a result of abnormal collagen fibres resulting in ligamentous insufficiency. The soft-tissue microtrauma caused by this instability is one accepted explanation for the joint and muscle pains (Gedalia & Brewer 1993). It follows then that improving the dynamic muscle control to supplement the ligamentous insufficiency should minimize the trauma (Kerr et al 2000).

It is commonly recognized that children respond well to a muscle-strengthening programme, and while they may not improve their muscle bulk, they do improve strength and neuromuscular co-ordination, thereby making the muscles more effective (Finsterbush & Pogrund 1982, Biro et al 1983, Barton & Bird 1996). It appears clear that a muscle-strengthening programme, improving control into their full range of movement, including the hypermobile range, is the treatment of choice for children with JHS (Russek 1999, 2000, Kerr et al 2000).

When devising an exercise programme, all aspects of muscle function need to be considered, including isometric, isotonic, concentric and eccentric muscle strength, stamina and general function. It is ideal to start with a programme that isolates each muscle group individually and that considers all aspects of its function. It is particularly important to ensure that all muscle groups around the joint are strengthened equally, for example, in the knee joint both quadriceps and hamstrings need to be strong to ensure physiological balance.

The principles for training muscles in children are well supported by evidence and should follow the guidelines of high repetitions and low weights (Augustsson & Thomee 2000, Bernhardt et al 2001, Bilkey et al 1981, Bundonis 2007, Christou et al 2006, Faigenbaum et al 1999, Faigenbaum 2000, Faigenbaum et al 2001, Faigenbaum et al 2002, Flanagan et al 2002, Hakkinen et al 1989, Hoffman et al 2005, Kaufman & Schilling 2007, Logsdon 2007, McCambridge & Stricker 2008, McNee et al 2009, Purcell & Hergenroeder 1994, Schnizer 1993, Vaughn & Micheli 2008, Webb 1990, Yamamoto et al 2008). The muscles should be strengthened using a programme of open-chained individual and specific exercises with some closed chain and functional exercises included. It is not effective if functional and closed chain exercises are used exclusively, as the body will continue to favour the stronger and pain-free range and this needs to be challenged in order to resolve the resulting pain (Maillard et al 2004, Yamamoto et al 2008, McNee et al 2009). For example, in the knee it is usually the muscles that flex the joint that are strong and the extensors, particularly vastus medialis obliquus (VMO), which are weak and require strengthening. However, while performing squats or sit-to-stand exercises, this muscle is usually not used, therefore to strengthen VMO an exercise such as straight leg raise with no quadriceps lag is a very effective

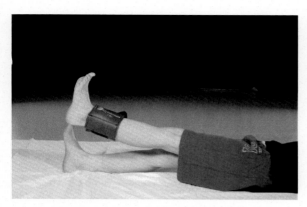

Fig. 11.2 Straight leg raise performed in supine lying with no quadriceps lag. The exercise should be completed slowly with a hold of 2 seconds and a controlled ascent and descent

open chained exercise that can be progressed well using increasing repetitions and weights (Fig. 11.2). It is usually necessary to strengthen VMO into the hypermobile range in order to correct the muscle balance and improve joint stability. If the child is experiencing significant pain, isometric exercises in the hypermobile range should be used. This is progressed to dynamic work and then on to resisted work (Borms 1986) and from non-weight-bearing work to weight-bearing work.

The same can be applied to hip abduction completed in side lying, ensuring the hip is slightly extended to avoid psoas major taking over (Fig. 11.3). Hip extension is also more effective if

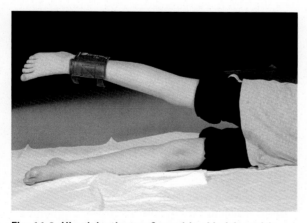

Fig. 11.3 Hip abduction performed in side lying with the hips in slight extension and rolled slightly forward. The top leg is to be lifted above the midline and held for 2 seconds with a controlled ascent and descent

done in prone lying. Upper limb muscle strengthening works well with this principle too, however closed chain exercises such as press ups are also effective in strengthening scapular stability.

Stamina training is also very important for the muscles, since it is important not only to have strong muscles but muscles that will not fatigue easily. The most effective training programme is one that is completed at least four times a week, and though it may be started very gently with low repetitions, these must be progressed regularly (once a day or a minimum of once a week) to a maximum of 30 repetitions, though less than 15 repetitions is not effective. Also, when the repetitions have been progressed to a maximum, the resistance should be increased from antigravity to applying weights in order to build both strength and stamina further. The recommended maximum weight for young children is age- and size-dependent but should be between 0.5 kg to a maximum of 5 kg with 30 repetitions. Even the youngest child should be able to progress to 1 kg weights.

The exercise programme in chronic pain syndrome should be completed daily in order to avoid the boom-and-bust cycle, however it should be simple and not too time-consuming so that normal activity and independent function can be completed as well.

A common pattern of muscle weakness has been observed in children with JHS, with hip abductors, hip extensors, inner range quadriceps, especially into the hypermobile range, and plantar flexors being most affected. Therefore it is often very effective to start with a programme for these four muscle groups, starting with 5 repetitions for 1 week and increasing by 5 repetitions each week to a maximum of 30 repetitions before adding resistance (weights). The weights should be increased regularly by 0.5 kg until at least 1–5 kg is being lifted, depending upon age, size and activities of the young person. An example of an exercise programme is given in Box 11.1.

A muscle-strengthening programme can be prescribed for the hand to help with the pain and fatigue often experienced by young people during handwriting. The use of therapeutic putty with increasing strengths can be very effective and a fun way to exercise. The young person is encouraged to change the shape of the putty using different grips to work different hand muscles, using one hand and no surface for support.

> **BOX 11.1   An example of a home exercise programme**
>
> Exercise 1. Straight leg raise performed in supine lying with no quadriceps lag. The exercise should be completed slowly with a hold of 2 seconds and a controlled ascent and descent.
>
> Exercise 2. Hip abduction performed in side lying with the hips in slight extension and rolled slightly forward. The top leg is to be lifted above the midline and held for 2 seconds with a controlled ascent and descent.
>
> Exercise 3. Hip extension performed in prone lying with legs slightly apart and with full knee extension maintained during the lift. Each lift is held for 2 seconds with a controlled ascent and descent.
>
> Exercise 4. Plantarflexion and balance. Standing on one leg, initially with support if necessary, lift up the heel to rise onto tiptoes with maximum arch development. Performed with a controlled ascent and descent.

The efficiency of writing can be addressed by recommending the use of thick, fat pens and pencils (Chapter 12.2 and Figure 12.2.2).

GAIT RE-EDUCATION AND BALANCE

A combination of hypermobile joints, reduced proprioception, weak muscles and reduced stamina can profoundly affect the gait of a child with JHS. Retraining balance and proprioception is therefore a very important part of the rehabilitation process to reduce abnormalities in gait and to try to minimize injury in the future. Using a simple exercise such as standing on one leg, without shoes and socks on and without support, can be progressed further by encouraging the child to go up and down onto tiptoes. This is an effective way to strengthen gastrocnemius and improve the balance and proprioception of each leg. Items such as balance boards and uneven surfaces are also very effective.

'Rhythmical stabilizations' are also a useful method for improving postural stability both globally and specifically. Weight-bearing exercises can be used to progress this further for both upper limbs (four-point kneeling) and lower limbs. Vibration plates can be helpful in improving muscle strength needed for balance in some individuals.

In order to correct gait, the causes of the abnormalities need to be identified and worked on separately, before the gait will improve. The use of crutches and wheelchairs should be avoided as these promote muscle weakness, loss of stamina and reduced activity. However, it is important that the child recognizes the abnormalities in their gait and learns to correct them; the use of biofeedback through video recording and mirrors can aid this and help to give the child positive feedback as they work on improving their gait.

FUNCTIONAL TASKS

Children with JHS often adapt to their hypermobility by altering the mechanics of how they function. This often leads to increased pain, pain in other locations and increased fatigue. It is therefore important to work on specific functional activities and to develop with the child energy-saving, biomechanically correct, safe and pain-free ways of approaching these activities.

Practising these functional movements can be included into their rehabilitation programme, for example, step-ups on a stair and repeated sit-to-stand from a chair.

HYDROTHERAPY

Hydrotherapy can be used in the treatment of JHS. The heat will provide pain relief and help reduce muscle spasm. Because water is an unstable medium which makes it more difficult for children with hypermobility to co-ordinate their movements effectively and control strengthening exercises into the hypermobile range, it should not be the only treatment modality advocated.

AIDS AND SUPPORTS

Splinting of hypermobile joints should rarely be recommended, since this is likely to exacerbate the ineffective use of the muscles causing them to become weaker still and more prone to injury. In addition, it can inhibit the rehabilitation programme and imply that there is a more serious medical disorder requiring therapy rather than home management. However, limited use of other supports, such as orthotics (see below) or aids such as pen grips (Chapter 12.8) can be a useful adjunct to a hand muscle-strengthening programme. They reduce the force required to sustain the gripping of a pen, therefore reducing the pain and fatigue experienced in fingers and wrists during school work for example. Writing can cause considerable difficulties and it may be advisable to discuss with the school and young person the use of a computer to type longer pieces of work and at exam time. The child can be helped further through support for training in touch typing. However, writing should be encouraged in subjects where less writing is required, such as maths and science, to ensure that writing ability is not lost. During exam time it may be necessary to ask for extra time to allow the young person to get up and move around and stretch all their joints, but particularly their hands, to minimize the gradual increase in pain and discomfort that exams can induce.

ORTHOTICS AND FOOTWEAR

Children with JHS often present with very pronated flat feet as a result of their hypermobility (Chapter 12.5). This can contribute to lower limb symptoms and often responds very well to the use of orthotics. These often take the form of heel cups or arch supports that support the position of the subtalar joint and medial arch, therefore helping to correct the foot position. Though it can be argued that this may be encouraging weaker foot muscles, in practise, the benefits of correcting the biomechanics of the foot has such a positive effect upon the whole gait pattern that it is considered a preferential course of treatment (Agnew 1997). In many cases, correcting the biomechanics of the feet significantly reduces the abnormal forces throughout the other joints, therefore reducing the pain experienced (such as an anterior knee pain).

Good supportive footwear should also be encouraged and ankle boots with laces are ideal. These boots often have good shock-absorbing soles which reduce the forces through the lower limbs. They should also be very sturdy at the heel and along the ankle with the laces tied tightly so that the whole foot and ankle are supported to prevent over-pronation. Supporting the foot and ankle in a good position will also improve the functional position of the knees and hips. For very young children who are slow to walk or who are tiptoe-walking, the use of boots very early is often an effective way of encouraging confident walking.

GENERAL FITNESS AND SPORT

Children with JHS will often have become very sedentary due to their pain, fatigue and muscle weakness and present in a deconditioned and generally unfit state. It is therefore important to incorporate aerobic exercise into the rehabilitation programme. Care needs to be taken early on in the programme, when there is still sub-optimal muscle strength, to ensure that the fitness aspect of the programme is of low impact to the joints to prevent symptom exacerbation and a consequent loss of faith by the child and family in the programme. The authors have commonly seen resistance by the child and family to sport and physical activity as it has previously increased pain. However it is important to re-assure the family that the strengthening programme is tailored to ensure the body is 'fit for purpose' and that when the muscles are effectively protecting the joints, the child can participate in sport without symptom exacerbation.

Swimming is a highly desirable method of exercise, because it is usually 'low stress' for the joints and is a good aerobic activity. It is preferable that a normal swimming pool is used for ongoing management, since hydrotherapy pools are too hot for distance swimming.

Bicycling is also very good for aerobic work and again does not over-stress the other joints. As soon as strength and stamina are improving, normal aerobic and sporting activities should be gradually included. It is often advisable to restart a sport that the child really enjoys first, because pain after new physical activity is normal and it is easier to cope with if the activity has been enjoyed. Young people need to be reassured that some muscle pain after sport is normal and just indicates that more training is necessary to get fitter and stronger to be able to cope with that level of activity.

In the author's opinion, trampolining should be avoided initially, because it is a high-impact activity with an unstable landing area on which it is easy to twist and strain joints and thereby increase pain.

PACING

Pacing is an extremely important part of the rehabilitation of a child with JHS (Chapter 8).

It is very often the case that the child will report that they will play football, go swimming, go out with their friends and dance at the weekend. They are then very sore on Monday and are unable to attend school, but by the weekend they have recovered enough to be able to do many activities again, and the cycle continues. This causes a constant 'peaking and troughing' of symptoms and causes a major disruption to life. Eventually this may form part of a 'school refusal' pattern.

The aim of pacing is to stop this cycle by evening out activities and to build them up again slowly. Therefore, specific tasks are set to be completed each day, no more and no less, and they must be done whether there is a lot of pain or just a little. This is decided according to the level of disability experienced by the child and by their level of fitness at the initial phase of the programme. This is gradually increased weekly until they are able to do everything. This technique must include attendance at school as one of the tasks, and must limit the activities at the weekend. There is then an evening out of tasks over the whole week, and a reduction of the peaking of pain as before.

For this programme to work effectively, everyone involved in the care of the child should be included in planning the pacing. This should include the child, parents, school and therapist as a minimum. A written agreement may be used to facilitate progression and to ensure that the programme is developed between the therapist and the family. It is also often useful to develop a 'back-up' plan if problems arise, so that the original problems do not develop again or can be brought under control more rapidly.

Many young people may miss school due to JHS and chronic pain syndromes. Initially, a structured and graduated return to school is required in order to ensure an eventual full return to school. The return to school should be a priority and the aim is to achieve this before returning to full socialization and fun activities. There may be aspects of school that are causing the young person some anxieties which in turn will increase their pain levels and these should be explored and a plan devised in order to manage them. There should not be a period longer than 2 weeks in between increasing attendance at school. Physical education should be the last thing returned to the school timetable to ensure all academic subjects are regained first. Planning for the day is useful to avoid carrying too many heavy books and equipment. The provision of lockers, with time to store and fetch things from the locker, can be arranged with the school. It may be necessary to provide transport to and from the school initially to avoid the journey causing fatigue and preventing the return to school being successful.

PSYCHOLOGY

In some cases where pain and loss of independent function are profound, it is important to include the clinical psychologist in the management team. They will be able to help develop pain management skills for the child, as well as generally help the family cope with the condition and to understand its impact on the whole family. Many families find this support invaluable and are able to change many unhelpful coping strategies into helpful ones, leaving behind the 'chronic pain cycle' that may have developed in the preceding phase.

CHRONIC PAIN SYNDROME

The diagnosis of chronic pain syndrome is complex. However, there are some characteristic features that would alert the clinician.

OVER-REACTION

This is defined as excessive wincing, muscle tremors, screaming, collapsing with pain, reporting pain as a level above 10/10. This may occur even during discussion of the pain symptoms without any physical examination. This is however subjective and may vary with age, mental status, cultural influences and fear.

ALLODYNIA

This is defined as reported pain to touch or gentle pinching. This can include the touch of clothes or gentle normal touch such as a cuddle.

FIXED JOINTS

This is where the patient will not only be reluctant for the joints to be touched but will either not move the joint themselves or will not allow the joint to be moved by anyone else. This may be accompanied by anticipated withdrawal.

ANTICIPATED WITHDRAWAL

This is when the child will either react before the examiner has touched the affected area or instantly it is touched. The limb is withdrawn very quickly and often in an exaggerated fashion.

FUNCTION IS LIMITED BY PAIN

This however is to an extreme level where the children are not only missing out on physical activities such as sport but are often not attending school and in many cases are not enjoying any social activity either.

ANXIETY

It is common for young people with hypermobility to be more anxious and anxiety has been linked with increasing the experience of pain (Bulbena et al 1993, 2004, 2006a, 2006b, Martin-Santos et al 1998) (Chapter 4).

COMPLEX REGIONAL PAIN SYNDROME

CRPS is a very specific pain syndrome and is characterized by the individual presenting with a limb (usually, but can affect any area of the body) that has severe allodynia. The limb will be fixed in an abnormal position and will not be used functionally. The area will be colder than the other limb and the surrounding unaffected skin and is usually a purple/blue mottled colour. There may be excessive hair growth in the area and the skin may be dry and scaly depending upon the time it has been since it has been washed or touched (Fig. 11.4). The limb is often swollen, though this is global and not related to a joint effusion (Wilder et al 1992, Veldman et al 1993, Harden et al 1999, Stanton-Hicks 2000, Bruehl et al 2002, Maillard et al 2004).

Assessment

The assessment follows the guidelines above, but with some particular modifications. While it is important to assess carefully and objectively in all cases, it is particularly important, in the case of

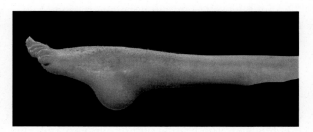

Fig. 11.4 Appearance of the lower limb of a child with CRPS

CRPS, that the level of pain reported by the child and family is never questioned. The goal is to gain facts and not to make initial judgements as to the level of pain reporting. It is vital to believe the amount of pain they are experiencing at all times.

Subjective

For these patients it is vital that they feel the clinician has heard what they have to say and that they have been believed. It is often better to spend a little more time allowing the patient and family to describe the pain, examinations, investigations and explanations they have previously experienced. This time is often well spent, because a family who feels that they have been heard and understood is much more likely to respect what the clinician has to say and will be able to work with the suggested treatment more effectively.

It is helpful to ask the child and family about their beliefs and expectations, such as what they think is happening, what has caused the pain and what they think might make the pain better. It is advisable to ask the child first so that they are not influenced by their parents' answer.

Discussing the activities of daily living (ADL) that are causing difficulties is helpful to see what level of help they require on a regular basis. Areas to be explored should include hygiene, dressing, eating, school, sport, play and social interactions. Barriers preventing full participation at school are a particularly important topic to explore. A young person with severe pain may have significant difficulties even getting to school. Finding out about the specific difficulties, such as public transport being too painful and difficult to use may be resolved by involving the local educational authority providing better transport on a temporary basis to enable the child to attend school. Asking what a child feels about school is a difficult question, because it is not helpful to suggest that the pain is linked to being unhappy at school, however, there may be many issues at school that could be improved that would make school easier and more enjoyable.

Objective

This may be very difficult as the level of pain may be too great at the time of initial assessment to allow much movement and touch. But there should be some discussion about why the examination needs to happen, what is being looked for and reassurance that the examination will be very gentle to ensure no damage is done despite the pain.

Assessing the area the pain affects is vital, looking at temperature, skin texture and colour changes present. Observing the reaction of the child and their parents as you examine the painful area is important to help define the pain reactions present.

As previously discussed, the assessment should include examination of range of movement of all joints in order to examine the level of hypermobility present or joint limitation due to muscle spasm and pain, as well as specific and individual muscle strength, focusing on antigravity muscles and especially into hypermobile range. The assessment of function should include an examination of general mobility, balance, proprioception and gait to identify what muscles and joints are being used in a weight-bearing activity and so guide the treatment plan.

MANAGEMENT OF CHRONIC PAIN SYNDROMES

The principles are similar to those for managing JHS, with the inclusion of some important additional therapy interventions such as desensitization.

The most important message to convey to the child and their family is that medical pain relief has a very limited role in the management of this severe biomechanically driven pain and that the goal of any future intervention is to regain normal function and activity despite the pain. The family need to realize that waiting for the pain to go before returning to physical activity is not going to work, because inactivity and abnormal movement are the two most significant driving forces for the pain. The philosophy of this approach is to correct the abnormal biomechanics involved in their movements and gait, address the inactivity, weakened muscles and reduced movement of a specific limb which are all responsible for increasing the pain.

An explanation that families can often identify with is that of 'pins and needles'. When this occurs it is usually due to a limb being held in an unusual position for a period of time without any movement. Constant movement is normal. But in managing 'pins and needles' the sensation is not really noticeable if not moving and the area often feels numb, however a small amount of movement makes the sensation very uncomfortable. However, the quickest way to get rid of 'pins and needles' is to move a lot and get back to normal movement and activity as quickly as possible. Often during this process the pain increases temporarily, but then it dramatically decreases and goes away. Managing this type of pain syndrome, especially CRPS, follows the same approach.

The children and the families need to appreciate that the management of chronic pain syndrome requires a combined approach, both physical and psychological, and that they cannot be separated.

Desensitization

The principles of desensitization have changed over the years. It used to be understood that using different textures to rub the skin with regularity was an effective way of helping reduce the sensitivity of the skin. However, this approach rarely works, and children and families become despondent and often give up because the pain continues to escalate. An alternative suggestion is to adopt a functional desensitization approach with the focus on 'function despite pain'. The approach starts with attempts to regain normal movement, even a small amount of movement in the case of a limb with CRPS. This can be done by passive movement supported by active assisted movement and progressed to totally active movement before the treatment session is completed. The active independent function is maintained and used by the young person until the next treatment session where it is progressed further.

The most important aspect to reducing the pain is regaining normal movement patterns and independent function. This is supported by efficient muscle control of all joints and throughout full range of movement. These measures will start to bring the pain under control and when combined with psychological pain management strategies the young person should be able to return to full and active function.

SUMMARY

Joint hypermobility syndrome is a condition with many forms of clinical presentation in young people. If undiagnosed or untreated it can result in the development of a chronic pain cycle, or chronic pain syndrome, with a high level of disability. This requires an intensive, but paced, musculoskeletal rehabilitation programme to manage the symptoms effectively. It is vital that the child and family are clear in their understanding of the condition and that a self-management programme is the most appropriate long-term treatment approach for this condition.

References

Acasuso-Diaz M, Collantes-Estevez E: Joint hypermobility in patients with fibromyalgia syndrome, *Arthritis Care Res* 11(1):39–42, 1998.

Agnew P: Evaluation of the child with ligamentous laxity, *Clin Podiatr Med Surg* 14(1):117–130, 1997.

Al Rawi Z, Nessan AH: Joint hypermobility in patients with chondromalacia patellae, *Br J Rheumatol* 36(12):1324–1327, 1997.

Augustsson J, Thomee R: Ability of closed and open kinetic chain tests of muscular strength to assess functional performance, *Scandanavian Journal of Medicine and Science in Sports* 10(3):164–168, 2000.

Barron DF, Cohen BA, Geraghty MT, et al: Joint hypermobility is more common in children with chronic fatigue syndrome than in healthy controls, *J Pediatr* 141(3):421–425, 2002.

Barton LM, Bird HA: Improving pain by the stabilization of hyperlax joints, *Journal of Orthopaedic Rheumatology* 9:46–51, 1996.

Beighton P, Solomon L, Soskolne CL: Articular Mobility in an African Population, *Annals of Rheumatic Diseases* 32:413–418, 1973.

Bernhardt DT, Gomez J, Johnson MD, et al: Strength training by children and adolescents, *Pediatrics* 107(6):1470–1472, 2001.

Bilkey WJ, Baxter TL, Kottke FJ, et al: Muscle formation in Ehlers-Danlos syndrome, *Arch Phys Med Rehabil* 62(9):444–448, 1981.

Biro F, Gewanter HL, Baum J: The hypermobility syndrome, *Pediatrics* 72(5):701–706, 1983.

Birrell FN, Adebajo AO, Hazleman BL, et al: High prevalence of joint laxity in West Africans, *Br J Rheumatol* 33(1):56–59, 1994.

Boardman DL, Dorey F, Thomas BJ, et al: The accuracy of assessing total hip arthroplasty outcomes: a prospective correlation study of walking ability and 2 validated measurement devices, *J Arthroplasty* 15(2):200–204, 2000.

Borms J: The child and exercise: an overview, *J Sports Sci* 4(1):3–20, 1986.

Bruehl S, Harden RN, Galer BS, et al: Complex regional pain syndrome: are there distinct subtypes and sequential stages of the syndrome? *Pain* 95(1–2):119–124, 2002.

Bulbena A, Duro JC, Porta M, et al: Anxiety disorders in the joint hypermobility syndrome, *Psychiatry Res* 46(1):59–68, 1993.

Bulbena A, Agullo A, Pailhez G, et al: Is joint hypermobility related to anxiety in a nonclinical population also? *Psychosomatics* 45(5):432–437, 2004.

Bulbena A, Gago J, Sperry L, et al: The relationship between frequency and intensity of fears and a collagen condition, *Depress Anxiety* 23(7):412–417, 2006a.

Bulbena A, Sperry L, Pailhez G, et al: Anxiety, temporomandibular disorders, and joint hypermobility syndrome. Response to 'Psychological assessment of patients with temporomandibular disorders: confirmatory analysis of the dimensional structure of the Brief Symptoms Inventory 18', *J Psychosom Res* 61(6):851, 2006b.

Bundonis J: Pediatric strength training, *Rehab Manag* 20(3):22–24, 2007.

Cheng JC, Chan PS, Hui PW: Joint laxity in children, *J Pediatr Orthop* 11(6):752–756, 1991.

Christou M, Smilios I, Sotiropoulos K, et al: Effects of resistance training on the physical capacities of adolescent soccer players, *J Strength Cond Res* 20(4):783–791, 2006.

Davidovitch M, Tirosh E, Tal Y: The relationship between joint hypermobility and neurodevelopmental attributes in elementary school children, *J Child Neurol* 9(4):417–419, 1994.

Decoster LC, Vailas JC, Lindsay RH, et al: Prevalence and features of joint hypermobility among adolescent athletes, *Archives of Pediatric and Adolescent Medicine* 151(10):989–992, 1997.

Dinos S, Khoshaba B, Ashby D: A systematic review of chronic fatigue, its syndromes and ethnicity: prevalence, severity, co-morbidity and coping, *Int J Epidemiol* 38(6):1554–1570, 2009.

El Garf AK, Mahmoud GA, Mahgoub EH: Hypermobility among Egyptian children: prevalence and features, *J Rheumatol* 25(5):1003–1005, 1998.

El-Shahaly HA, El-Sherif AK: Is the benign joint hypermobility syndrome benign? *Clin Rheumatol* 10(3):302–307, 1991.

Engelbert RH, van Bergen M, Henneken T, et al: Exercise tolerance in children and adolescents with musculoskeletal pain in joint hypermobility and joint hypomobility syndrome, *Pediatrics* 118(3):e690–e696, 2006.

Faigenbaum AD, Westcott WL, Loud RL, et al: The effects of different resistance training protocols on muscular strength and endurance development in children, *Pediatrics* 104(1):e5, 1999.

Faigenbaum AD: Strength training for children and adolescents, *Clin Sports Med* 19(4):593–619, 2000.

Faigenbaum AD, Loud RL, O'Connell J, et al: Effects of different resistance training protocols on upper-body strength and endurance development in children, *Journal of Strength and Conditioning.Research* 15(4): 459–465, 2001.

Faigenbaum AD, Milliken LA, Loud RL, et al: Comparison of 1 and 2 days per week of strength training in children, *Res Q Exerc Sport* 73(4):416–424, 2002.

Finsterbush A, Pogrund H: The hypermobility syndrome. Musculoskeletal complaints in 100 consecutive cases of generalized joint hypermobility, *Clinical Orthopaedics* 168:124–127, 1982.

Flanagan SP, Laubach LL, De MG Jr, et al: Effects of two different strength training modes on motor performance in children, *Res Q Exerc Sport* 73(3):340–344, 2002.

Forleo LH, Hilario MO, Peixoto AL, et al: Articular hypermobility in school children in Sao Paulo, Brazil, *J Rheumatol* 20:916–917, 1993.

Garofano RP, Barst RJ: Exercise testing in children with primary pulmonary hypertension, *Pediatr Cardiol* 20(1):61–64, 1999.

Gedalia A, Person DA, Brewer EJ, et al: Hypermobility of the joints in juvenile episodic arthritis/ arthralgia, *J Pediatr* 107(6):873–876, 1985.

Gedalia A, Brewer EJ: Joint hypermobility in pediatric practice–a review, *J Rheumatol* 20(2):371–374, 1993.

Gedalia A, Garcia CO, Molina JF, et al: Fibromyalgia syndrome: experience in a pediatric rheumatology clinic, *Clin Exp Rheumatol* 18(3):415–419, 2000.

Grahame R: Joint hypermobility and genetic collagen disorders: are

they related? *Archives of Diseases in Childhood* 80(2):188–191, 1999.

Grahame R, Bird HA, Child A, et al: The revised (Brighton 1998) criteria for the diagnosis of benign joint hypermobility syndrome (BJHS), *J Rheumatol* 27(7):1777–1779, 2000.

Hagroo GA, Zaki HM, Choudhary MT, et al: Pulled elbow - not the effect of hypermobility of joints, *Injury* 26(10):687–690, 1995.

Hakkinen K, Mero A, Kauhanen H: Specificity of endurance, sprint and strength training on physical performance capacity in young athletes, *J Sports Med Phys Fitness* 29(1):27–35, 1989.

Hall MG, Ferrell WR, Sturrock RD, et al: The effect of the hypermobility syndrome on knee joint proprioception, *Br J Rheumatol* 34(2):121–125, 1995.

Hamilton DM, Haennel RG: Validity and reliability of the 6-minute walk test in a cardiac rehabilitation population, *J Cardiopulm Rehabil* 20(3):156–164, 2000.

Harden RN, Bruehl S, Galer BS, et al: Complex regional pain syndrome: are the IASP diagnostic criteria valid and sufficiently comprehensive? *Pain* 83(2): 211–219, 1999.

Hoffman JR, Ratamess NA, Cooper JJ, et al: Comparison of loaded and unloaded jump squat training on strength/power performance in college football players, *J Strength Cond Res* 19(4):810–815, 2005.

Hudson N, Fitzcharles MA, Cohen M, et al: The association of soft-tissue rheumatism and hypermobility, *Br J Rheumatol* 37(4):382–386, 1998.

Jaffe M, Tirosh E, Cohen A, et al: Joint mobility and motor development, *Arch Dis Child* 63(2):159–161, 1988.

Kaufman LB, Schilling DL: Implementation of a strength training program for a 5-year-old

child with poor body awareness and developmental coordination disorder, *Phys Ther* 87(4):455–467, 2007.

Kendall FP, McCreary EK, Provance PG: *Muscles Testing and Function*, ed 4, Baltimore, 1993, Williams & Wilkins, p 188.

Kerr A, Macmillan CE, Uttley WS, et al: Physiotherapy for Children with Hypermobility Syndrome, *Physiotherapy* 86(6):313–317, 2000.

King MB, Judge JO, Whipple R, et al: Reliability and responsiveness of two physical performance measures examined in the context of a functional training intervention, *Phys Ther* 80(1):8–16, 2000.

Kirby A, Davies R: Developmental Coordination Disorder and Joint Hypermobility Syndrome– overlapping disorders? Implications for research and clinical practice, *Child Care Health Dev* 33(5):513–519, 2007.

Kirk JA, Ansell BM, Bywaters EG: The hypermobility syndrome. Musculoskeletal complaints associated with generalized joint hypermobility, *Ann Rheum Dis* 26(5):419–425, 1967.

Larsson LG, Baum J, Mudholkar GS: Hypermobility: features and differential incidence between the sexes, *Arthritis Rheum* 30:1426–1430, 1987.

Logsdon VK: Training the prepubertal and pubertal athlete, *Curr Sports Med Rep* 6(3):183–189, 2007.

McCambridge TM, Stricker PR: Strength training by children and adolescents, *Pediatrics* 121(4):835–840, 2008.

McGrath P: Annotation: aspects of pain in children and adolescents, *J Child Psychol Psychiatry* 36(5): 717–730, 1995.

McNee AE, Gough M, Morrissey MC, et al: Increases in muscle volume after plantarflexor strength training in children with spastic cerebral palsy, *Dev Med Child Neurol* 51(6):429–435, 2009.

Maillard S, Murray KJ: Hypermobility syndrome in children. In Keer R, Grahame R, editors: *Hypermobility Syndrome: Recognition and Management for Physiotherapists*, Edinburgh, 2003, Butterworth Heinmann, pp 33–50.

Maillard SM, Davies K, Khubchandani R, et al: Reflex sympathetic dystrophy: a multidisciplinary approach, *Arthritis Rheum* 51(2):284–290, 2004.

Malleson PN, Beauchamp RD: Rheumatology: 16, Diagnosing musculoskeletal pain in children, *Can Med Assoc J* 165(2):183–188, 2001.

Mallik AK, Ferrell WR, McDonald AG, et al: Impaired proprioceptive acuity at the proximal interphalangeal joint in patients with the hypermobility syndrome, *Br J Rheumatol* 33(7):631–637, 1994.

Martin-Santos R, Bulbena A, Porta M, et al: Association between joint hypermobility syndrome and panic disorder, *Am J Psychiatry* 155(11):1578–1583, 1998.

Mato H, Sian S, Hasson N, et al: A review of the management of complex regional pain syndrome; an experience of an inpatient rehabilitation unit, *Pediatric Rheumatology* 6(suppl 1):171, 2008.

Mishra MB, Ryan P, Atkinson P, et al: Extra-articular Features of Benign Joint Hypermobility Syndrome, *Br J Rheumatol* 35:861–866, 1996.

Moreira A, Wilson J: Non-progressive paraparesis in children with congenital ligamentous laxity, *Neuropediatrics* 23(1):49–52, 1992.

Nixon PA, Joswiak ML, Fricker FJ: A six-minute walk test for assessing exercise tolerance in severely ill children, *J Pediatr* 129(3):362–366, 1996.

Pankoff B, Overend T, Lucy D, et al: Validity and responsiveness of the 6 minute walk test for people with fibromyalgia, *J Rheumatol* 27(11):2666–2670, 2000.

Purcell JS, Hergenroeder AC: Physical conditioning in adolescents, *Curr Opin Pediatr* 6(4):373–378, 1994.

Qvindesland A, Jonsson H: Articular hypermobility in Icelandic 12-year-olds, *Rheumatology Oxford* 38:1014–1016, 1999.

Russek LN: Hypermobility syndrome, *Phys Ther* 79 (6):591–599, 1999.

Rikken-Bultman DG, Wellink L, van Dongen PW: Hypermobility in two Dutch school populations, *Eur J Obstet Gynecol Reprod Biol* 73:189–192, 1997.

Russek LN: Examination and treatment of a patient with hypermobility syndrome, *Phys Ther* 80(4):386–398, 2000.

Scharf Y, Nahir AM: Case report: hypermobility syndrome mimicking juvenile chronic arthritis, *Rheumatol Rehabil* 21(2):78–80, 1982.

Schnizer W: Therapeutic muscle training, *Wien Klin Wochenschr* 105(8):232–238, 1993.

Seow CC, Chow PK, Khong KS: A study of joint mobility in a normal population, *Ann Acad Med Singapore* 28:231–236, 1999.

Silverman S, Constine L, Harvey W, et al: Survey of joint mobility and in vivo skin elasticity in London schoolchildren, *Annals of Rheumatic Diseases* 34(2):177–180, 1975.

Stanton-Hicks M: Reflex sympathetic dystrophy: a sympathetically mediated pain syndrome or not? *Curr Rev Pain* 4(4):268–275, 2000.

Sugden DA, Kirby A, Dunford C: Children with developmental coordination disorder. Special Edition of International Journal of

Disability, Development and Education, 55(2):93–187, 2008.

Tirosh E, Jaffe M, Marmur R, et al: Prognosis of motor development and joint hypermobility, *Arch Dis Child* 66(8):931–933, 1991.

van de Putte EM, Uiterwaal CS, Bots ML, et al: Is chronic fatigue syndrome a connective tissue disorder? A cross-sectional study in adolescents, *Pediatrics* 115(4):e415–e422, 2005.

Varni JW, Limbers CA: The PedsQL Multidimensional Fatigue Scale in young adults: feasibility, reliability and validity in a university student population, *Qual Life Res* 17(1):105–111, 2008.

Vaughn JM, Micheli L: Strength training recommendations for the young athlete, *Phys Med Rehabil Clin N Am* 19(2):235–245, viii, 2008.

Veldman PH, Reynen HM, Arntz IE, et al: Signs and symptoms of reflex sympathetic dystrophy: prospective study of 829 patients, *Lancet* 342 (8878):1012–1016, 1993.

Vougiouka O, Moustaki M, Tsanaktsi M: Benign hypermobility syndrome in Greek schoolchildren, *Eur J Pediatr* 159(8):628, 2000.

Webb DR: Strength training in children and adolescents, *Pediatric Clinics North America* 37(5):1187–1210, 1990.

Wilder RT, Berde CB, Wolohan M, et al: Reflex sympathetic dystrophy in children. Clinical characteristics and follow-up of seventy patients, *J Bone Joint Surg Am* 74(6):910–919, 1992.

Yamamoto LM, Lopez RM, Klau JF, et al: The effects of resistance training on endurance distance running performance among highly trained runners: a systematic review, *J Strength Cond Res* 22(6):2036–2044, 2008.

Chapter 12

Regional complications in joint hypermobility syndrome

12.1 The shoulder joint

Anju Jaggi and Simon M Lambert

INTRODUCTION

Laxity (or 'looseness') in the shoulder is defined as asymptomatic motion through a range which would be considered abnormal for the patient's age, gender or race. Laxity varies with age: adolescents have a greater overall range of motion than adults, and stiffness (reduced compliance of rotator cuff and capsular tissues) increases with age. Shoulder laxity can exist as part of the generalized hypermobility syndromes or in isolation. In the latter form, if one shoulder alone is affected then congenital bony architectural anomalies should be considered. If bilateral, isolated shoulder hypermobility is present and soft tissue anomalies are more prevalent.

LAXITY

APPROPRIATE LAXITY

Normal soft tissue laxity is influenced by oestrogen levels, the state of hydration, and training. Laxity is very useful in certain circumstances (for instance at child-birth), so selective biological advantage might be conferred on those who develop appropriate laxity. Similarly, degenerative arthritis is uncommon in those who have loose shoulders, unless there are associated morphological anomalies of the glenoid or proximal humerus, or inappropriate surgery.

INAPPROPRIATE LAXITY, ENERGY EXPENDITURE AND THE ROTATOR CUFF

Much greater energy expenditure is required to maintain shoulder stability in hyperlax individuals. These individuals must train consistently to protect their shoulders from overload; the capacity of the rotator cuff to generate a centralizing joint reaction force (to keep the humeral articular surface on the glenoid) is much less at the extreme ranges of motion. The rotator cuff is specifically organized from deep to superficial so that the shortest muscle fibres (the deepest fibres) take origin at the most lateral extent of their scapular attachment, and insert into the capsule of the shoulder. These fibres contribute the most to the centralizing or stability function; at the extremes of range of motion, their effectiveness as both stabilizers and controllers of motion is suboptimal. At these positions the activity of the rotator cuff becomes very asymmetric, so the stability and rapidity of response to motion are diminished. Greater muscle bulk increases the inertia of the joint (its 'passive' resistance to displacement), so that training to increase muscle bulk will improve stability, but will conversely require greater energy expenditure. If training ceases, muscle tone diminishes and the joints are less protected. If, in addition, microtraumatic structural surface damage has occurred as a result of previous activity, then the joint is at greater risk of degenerative change.

DOI: 10.1016/B978-0-7020-3005-5.00016-1

The quality of proprioception is reduced in shoulders with hyperlaxity, instability, and previous capsular trauma. Improvement in joint position and motion sense has been shown in trained shoulders and after anterior capsular reconstruction in those with traumatic structural instability (Myers et al 2006). It is not clear whether this is also the case for patients with atraumatic structural instability.

SHOULDER PATHOLOGY IN HYPERMOBILITY SYNDROMES

The shoulder can present the full range of shoulder pathologies according to the age of the patient, but the manifestation of pain is more profound in JHS. Muscular weakness and fatigue, maladaptive postural changes and subsequent chronic pain states are common. Pain of sclerotomal, neuroectodermal and mesodermal origin is prevalent in all shoulder conditions. This is particularly so in hypermobility conditions and patients appear readily precipitated into regional pain states. Recognition of the risk of developing a cascade of maladaptive responses to the initiating condition is of paramount importance and close supervision of rehabilitation of even simple shoulder conditions is vital. It is not clear whether rotator cuff degeneration is accelerated in hypermobility conditions. The incidence of new rotator cuff disease does not appear to be earlier or more likely, reflecting the generally younger age represented in this group.

COMMON DISEASE CONDITIONS

IMPINGEMENT

Given the greater range of motion available, and easier fatigue of stabilizing muscles, conditions characterized by surfaces rubbing together to create painful roughness or buckling of tissues (so-called 'impingement') are common. These include both external and internal anterosuperior and posterosuperior subacromial impingement. External impingement causes superior compartment mechanical pain during mid-range motion with sclerotomal radiation to the upper arm. It may also precipitate abnormal scapular posturing, so promoting the tendency to abnormal patterns of motion in the shoulder. The tendon of the long head of the biceps (LHBT) is then exposed to greater strain. Internal impingement causes mechanical joint cavity pain at the extremes of motion, which are rather more difficult to differentiate.

BICEPS TENDON PATHOLOGY

When the centralizing effect of the rotator cuff is insufficient, the LHBT becomes a more important restraint to forward motion; it is often a source of pain (having a huge autonomic nerve supply), even if apparently normal to imaging and at arthroscopy. Therefore, in external impingement syndromes, the LHBT can become a secondary source of pain. In turn, bicipital pain can confound attempts to rehabilitate the rotator cuff.

GLENOHUMERAL INSTABILITY

Classification

The clinical syndrome of glenohumeral instability is a disturbance of one or more of the following factors, in isolation or together:

- the capsulolabral proprioceptive mechanism (CLPM)
- the rotator cuff (RC)
- the surface arc or area of contact (SAC) between the glenoid and humeral head
- the central/peripheral nervous system (NS).

The relative importance of each factor to the syndrome can change over time. The pathologies causing instability comprise structural (RC, SAC, CLPM) and non-structural (NS) elements (Lewis et al 2004). The structural elements may be congenitally abnormal, comprise abnormal collagen, acquire microtraumatic lesions over time (atraumatic structural) or be damaged by extrinsic force (traumatic structural). The non-structural elements can be congenitally abnormal or acquired over time as perturbations of neuromuscular control, particularly at periods of skeletal growth.

The concept of instability (which may change over time) being caused by a combination of structural (traumatic and atraumatic) and neurological system disturbances, has led to the classification of instability as a continuum of pathologies, which can be graphically displayed as a triangle (Lewis et al 2004). The polar pathologies are labelled type I (traumatic instability), type II (atraumatic instability) and type III (neurological dysfunctional or muscle-patterning). Polar groups I and II and the axis I–II, representing the spectrum between the two poles, correspond to the TUBS-AMBRI classification (Thomas & Matsen 1989). This allows for a spectrum of structural shoulder pathology but does not admit those shoulders in which there is no structural (traumatic or atraumatic) cause for the instability. Personal observation has further subdivided polar group III into peripheral, central, protective and combination subtypes (A Jaggi, personal communication). The interpolar spectrum describes dual pathologies in which traumatic, atraumatic and muscle-patterning factors play a variable role in the emergence of instability. All groups can be represented in patients with JHS, but more commonly present in groups II and III.

Presentation

JHS patients may present with pain rather than overtly abnormal displacements. Anterior atraumatic instability is less common than posterior types (Malone et al 2006a). Posterior structural anomalies (including posterior glenoid dysplasia, excessive glenoid retroversion, glenoid hypoplasia and medialized posterior capsular attachment) create the environment in which obligatory positional posterior displacement may occur during elevation of the arm in the sagittal plane. If abnormal muscle activation appears clinically obvious, either at the onset of motion, or during the motion, then the diagnosis has a muscle patterning component (type III). If there is no clinically or electrophysiologically proven aberrant muscle activation then the condition is labelled type II (positional subtype).

Scapular dyskinesis is common, and reflects the attempt by the scapular postural muscles to maintain scapulohumeral homeostasis.

Assessment of the structural diagnosis is by magnetic resonance arthrography (MRA) and/or diagnostic arthroscopy. These are complementary, not alternative, techniques. MRA is useful to look for capsular detachments, bony defects and the bulk and quality of rotator cuff muscles, particularly subscapularis and infraspinatus. Arthroscopy is useful to look for the subtleties of internal lesions of occult instability, such as bicipital and deep surface cuff lesions, soft tissue Broca defects, internal impingement and external impingement lesions.

Muscle-patterning instability (MPI) comprises aberrant activation of large muscles and simultaneous suppression of the rotator cuff. Thus far, dynamic electromyography has characterized latissimus dorsi, pectoralis major and anterior deltoid among the large muscles, and only infraspinatus of the rotator cuff. It is as yet not clear whether suppression of infraspinatus reflects whole rotator cuff suppression or specific suppression of the infraspinatus. MPI can be clinically obvious in polar group III, but may be occult, requiring dynamic electromyography (DEMG) for confirmation in type II/III and III/II instabilities (Malone et al 2006b).

The patient with JHS has a tendency to experience symptoms of instability often unrelated to traumatic injury. Minor events can create recurring episodes of shoulder displacement and ongoing pain, cascading the patient into a cycle of increasing disability. Classifying the instability correctly will lead to appropriate management and avoid unnecessary surgery, which in certain cases can exacerbate symptoms and disability. Management also requires a multifaceted approach, not simply isolated to strengthening regimens or surgery, but training the motor control system that contributes to stability. More challenging cases may require input from a multidisciplinary team. The remainder of this chapter will address the conservative management of atraumatic shoulder instability pertinent to the JHS patient.

CLINICAL ASSESSMENT

Abnormal muscle patterning is the result of aberration in one or more of three sub-systems, which contribute to neuromuscular control. At a peripheral level, capsular laxity and abnormal collagen composition may affect proprioception and lead to injury and resultant instability (Blasier et al 1994, Myers & Lephart 2002). Furthermore, a proprioceptively deficient joint can disrupt movement at other joints along the kinetic chain by altering the motor programme, thereby affecting control at a central level (Myers & Lephart 2002). In addition, impaired central nervous motor programming due to stress, constrained movements, postures and/or chronic fatigue will influence muscle tone, creating the risk of instability. Assessment of all three systems is therefore necessary to aid appropriate management. (Chapter 3, Fig. 3.2 and Chapter 8, Fig. 8.1 & 8.2)

SUBJECTIVE ASSESSMENT

The mechanism of the event that causes the initial symptoms is key to classification. JHS patients will commonly describe atraumatic events. These can include an over-stretching manoeuvre or repetitive use, which causes initial displacement but with spontaneous relocation or relocation with minimal assistance. Impaired proprioception leads to a propensity to injury and the most minor incidents can cause easy displacement of the glenohumeral joint (GHJ) with minor or no resultant structural damage. Subsequently, the patient notices recurrent episodes of dislocation on simple manoeuvres often associated with daily activities. Some patients with a predominant muscle-patterning problem often describe an ability to voluntarily displace the shoulder, a 'party trick'. An initial childhood voluntary trick causing no problems, may develop after minor injury, into an involuntary problem creating a so-called habitual problem. On occasion, the shoulder can remain persistently displaced as a result of ongoing abnormal muscle activity. Patients may recall that emergency room staff had difficulty relocating the shoulder or keeping the joint located after cessation of anaesthesia. During muscular relaxation under anaesthesia, the shoulder reduces spontaneously, but on recovery of conscious function the shoulder re-dislocates readily, but, importantly, not voluntarily. How much of this ongoing abnormal muscle activation is a result of pain, fear and altered central inhibitory control (Barrett et al 2000) is difficult to ascertain, but points to the likelihood of a non-structural cause to the instability.

The dislocations themselves are often painless. However, patients can experience intense pain due to muscle spasm, or continued aching in or around the shoulder. JHS patients may exhibit heightened pain responses due to altered pain perception. They may additionally describe non-dermatomal, non-radicular paraesthesia and dysaesthesia in the upper limb, secondary to altered neural dynamics and autonomic disturbance associated with hypermobility syndrome, resembling sympathoparetic pain syndromes.

In adolescents, accelerated growth may be associated with exacerbation of symptoms (Chapter 10). The peak incidences of new-onset muscle-patterning instability occur at about 10, 15 and 20+ years, suggesting a coincidence with pubertal hormonal effects, especially within the female cohort (Malone et al 2006a). Leisure and sport activities should also be considered. The repetitive nature of an activity such as swimming may expose the predisposed joint to overuse, leading to peri-articular muscle fatigue. Certain activities, such as poorly supervised weight-training may cause asymmetric overuse in agonist muscle groups, thus exacerbating postural and motor imbalances. A common pattern involves a dominance of powerful internal rotators (pectoralis major and latissimus dorsi) over weaker, or suppressed, external rotators (infraspinatus) and aberrant trunk stability.

Psychological stress has been implicated in the production of symptoms. However, experience at our unit strongly suggests that the observed stress and anxiety is secondary to the persistent challenge of painful instability. Fear of using the upper limb or modification of activity compounds the problem, altering central motor control. Careful and sensitive history-taking allows the therapist to extract this information and avoid the implication that patients may be displacing their shoulder for a secondary gain, which has sometimes been implied by health professionals who do not appreciate that muscle patterning can contribute to shoulder instability. Involvement of clinical psychologists can be useful to help the patient acknowledge and manage their fear of, as well as the fact of, persistent and recurrent instability and prepare the path for active management of JHS (Chapter 8).

OBJECTIVE ASSESSMENT

A thorough clinical examination must not only assess the shoulder, but also include posture, global laxity, scapula dysrhythmia, general balance and proprioception (Chapter 6.4). The shoulder does not function in isolation, but provides the integral link in producing and transferring energy from the trunk to the arm (Kibler et al 2001). Lower limb and trunk stability has a resultant effect on the scapula and GHJ. Integrating multiple body segments (proximal to distal) rehabilitates the entire neuromuscular system, so optimizing shoulder function (McMullen & Uhl 2000).

Posture

An assessment of standing posture should be performed from all directions. The hypermobile patient typically adopts the sway-back posture as described by Kendall et al (1993), a tendency to hyperextend the hips and knees and cause forward displacement of the pelvis. This tendency to hang at the extreme of their hypermobile range results in poor core stability and may increase the use of more superficial torque muscles such as latissimus dorsi, having a resultant effect at the shoulder girdle (Gibson 2004).

A secondary thoracic kyphosis may develop to compensate for the sway posture. As a result the scapula adopts a protracted, laterally tilted position. The glenoid cavities face downwards and forwards, such that the humeral head 'hangs' from the glenoid, further challenging the joint reaction compression force. If the medial border or inferior pole of the scapula also wings, the combination of inhibition of the scapula stabilizers (serratus anterior and the lower fibres of trapezius) with increased activity in the pectoral and latissimus muscles (Kibler 2000a, Mottram 1997) should be assessed.

Quality of movement

Aberrant scapular mechanics are fundamental to the aetiology of instability and must be assessed both at rest and dynamically. The scapula is observed as the patient elevates the arm in both flexion and abduction planes. It is also useful to assess scapular stability in weight bearing by placing the patient in four-point kneeling. This may highlight scapula winging as well as poor trunk stability (Magarey & Jones 2003) (Figure 12.1.1). Movement faults are not always present on one manoeuvre and if symptoms tend to be present on overuse, it is helpful to ask the patient to repeat movements with varied speed to pick up abnormality.

In those patients who can demonstrate a party trick it is useful to observe the direction of displacement and any associated abnormal muscle activation. It is also important to observe the resting position of the GHJ prior to movement, to be sure it is not already displaced under the effect of abnormal resting tone in surrounding muscles.

A persistently inferiorly displaced GHJ can prove difficult to manage, because this indicates gross inhibition of rotator cuff and deltoid tone which is likely to be centrally driven (Figure 12.1.2).

Patients with MPI usually present with posterior instability (Takwale et al 2000, Kuroda et al 2001, Malone et al 2006a). The dominant pattern of elevation of the arm is in internal rotation (associated with overactivity in latissimus dorsi and/or pectoralis major), with resultant or associated inhibition of infraspinatus and posterior deltoid. As a result, posterior displacement of the GHJ occurs in ascent with an associated 'reverse-scapular' action, as the scapula is prevented from protracting and upwardly rotating in the normal way (Takwale et al 2000). As the arm descends, there may be an audible click or clunk as the GHJ relocates.

A useful clinical test to confirm whether posterior instability is a result of such imbalance is the external rotation facilitation test. The practitioner facilitates the action of infraspinatus by encouraging active external rotation against resistance as the limb is elevated. If the GHJ remains stable (located) then treatment should be focused towards restoring normal movement patterns (Takwale et al 2000) through biofeedback programmes, which facilitate infraspinatus and suppress pectoralis and latissimus activity.

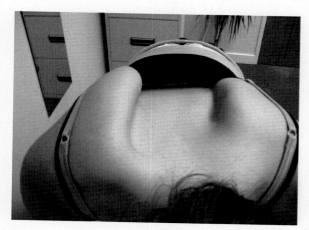

Fig. 12.1.1 Winging scapulae in 4-point kneeling

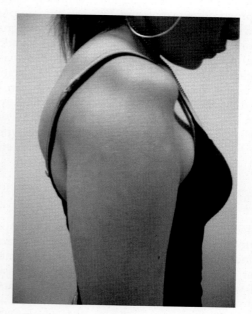

Fig. 12.1.2 Sulcus sign: persistent subluxation of the glenohumeral joint

Muscle activation

Conservative management of shoulder instability has concentrated on strengthening exercises to the rotator cuff (Aronen & Regan 1984, Burkhead & Rockwood 1992). However, it is now recognized that abnormal muscle activation in other muscle groups can contribute to instability. Experience at our specialist unit through the use of DEMG has indicated that abnormal activation patterns in latissimus dorsi, pectoralis major, anterior deltoid and infraspinatus contribute to shoulder instability (Malone et al 2006b). In the absence of electromyography equipment, the therapist can assess abnormal tone through palpation and observation as discussed above. Asking the patient to perform simple distal movements with the hand or elbow, and palpating for any increased activation of the pectoral or latissimus dorsi muscles, may indicate abnormal recruitment. Strengthening programmes may not always be fruitful in the presence of abnormal tone in other muscles and sometimes management may need to focus on inhibiting muscle activation to gain stability.

Standard instability tests for the shoulder may be useful in cases where observation alone does not indicate the direction of instability, but it must be recalled that asymptomatic translation of the glenohumeral joint simply indicates laxity of the joint. Instability can, by definition, only be present if the patient has recognizable symptoms during the provocative manoeuvre. JHS patients can present with clumsiness, poor co-ordination and gross motor maldevelopment (Adib et al 2005), so additional neurological tests to assess cerebellar, basal ganglia and dorsal (spinal cord) column functions are useful. General balance and stability can be tested by the single-leg balance test, both with eyes open and closed (Chapter 6.4). Poor control will highlight lower limb and trunk imbalances, which may be contributing to the instability (Kibler et al 2001, Gibson et al 2004).

MANAGEMENT

Correcting abnormal muscle patterns and appropriate strengthening are the key principles in management. Re-establishing neuromuscular control must integrate peripheral somatosensory, visual and vestibular afferent input and improve motor control through spinal reflex, brain stem and cognitive programming (Lephart & Henry 2000, Griffin and Letha 2003).

EARLY AND INTERMEDIATE STAGES

Initial management includes explanation and reassurance, as compliance is paramount for a successful outcome. A shoulder that is displacing primarily under the abnormal control of muscle activation is unlikely to cause structural harm. Often, fear and avoidance perpetuate the instability, so it is essential that the patient is reassured. Voluntary displacements should be discouraged to avoid a habitual pattern developing, as well as activities that are reinforcing abnormal muscle activation. However, general fitness should still be encouraged to maintain general tone and condition.

Postural awareness and correction is the foundation of early intervention. Improving core strength may directly influence abnormal muscle tone at the shoulder girdle. This can be achieved by simple postural exercises such as back flattening against a wall, challenging balance using a Swiss ball (Fig. 12.1.3) or balance board and single-leg stance to increase postural tone. Research has shown that preparatory trunk muscle activation accompanies limb motion (Zattara & Bouisset 1988, Hodges

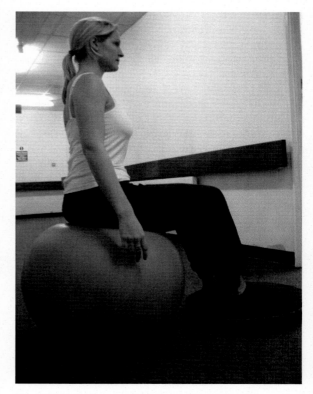

Fig. 12.1.3 Posture re-education on the Swiss ball

et al 2001) and supports the concept of working on posture prior to upper limb movement.

Many JHS patients lack joint awareness, so early feedback of posture and shoulder girdle position is important to avoid inappropriate patterning and strengthening. Postural tape, corsets or pressure garments are helpful in providing tactile feedback to aid correct sensory feedback (DeCarlo et al 1996, Chu et al 2002, Ide et al 2003, Ulkar et al 2004). (Fig. 12.1.4).

Additional biofeedback can be provided through the use of surface EMG, video and mirrors. Experience at our unit has found the use of surface EMG helpful in training appropriate activation patterns in shoulder movement (Malone et al 2006a) and has been shown to be more effective in regaining normal stability then strengthening exercises alone (Beall et al 1987, Reid et al 1996, Kiss et al 2001, Magarey & Jones 2003) (Fig. 12.1.5). Biofeedback techniques appear to facilitate the feed forward learning process at a cortical level, which may help to achieve more efficient motor patterns.

Weight-bearing exercises enhance joint stability, stimulate muscular co-activation and facilitate proprioception (Wilk et al 1993, Dines & Levinson 1995, Lephart & Henry 1996, Kibler 2000b). These can initially be done on a fixed base of support, progressing to stabilizing on a ball or balance board, enhancing neuromuscular control at a reflex level (Fig. 12.1.6). Strengthening exercises to the rotator

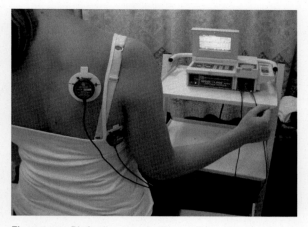

Fig. 12.1.5 Biofeedback to facilitate infraspinatus and inhibit latissimus dorsi

cuff and deltoid can be introduced once the patient has achieved postural correction and the GHJ is located. The load applied must be graded appropriately to ensure that the correct muscles are strengthened. It is often unnecessary to use a Cliniband greater than yellow for cuff strengthening, where the emphasis should be placed on repetition rather than load to help build on endurance of the muscle.

The grades of Cliniband are:

- Yellow – light
- Red – medium
- Green – heavy
- Blue – extra heavy
- Black – special heavy.

ADVANCED STAGE

End-stage rehabilitation should focus on retraining patterns of movement biased towards functional tasks. Functional exercises, such as throwing, require co-ordination among multiple muscle groups, so it is important to address the entire kinetic chain (Dines & Levinson 1995, Kibler et al 2001). Repetition, speed and load may be varied in relation to the desired task, facilitating feed forward processing (Griffin & Letha 2003).

Proprioceptive neuromuscular facilitation (PNF) is useful to gain stability and control into functional patterns, strengthening through range (Voss et al 1953), while emphasis is placed on eccentric loading of the rotator cuff. It is important not to bombard the patient with numerous exercises, but to build on two or three sequentially.

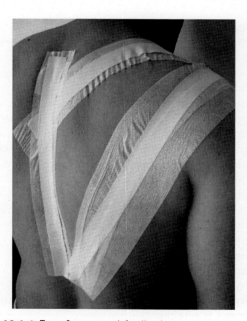

Fig. 12.1.4 Tape for postural feedback

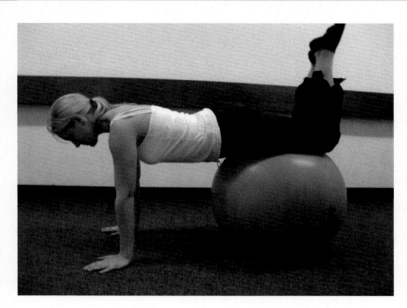

Fig. 12.1.6 Closed chain exercise on the Swiss ball

The frequency of exercise should be little-and-often, guided by fatigue and pain. Wherever possible, they should be made simple so they can easily be performed throughout the day. Patients who have particular problems with pain, will have to pace their activities, to gain a balance between appropriate use and exercise. The duration of management will vary amongst patients; on occasion, correction of a movement fault can be immediate, but it can take several months for the corrected pattern to become established at an unconscious level. It is also important to note that relapses may occur if a new task is undertaken, a growth spurt occurs, or the patient fails to adapt motor responses (Shumway-Cook & Woollacott 2001).

SUMMARY

Patients with JHS comprise a particularly challenging group, in which shoulder problems can include the entire spectrum of common shoulder pathology, but in which specific forms of shoulder conditions occur with peculiar characteristics. It follows that rehabilitation for these patients is complex, time-consuming and prolonged. Successful rehabilitation of the unoperated shoulder, for example, for posterior atraumatic (group II) with

muscle-patterning (group III), is achieved in excess of 85% of cases. Relapses occur, and 25% of patients with initially successful rehabilitation, will return for top-up therapy within 2 years. Success rates fall off for anterior forms of instability and are severely affected by ill-judged operations.

IMPORTANT MESSAGES

- Patients with JHS have a full spectrum of shoulder disorders with profound instability and pain.
- Physiotherapy-based rehabilitation is appropriate, but is prolonged and should be undertaken under the remit of a multidisciplinary team and within the context of pain management, psychological assessment and occasional surgical intervention.
- Rehabilitation is successful in controlling symptoms in the majority of cases, but relapses are common, so patients should be regularly monitored.
- Long-term management of the condition requires lifestyle modification, pacing of physical activity and maintainence of good physical condition to ensure postural muscular control is retained.

References

Adib N, Davies K, Grahame R, et al: Joint Hypermobility syndrome in childhood. A not so benign multisystem disorder? *Rheumatology* 44:744–750, 2005.

Aronen JG, Regan K: Decreasing the incidence of recurrence of first time anterior shoulder dislocations with rehabilitation, *Am J Sports Med* 12(4):283–291, 1984.

Barrett C, Emery R, Wallace A, et al: *Altered corticospinal control of shoulder musculature in shoulder instability – a case study*, Proceedings of the third conference of the International Shoulder group. Newcastle-upon-Tyne, Sept 4–6, 2000.

Beall MS, Diefenbach G, Allen A: Electromyographic biofeedback in the treatment of voluntary posterior instability of the shoulder, *Am J Sports Med* 15(2): 175–178, 1987.

Blasier RB, Carpenter JE, Huston IJ: Shoulder proprioception: Effects of joint laxity, joint position and direction of motion, *Orthop Rev* 23:45–50, 1994.

Burkhead WZ, Rockwood CA: Treatment of Instability of the Shoulder with an exercise program, *J Bone Joint Surg Am* 74:890–896, 1992.

Chu JC, Kane EJ, Brent AL, et al: The Effect of a Neoprene Shoulder Stabilizer on Active Joint-Reposition Sense in Subjects With Stable and Unstable Shoulders, *Journal of Athletic Training* 37(2): 141–145, 2002.

DeCarlo M, Malone K, Gerig B, et al: Evaluation of Shoulder instability braces, *Journal of Sports Rehabilitation* 5:143–150, 1996.

Dines DM, Levinson M: The Conservative Management of the Unstable Shoulder including Rehabilitation, *Clin Sports Med* 14(4):797–816, 1995.

Gibson JC: Mini-Symposium: Shoulder Instability (iii) Rehabilitation after shoulder instability surgery, *Current Orthopaedics* 18:197–209, 2004.

Gibson JC, Rayner VS, Frostick S: *Expanded Assessment in Multidirectional instability: An aid in planning effective rehabilitation?* 9th International Congress on the Surgery of the Shoulder, 2004. Washington USA, May 2004.

Griffin E, Letha Y: Neuromuscular Training and Injury Prevention in Sports, *Clinic Orthopaedics and Related Research* 409:53–60, 2003.

Hodges PW, Cresswall AG, Thorstensson A: Perturbed Upper Limb Movements Cause Short-Latency Postural Responses in Trunk Muscles, *Exp Brain Res* 138:243–250, 2001.

Ide J, Maeda S, Yamaga M, et al: Shoulder strengthening exercise with an orthosis for multidirectional shoulder instability: Quantitive evaluation of rotational shoulder strength before and after the exercise program, *J Shoulder Elbow Surg* 12(4):342–345, 2003.

Kendall FP, McCreary EK, Provance PG, et al: *Muscles: Testing and Function with Posture and Pain*, ed 4, Baltimore, 1993, Williams & Wilkins.

Kibler WB: Evaluation and Diagnosis of Scapulothoracic Problems in the Athlete, *Sports Med Arthrosc* 8:192–202, 2000a.

Kibler WB: Closed Kinetic Chain Rehabilitation for Sports Injuries, *Phys Med Rehabil Clin N Am* 11(2): 369–384, 2000b.

Kibler WB, McMullen J, Uhl T: Shoulder rehabilitation strategies, guidelines and practice, *Orthopaedic Clinics of North America* 32(3):527–538, 2001.

Kiss J, Damrel D, Mackie A, et al: Non-operative treatment of multidirectional shoulder instability, *International Orthopaedics (SICOT)* 24:354–357, 2001.

Kuroda S, Sumiyoshi T, Moriishi J, et al: The natural course of shoulder instability, *J Shoulder Elbow Surg* 10(2):100–104, 2001.

Lephart SM, Henry TJ: The Physiological basis for open and closed kinetic chain rehabilitation for the upper extremity, *Journal of Sports Rehabilitation* 5:71–87, 1996.

Lephart SM, Henry TJ: Restoration of proprioception and neuromuscular control of the unstable shoulder. In Lephart SM, Fu FH, editors: *Proprioception and Neuromuscular Control in Joint Stability*, USA, 2000, Human Kinetics, pp 405–413.

Lewis A, Kitamura T, Bayley JIL: Mini symposium: Shoulder instability (ii) The classification of shoulder instability: New light through old windows, *Current Orthopaedics* 18:97–108, 2004.

Magarey ME, Jones MA: Dynamic evaluation and early management of altered motor control around the shoulder complex, *Man Ther* 8(4):195–206, 2003.

Malone AA, Jaggi A, Calvert PT, et al: Muscle patterning instability – classification and prevalence in a reference shoulder service, In Norris TR, Zuckerman JD, Warner JJP, Lee QT, editors: *Surgery of the Shoulder and Elbow: An International Perspective*, Rosemont, Illinois, USA, 2006a, American Academy of Orthopaedic Surgeons, section 7.

Malone AA, Noorani A, Jaggi A, et al: *The role of dynamic electromyography in muscle patterning instability*, Abstract proceedings, British Elbow & Shoulder Society 17th Annual Scientific Meeting, Edinburgh, 2006b.

McMullen J, Uhl TL: A Kinetic Chain Approach for Shoulder

rehabilitation, *Journal of Athletic Training* 35(3):329–337, 2000.

Mottram SL: Dynamic Stability of the Scapula, *Man Ther* 2(3):123–131, 1997.

Myers JB, Lephart SM: Sensorimotor deficits contributing to glenohumeral instability, *Clin Orthop Relat Res* (400):98–104, 2002.

Myers JB, Wassinger CA, Lephart SM: Sensorimotor contribution to shoulder stability: effect of injury and rehabilitation, *Man Ther* 11:197–201, 2006.

Reid DC, Saboe LA, Chepeha JC: Anterior Shoulder Instability in Athletes: Comparison of isokinetic resistance exercises and an electromyographic biofeedback re-education program – A pilot program, *Physiotherapy Canada* 48(4):251–256, 1996.

Shumway-Cook A, Woollacott MH: Abnormal Postural Control. In: *Motor Control Theory and Practical Applications*, ed 2, Philadelphia, 2001, Lippincott Williams & Wilkins.

Takwale VJ, Calvert P, Rattue H: Involuntary positional instability of the shoulder in adolescents and young adults, *J Bone Joint Surg* 82B:719–723, 2000.

Thomas SC, Matsen FA: An approach to the repair of avulsion of the glenohumeral ligaments in the management of traumatic anterior glenohumeral stability, *J Bone Joint Surg* 71A:506–513, 1989.

Ulkar B, Kunduracioglu B, Cetin C, et al: Effect of positioning and bracing on passive position sense of shoulder joint, *Br J Sports Med* 38(5):549, 2004.

Voss DE, Knott M, Kabat M: Application of Neuromuscular Facilitation in the Treatment of Shoulder Disabilities, *Phys Ther Rev* 33:536–541, 1953.

Wilk KE, Arrigo C: Current Concepts in the Rehabilitation of the Athletic Shoulder, *J Orthop Sports Phys Ther* 18(1):365–378, 1993.

Zattara M, Bouisset S: Posturo-kinetic organization during the early phase of voluntary upper limb movement. 1 Normal Subjects, *J Neurol Neurosurg Psychiatry* 51:956–965, 1988.

12.2 The hand

Katherine Butler

INTRODUCTION

Hand dysfunction is commonly linked to ligamentous laxity (Murray 2006). The carpometacarpal joint (CMCJ) of the thumb may be particularly susceptible to weakened ligamentous constraints in the Ehlers-Danlos syndrome (Moore et al 1985). Symptoms may only present if the joint has been subject to excessive trauma, overuse or misuse and thus strains of the surrounding muscles and ligaments may have developed (Wynn Parry 2000).

In this chapter, assessment and treatment principles for the hypermobile hand will be discussed, including joint protection advice, energy conservation techniques, strengthening exercises, proprioceptive retraining and surgical principles. In particular, the impact of hypermobility in the hand is explored in relation to musicians, who are often hypermobile, and in relation to writing, which can also be significantly affected by the presence of hypermobility in both adults and children. Musical instrument modifications, writing retraining and the relationship between hypermobility and the development of osteoarthritis will be presented.

ASSESSMENT OF THE HAND

If appropriate and safe to do so, hand therapy patients are routinely assessed for hypermobility utilizing the 9-point Beighton score (Chapter 1). Other relevant joints are assessed using passive and active range of motion measurements, and appropriately recorded utilizing the standardized goniometry guidelines established by the American Society of Hand Therapists. It is important not to limit the assessment to the joints examined in the Beighton Scale, since the patient may be hypermobile in other joints. The scale is not all-encompassing and should be used only as a guide to the level of hypermobility displayed by an individual.

Circumferential measurements of joints using finger tape measures that are provided by Jobst™ are taken as appropriate. The modified Oxford Scale of manual muscle testing (Kendall et al 1993) is used to assess relevant muscle groups and as a way of assessing if the treatments are having an effect in increasing muscle strength and, in turn, joint stability. Maximal grip and pinch strength are measured using a hydraulic hand dynamometer and pinch meter, such as Jamar dynamometer and the pinch gauge by B&L Engineering (Mathiowetz 2002, Massy-Westropp et al 2004, Coldham et al 2006) and these again can map the patient's progress and provide feedback as to the tolerance to exercises and functional activities.

As mentioned previously, hypermobility may only be present in one specific joint, and not global, and thus careful assessment is required in order to fully ascertain the patient's symptoms and why the pain or functional difficulties are occurring. Assessment whilst performing functional tasks such as playing a musical instrument, writing or using cutlery is imperative, as hyperlaxity may be more evident whilst doing these activities (Fig. 12.2.1). It is important to distinguish between finger joint hyperextension, which can be a normal phenomenon, and lateral instability, which is often acquired or pathological (Tubiana 2000). Some level of hyperextension can be useful and assistive with certain task performance and the individual may have been born with a certain amount of hyperextension. If, however, the instability is acquired or pathological, the mechanisms and reasons why the phenomenon is occurring need to be analysed and addressed appropriately, in order to decrease progression of the condition.

TREATMENT PRINCIPLES

Symptom management is the key factor in this patient group. Initially, treatment may focus on decreasing an acute episode of pain through resting the affected area. Splinting is particularly important in this respect. In time, treatment must focus on joint stability, muscle strengthening, sensorimotor retraining to improve proprioception and patient education regarding healthy joint use (Warrington 2003).

The assessment and treatment of symptoms and dysfunction in the hand due to hypermobility should be considered in the context of the whole

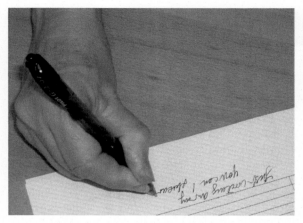

Fig. 12.2.1 Assessment of hypermobility while handwriting

person. This will include attention to other areas of the body with symptoms, in particular the shoulder (Chapter 12.1) and cervical spine (Chapter 12.7), as well as considering postural alignment (Chapter 9) and general fitness (Chapter 13).

JOINT PROTECTION AND ENERGY CONSERVATION

Whether or not hypermobility is the primary cause of symptoms, joint protection advice and energy conservation techniques are always provided to patients with this condition. There are specific exercises and many adaptive ways of performing tasks that can be helpful and easily incorporated into the patient's lifestyle.

These principles can be employed to preserve the patient's joints and reduce pain levels. They are a 'style of life' that once learned becomes second nature and rather than complicating life are designed to encourage independence.

Hand therapists can assist in giving advice about joint protection and energy conservation techniques. These principles have been modified from those utilized for patients with rheumatoid arthritis (Boxes 12.2.1 and 12.2.2).

STRENGTHENING EXERCISES

Patients can benefit greatly from a rehabilitation programme to improve joint control, muscle power (Wynn Parry 2003) and stamina (Wynn Parry 2000). Initially, stability exercises include isometric muscle contraction in a pain-free range (with a support on if being used) to encourage co-

contraction of the muscles surrounding a joint. Involving the target object can be a useful progression to develop isometric strength and proprioceptive awareness, by maintaining the neutral joint position while holding a pen, violin bow or clarinet (Warrington 2003) and while performing the functional task. Later, exercises can be progressed to include concentric and eccentric strengthening.

The intrinsic and extrinsic muscles of the hand are frequently stressed in an attempt to compensate for joint instability (Brandfonbrener 1990). Therapeutic putty exercises can be useful for specific muscle strengthening and in turn joint stability. Intrinsic muscle strength is very important and, because these muscles fatigue quickly, short pain-free sessions of exercise are efficient and encouraged (Davis & Rogers 1998). It is imperative that the exercises are performed with slightly flexed joints, rather than collapsing into hypermobile positions (Fig. 12.2.2). The use of graded rubber bands to assist in strengthening the interossei and lumbricals of the hands is also recommended (Wynn Parry 1998).

Strength gains are slower in the hypermobile patient, possibly due to alterations in central and peripheral neuromuscular physiological processes. It may therefore take many months for stability and strength to improve enough for the patient to be able to perform the task in a modified way and so a graded return to task performance is often required (Simmonds & Keer 2007). A diary of writing retraining times or musical practice schedule may be necessary to monitor symptoms and tolerable time of task performance. Exercises must be continued until sufficient muscle strength has been gained so a neutral joint position can be maintained whilst performing the required task.

PROPRIOCEPTIVE RETRAINING

Proprioception exercises and retraining, such as tapping exercises and weight-bearing exercises in a neutral position should be performed first with the eyes open and then with the eyes closed. After several months of performing strengthening exercises symptoms can improve and it is not uncommon to detect an improvement in ligament tautness with joint translation testing. It is encouraging for the hypermobile patient to be told that biomechanical dysfunction can be improved.

The product 3M™ Coban™ can be wrapped around a pencil, a bow of a stringed instrument,

---

BOX 12.2.1 Methods of joint protection

1. Use joints in a good position

Joints work best in certain positions. When they are used in the wrong position, such as when twisting, extra force is placed through the joint and the muscles are unable to work as well, eventually causing pain and deformity.

2. Avoid activities that don't let you change the position of your hand

When you are in a position for a long time your muscles get stiff and pull the joint into a bad position. The muscles also get tired quickly so the force is taken up by the joint and not the muscles, leading to pain and damage.

3. Respect pain

If pain continues for hours after an activity has stopped, this means that the activity was too much and should have been changed or stopped sooner.

4. Avoid tight grips or gripping for long periods

Gripping tightly may increase your pain. If you grip something that is small or narrow it can require greater power to hold and manipulate it. Some examples of how to decrease strain on joints include:
- Using thicker or padded pens for writing.
- Resting books on a table or book rest.
- Using a chopping board with spikes to secure vegetables.
- Using non-slip mats under bowls to hold them.
- Allowing hand washing to drip-dry rather than wringing it out.
- Relaxing your hands regularly during activities such as knitting or writing.

- Building up objects using foam tubing or special grip aids.
- Increasing the grip ability on a slippery object such as a shiny pen or toothbrush by using elastoplast or Coban tape.
- Many items have been ergonomically designed and can be purchased from supermarkets and department stores.

5. Avoid activities that could lead to over-extension

Some directions of force can lead to over-extension at the joints.
- Use a flat hand where possible such as when dusting or wiping.
- Try to use lightweight mugs with large handles rather than small teacups so pressure is not put on just one or two fingers.

6. Use one large joint or many joints

Stronger muscles protect large joints so it is better to use large joints where possible, or try to spread the force over many joints.
- Use the palms of your hands and not your fingers when you carry plates or dishes.
- When standing up from a chair, try to rock gently forward and use your leg muscles to stand up rather than pushing from your knuckles or wrists.
- Carry light bags from a strap on your shoulder rather than your hands.
- Use your bottom or hips to close drawers or move light chairs.
- Use your forearms to take the weight of objects when carrying, not your hands.

---

a stick of a drum or directly onto the finger to assist in retraining appropriate amounts of pressure applied when holding these items, and in turn facilitate an increase in proprioceptive awareness. This can lead to a decrease in the amount of muscle energy exerted to perform the task and thus fatigue and pain levels can be significantly decreased. Research performed by Lowell et al (2003) found that 3M™ Coban™ was effective in decreasing oedema in the skin-grafted burnt hand, and that this contributed to improved hand function, range of motion and strength levels with no impact on hand mobility, grip strength or function.

The use of a foam pad, lycra or silicon sleeve such as Silipos® can assist with proprioceptive retraining while performing a task such as playing a musical instrument (Fig. 12.2.3).

SPLINTING

Splints are a useful tool for supporting a joint in a neutral position to assist in decreasing joint strain and allow functional activities without pain. They are also thought to retrain proprioceptive awareness. Brandfonbrener (2003) comments that the use of ring splints for musicians with unstable

BOX 12.2.2 Methods of energy conservation

1. Balance, rest and activity

It is important to balance your rest and activity to allow your joints to rest and repair. Stop before you feel tired or are in pain and avoid activities that you cannot stop when you need to.

- Try to plan ahead. Write a weekly or daily diary with activities in red and rest times in blue. Think about what you need to do and space the harder activities out over time.
- Activities such as vacuuming, ironing and cleaning windows mean that you are doing the same movement lots of times and keeping the hand in the same position for long periods of time. Try to do them for very short periods, or where possible get someone else to do them for you.

2. Organize and arrange space

Prepare your work areas so that everything you need for that activity is there. Store items you use often in places that are easy to reach and keep things in small refillable containers, rather than large, heavy jars.

3. Stop activities or parts of them

- Use clothes that are easy to care for.
- Make the bed on one side and then the other.
- Soak dishes before washing them and let them drip dry.
- Where possible use tinned, frozen or prepared foods.
- Hang items within easy reach.
- Where possible get someone else to help with activities.

4. Reduce the amount of weight you take through your joints

- Consider wheeled trolleys rather than carrying things.
- Slide pans where possible and use a wire basket or slotted spoon to drain vegetables.
- When you buy new equipment, make sure it is lightweight.
- Use a teapot and/or kettle tipper and fill the kettle with a lightweight jug.

5. Use equipment that reduces effort

Automatic washing machines, frost-free freezers and food processors are all energy-saving devices and sharp knives enable less pressure and effort to be exerted.

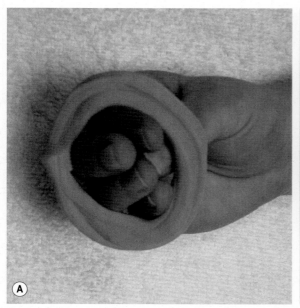
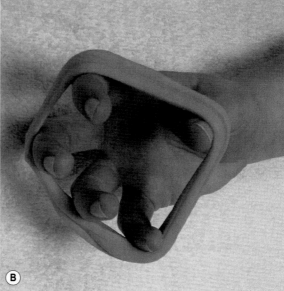

Fig. 12.2.2a, b Therapeutic putty exercises. Exercising between extension (a) and relaxation (b) without allowing hyperextension to occur at the fingers and thumb

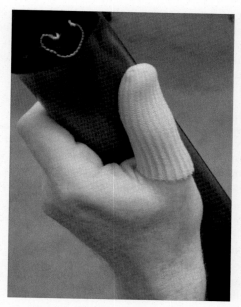

Fig. 12.2.3 A Silipos® digital sleeve can be useful in decreasing the pressure exerted through a finger or thumb and in retraining positioning on the instrument

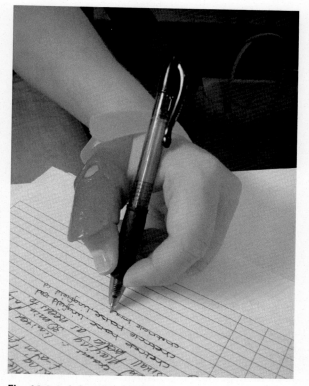

Fig. 12.2.4 A functional thumb metacarpal extension blocking splint (Butler & Svens 2005)

fingers caused by ligamentous laxity helps prevent hyperextension but also helps retrain proprioceptivity in how they position their fingers.

They may need to be worn for some time with a gradual reduction in their use as strength levels increase and symptoms decrease. There are a wide variety of splints that can be made individually for the patient and it may be appropriate to have one or more during the day, depending on the activity being performed, and a different splint when sleeping. Supports can include light thermoplastic splints, neoprene wraps, wrist braces, lycra finger sleeves or Coban™ wrap. There are also many pre-fabricated splints available which require assessment to ensure correct fit and functionality.

Hyperextension of the first metacarpal joint (MCPJ) is commonly observed in people with hypermobility, arthritis and in professionals such as musicians (Wynn Parry 2004) and hand therapists (Bozentka 2002). This may be due to decreased stability of the first carpometacarpal joint (CMC) and/or MCPJ (Alter et al 2002), which subsequently leads to degenerative changes. Butler and Svens (2005) present an alternative splint based on Van Lede's (2002) anti-swan neck splint for fingers, which restricts MCPJ extension of the thumb (Fig. 12.2.4). There are many other bespoke

splinting options such as the (Galindo-Lim 2002), which allows for maximum functional use of the hand, stabilizes the MCPJ of the thumb and does not cross the wrist crease therefore allowing fairly full wrist motion.

SURGICAL PRINCIPLES

There are a wide range of surgical procedures for the reconstruction of the osteoarthritic basal thumb joint: ligament reconstruction, hemiarthroplasty, trapezial resection with or without replacement and arthrodesis (Eaton & Glickel 1987). The option chosen depends on the pain experienced by the patient, the degree of hypermobility, the quality of the articular cartilage and the stiffness and degeneration in the trapezium. Radiographic evaluation of the trapezial articulations and open-mindedness when directly inspecting the articular surfaces at surgery influence the decision as to what procedure to apply to individual patients (Eaton & Glickel 1987).

Specific surgical stabilizing procedures for the unstable MCPJ should be considered, in order to increase levels of hand function, although Butler and Winspur (2009) conclude from their study of 130 professional musicians who underwent surgery, that conservative management and splinting achieve greater benefit than surgery in those with painful hypermobile joints.

HYPERMOBILITY AND MUSICIANS

There is evidence to suggest that a higher incidence of hypermobility exists in musicians than in the population at large (Wynn Parry 2004). There remains debate as to whether this is an advantage or disadvantage for instrumentalists; an advantage in that it adds to the ability; a disadvantage in that injury may be more likely and take longer to resolve.

Increased range in the fingers, thumb and wrist may be an asset when playing repetitive motions on instruments such as the flute, violin or piano. Larsson et al (1993) found that 5% of musicians with hypermobility in their fingers and wrist joints presented with musculoskeletal problems, compared to 18% in those without hypermobility. Grahame (1993) showed a similar correlation and indeed, some very virtuosic players such as Paganini and Liszt were hypermobile.

However, Brandfonbrener (1990) consistently found a correlation between musicians with hand and arm pain and the presence of joint laxity. Jull (1994) and Hoppmann (1998) state that for many musicians hypermobility is an impediment and detrimental. Muscle weakness and increased vulnerability of the associated joint can lead to an increased propensity for the hypermobile musician to develop injuries or chronic 'overuse' syndromes. Ulnar nerve entrapment, known as cubital tunnel syndrome, is more likely in the musician with hypermobility of the elbow (Lambert 1992). Larsson et al (1993) concluded that hypermobility was a liability when the joints are required to be stabilizers, such as the knee or spine for timpanists who stand to play. In addition, there is evidence to suggest that hypermobile joints have a decreased sensitivity to proprioception (Chapter 6.4) so musicians may exert more force than necessary on keys or strings to provide greater security to that finger, thus increasing the possibility of chronic strain (Brandfonbrener 2003).

Particular attention must be paid to technique if the patient is hypermobile, with education, adaptive devices for the instrument and exercises to strengthen the muscles of the hand and wrist being implemented (Patrone et al 1988). Success has been reported in treating the hypermobile musician for conditions such as synovitis (Bird & Wright 1981) and digital nerve compression (Patrone et al 1988, 1989).

INSTRUMENT MODIFICATIONS

Many instruments can be modified to make playing them more comfortable and safer. Reducing the load to the musculoskeletal system can have an immediate beneficial effect. For example:

- The levers that operate the valves on the French horn can be lengthened and widened to provide greater leverage and increased contact area.
- Decreasing the load on the right thumb of a clarinet or oboe by using a splint (Fig. 12.2.5), a neck strap or a post that rests on the chest can alter right upper extremity loading (Hoppmann 2001).
- Adding an end pin to the cello relieves the player from supporting the instrument by grasping it with the legs. End pins have also been successfully employed in the bassoon, English horn and tuba. The end pin for the last two instruments has been modified into a ball that rests on the chair between the thighs. There are several devices on the market that relieve the right thumb strain so common to oboe and clarinet players (Markison 1993, Smutz et al 1995).
- The location of the flute keys can be customized to fit the player's hand. The cluster of keys worked by the right little finger can be angled inwards which reduces the strain between the fourth and fifth fingers. The keys operated by the left fourth and fifth fingers can be lengthened to achieve a more neutral left wrist position. A flute with a 'U' head can be useful for children.
- There are many adaptive devices and cases that have been specifically designed to decrease joint strain and distribute the load of the instrument. An example of a support is shown in Figure 12.2.5.

HYPERMOBILITY AND WRITING

Finger hyperextension is commonly seen in patients with hypermobility of the upper limbs, and as a result handwriting is often affected. Prolonged

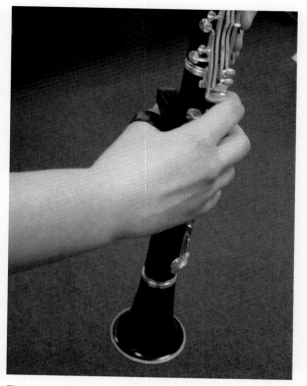

Fig. 12.2.5 Right hand 'Bo-Pep' assisting the support of the left index finger and maintaining the MCPJ in a more neutral position

periods of writing can be fatiguing and painful, due to joint strain and muscle overactivity producing aches and cramp. Frequently, children have been told their handwriting is messy and may have been labelled as lazy or not interested in their work.

Assessing the patient as they write will give the clinician many clues as to whether a positional retraining splint, built up pen, writing aids (Davis & Rogers 1998) or strengthening exercises are the most appropriate treatment option. There are many adaptations to the pen and the pen hold that can be taught to reduce pressure and encourage larger movements of the wrist and elbow when writing (Fig. 12.2.6). It is also important that the individual supports the page with their other hand whilst writing, to decrease any pressure being exerted through the writing hand in order to hold the page in place. It is important that the chair, table and other equipment being used at school or home is considered so that the patient is able to position themselves optimally when writing (Murray 2006). Sloping writing surfaces and the use of a laptop computer may assist in increasing functional levels in this patient group.

Witt and Jäger (1984) present a case of a 26-year-old man whom they believe developed writer's cramp as a result of congenital subluxation of the first metacarpophalangeal joint. They comment that after a stabilizing procedure on the patient's

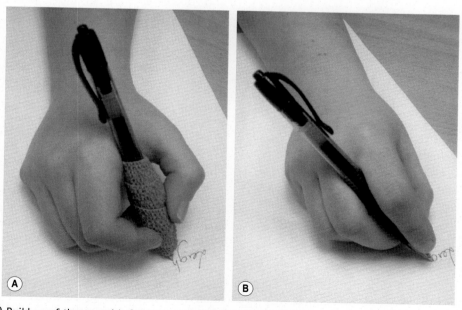

Fig. 12.2.6 (a) Build up of the pen with Coban tape; (b) Adaptive pen hold between middle and index finger

thumb to eliminate the pathological hypermobile first metacarpophalangeal joint, hand function was normalized.

OSTEOARTHRITIS

Some believe that hyperextension may be a risk factor for the evolution of osteoarthritis (Klemp & Learmonth 1984, Bridges et al 1992, Mikkelsson et al 1996, Jónsson et al 2009) whilst others do not support this view (Dolan et al 2003, Kraus et al 2004, Chen et al 2008).

Generalized ligamentous laxity has been seen for some time as a predisposing factor for development of idiopathic osteoarthritis of the trapeziometacarpal joint (Pelligrini 1991, Jónsson & Valtýsdóttir 1995, Jónsson et al 1996). It has been believed that hyperextension of the thumb metacarpophalangeal joint is secondary to degenerative subluxation of the trapeziometacarpal joint that occurs in osteoarthritis (Fig. 12.2.7).

Metacarpophalangeal joint flexion effectively unloads the palmar surfaces of the trapezio-metacarpal joint, regardless of the presence or severity of arthritic disease in this joint. Moulton et al (2001) postulate that hyperextension laxity of the

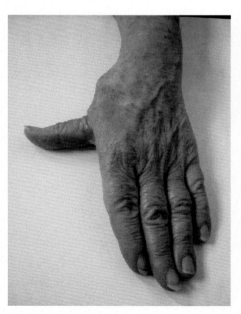

Fig. 12.2.7 Thumb MCPJ hyperextension when actively extending the thumb

metacarpophalangeal joint may identify individuals who are predisposed to development of osteoarthritis of the trapeziometacarpal joint, and that such individuals could benefit from intervention that assists in the stabilization of the MCPJ, thus reducing the progression of OA disease development at the base of the thumb. They also comment that in the symptomatic hypermobile MCPJ, fixation of this joint in flexion, by a splint or surgical stabilization, may decrease basal joint symptoms by redirecting trapeziometacarpal joint forces from the palmar compartment onto the healthier dorsal aspect of the joint.

A further study (Kraus et al 2004) assessed hypermobility and its relationship to radiographic hand OA in a family-based study. A total of 1043 individuals were enrolled into the study and the results showed no association of hypermobility and CMC OA, and indeed there was no evidence of increased chances of OA in any joint group of the hand due to associated articular hypermobility.

Rogers and Wilder (2007) present the effects of strength training among people with osteoarthritis. They set out to determine the effects of 2 years' whole-body strength training and grip exercises on hand strength, pain and functional levels in adults with radiographic evidence of hand OA. The results suggest that strength training increases both dynamic and static grip strength and decreases pain in older persons affected with OA.

SUMMARY

The hypermobile patient provides the hand therapist with great challenges, many rewards and the possibility of developing new splintage and therapeutic techniques. Thorough assessment both while performing functional tasks and at rest is required in order to formulate an appropriate and assistive treatment programme. Symptoms must be managed, and splints can be a useful way to initially assist in decreasing pain levels. Joint stability must be the focus when treating this patient group, and exercises and functional task performance that enhances proprioceptive awareness and muscle strengthening are paramount. The patient's joints must be protected and often their lifestyles have to be modified in order to decrease joint degeneration or strain. Surgery is not always the treatment of choice for this patient group; however, if it is required then it is imperative to select a surgeon with experience in treating patients with hypermobility. There are many ways of modifying equipment and task performance in order to enhance independence and confidence and enable a more normal and less painful existence.

References

Alter S, Feldon P, Terrono AL: Pathomechanics of deformities in the arthritic hand and wrist. In Mackin EJ, Callahan AD, Skirven TM, et al, editors: *Evaluation of the Hand and Upper Extremity*, ed 5, St Louis, 2002, Mosby, pp 1545–1554.

Bird HA, Wright V: Traumatic synovitis in a classical guitarist: A study of joint laxity, *Annals of Rheumatic Diseases* 40:161–163, 1981.

Bozentka DJ: Pathogenesis of osteoarthritis. In Mackin EJ, Callahan AD, Skirven TM, et al, editors: *Evaluation of the Hand and Upper Extremity*, ed 5, St Louis, 2002, Mosby, pp 1637–1645.

Brandfonbrener AG: The epidemiology and prevention of hand and wrist injuries in performing artists, *Hand Clin* 6(3):365–377, 1990.

Brandfonbrener AG: Musculoskeletal problems of instrumental musicians, *Hand Clinics: The Musician's Hand* 19:231–239, 2003.

Bridges AJ, Smith E, Reid J: Joint hypermobility in adults referred to rheumatology clinics, *Annals of Rheumatic Diseases* 51:793–796, 1992.

Butler K, Svens B: A functional thumb metacarpal extension blocking splint, *J Hand Ther* 18(3):375–377, 2005.

Butler K, Winspur I: A retrospective case review of time taken for 130 professional musicians to fully return to playing their instruments, following hand surgery, *Hand Therapy* 14: (In Print), 2009.

Chen HC, Shah SH, Li YJ, et al: Inverse association of general joint hypermobility with hand and knee osteoarthritis and serum cartilage oligomeric matrix protein levels, *Arthritis Rheum* 58(12): 3854–3864, 2008.

Coldham F, Lewis J, Lee H: The reliability of one vs. three grip trials in symptomatic and asymptomatic subjects, *J Hand Ther* 19:318–326, 2006.

Davis AT, Rogers G: The physical therapist's contribution. In Winspur I, Wynn Parry CB, editors: *The Musician's Hand: A Clinical Guide*, London, 1998, Martin Dunitz, pp 123–142.

Dolan AL, Hart DJ, Doyle DV, et al: The relationship of joint hypermobility, bone mineral density, and osteoarthritis in the general population: The Chingford Study, *J Rheumatol* 30:799–803, 2003.

Eaton RG, Glickel SZ: Trapeziometacarpal osteoarthritis degenerative arthritis II, *Hand Clin* 3(4):455–469, 1987.

Galindo A, Lim SA: Metacarpophalangeal joint stabilisation splint, *Journal of Hand Therapy Practice Forum* 83–84, 2002.

Grahame R: Joint hypermobility and the performing musician, *N Engl J Med* 329:1120–1121, 1993.

Hoppmann RA: Musculoskeletal problems in instrumental musicians. In Sataloff RT, Lederman RJ, Brandfronbrener AG, editors: *Performing Arts Medicine*, San Diego, 1998, Singular, pp 221–224.

Hoppmann RA: Instrumental Musicians' Hazards, *Occup Med* 16(4):619–631, 2001.

Jónsson H, Valtýsdóttir S: Hypermobility features in patients with hand osteoarthritis, *Osteoarthritis Cartilage* 3:1–5, 1995.

Jónsson H, Valtýsdóttir S, Kjartansson O, et al: Hypermobility associated with osteoarthritis of the thumb base: a clinical and radiological subset of hand osteoarthritis, *Annals of Rheumatic Diseases* 55:540–543, 1996.

Jónsson H, Elíasson GJ, Jónsson A, et al: High hand joint mobility is associated with radiological CMC1 osteoarthritis: the AGES-Reykjavik study, *Osteoarthritis Cartilage* 17(5):592–595, 2009.

Jull JA: Examination of the articular system. In Boyling J, Palastanga N, editors: *Grieve's Modern Manual Therapy*, ed 2, Edinburgh, 1994, Churchill Livingstone, pp 511–524.

Kendall FP, McCreary EK, Provance PG, et al: *Muscles: Testing and Function with Posture and Pain*, ed 4, Baltimore, 1993, Williams & Wilkins.

Klemp P, Learmonth ID: Hypermobility and injuries in a professional ballet company, *British Journal Sports Medicine* 18:143–148, 1984.

Kraus VB, Li YJ, Martin ER, et al: Articular hypermobility is a protective factor for hand osteoarthritis, *Arthritis Rheum* 50(7):2178–2183, 2004.

Lambert CM: Hand and upper limb problems of instrumental musicians, *Medical Problems of Performing Artists* 1:45–48, 1992.

Larsson LG, Baum J, Mudholkar GS, et al: Benefits and disadvantages of joint hypermobility among musicians, *N Engl J Med* 329:1079–1082, 1993.

Lowell M, Pirc P, Ward R, et al: Effect of 3M™ Coban™ Self-Adherent

Wraps on Edema and Function of the Burned Hand: A Case Study, *J Burn Care Rehabil* 253–258, 2003.

Markison RE: Treatment of musical hands: redesign of the interface, *Hand Clin* 6:525, 1993.

Massy-Westropp N, Rankin W, Ahern M, et al: Measuring grip strength in normal adults: reference ranges and a comparison of electronic and hydraulic instruments, *J Hand Surg Am* 29:514–519, 2004.

Mathiowetz V: Comparison of Rolyan and Jamar dynamometers for measuring grip strength, *Occup Ther Int* 9:201–209, 2002.

Mikkelsson M, Salminen JJ, Kautiainen H: Joint hypermobility is not a contributing factor to musculoskeletal pain in preadolescents, *J Rheumatol* 23:1963–1967, 1996.

Moore JR, Tolo VT, Weiland AJ: Painful subluxation of the carpometacarpal joint of the thumb in Ehlers-Danlos syndrome, *J Hand Surg Am* 10(5):661–663, 1985.

Moulton MJR, Parentis MA, Kelly MJ, et al: Influence of metacarpophalangeal joint position on basal joint-loading in the thumb, *J Bone Joint Surg* 83A (5):709–716, 2001.

Murray K: Hypermobility disorders in children and adolescents. Best Practice and Research, *Clin Rheumatol* 20(2):329–351, 2006.

Patrone NA, Hoppmann RA, Whaley J, et al: Benign hypermobility in a flutist, *Medical Problems of Performing Artists* 3:158–161, 1988.

Patrone NA, Hoppmann RA, Whaley J, et al: Digital nerve compression in a violinist with benign hypermobility, *Medical Problems Performing Artists* 4:91–94, 1989.

Pelligrini VD: Osteoarthritis of the trapeziometacarpal joint: The pathophysiology of articular cartilage degeneration II. Articular wear patterns in the osteoarthritic joint, *J Hand Surg* 16-A(6):975–982, 1991.

Rogers MW, Wilder FV: The effects of strength training among persons with hand osteoarthritis: a two-year follow-up study, *J Hand Ther* 20(3):244–249, 2007.

Simmonds JV, Keer RJ: Hypermobility and the hypermobility syndrome, *Man Ther* 12:298–309, 2007.

Smutz WP, Bishop A, Niblock H, et al: Load on the right thumb of the oboeist, *Medical Problems of Performing Artists* 10:94, 1995.

Tubiana R: Anatomy of the hand and upper limb. In Tubiana R, Amadio PC, editors: *Medical Problems of the Instrumentalist Musician*, ed 1, London, 2000, Martin Dunitz, pp 5–53.

Van Lede P: Minimalistic splint design: a rationale told in a personal style, *J Hand Ther* 15:192–201, 2002.

Warrington J: Hand Therapy for the musician: instrument-focused rehabilitation, *Hand Clinics The Musician's Hand* 19(2):287–301, 2003.

Witt TN, Jäger M: Congenital subluxation of the metacarpophalangeal joint of the thumb as the cause of writer's cramp, *Zeitschrift Fur Orthopaedie und ihre Grenzgebiete* 22(1):37–39, 1984.

Wynn Parry CB: Specific Conditions. In Winspur I, Wynn Parry CB, editors: *The Musician's Hand: A Clinical Guide*, London, 1998, Martin Dunitz, pp 53–76.

Wynn Parry CB: Clinical approaches. In Tubiana R, Amadio P, editors: *Medical Problems of the Instrumentalist Musician*, London, 2000, Martin Dunitz, pp 203–218.

Wynn Parry CB: Prevention of musician's hand problems, *Hand Clin* 19(2):317–324, 2003.

Wynn Parry CB: Managing the physical demands of musical performance. In Williamon A, editor: *Musical Excellence Strategies and techniques to enhance performance*, Oxford, 2004, Oxford University Press, pp 41–60.

12.3 The hip joint

Marc George and Marcus JK Bankes

INTRODUCTION

The hip, as a ball and socket joint, has a large range of movement even in the normal individual. In the hypermobile patient it can frequently be greater still. Whilst the hip is not specifically examined as part of the Beighton score for hypermobility, a number of conditions are frequently seen in the hips of hypermobile patients.

CLINICAL ASSESSMENT

Hip pain may be the first presentation of generalized joint hypermobility syndrome (JHS). Alternatively, patients who have already been diagnosed with JHS may present with hip pain as part of their condition. Activity-related groin, trochanteric and thigh pain, with or without mechanical symptoms, are the key features of hip joint pathology.

A painful hip, which develops stiffness as a consequence, may give rise to compensation in the lumbar spine. This occurs particularly into rotation and can lead to overuse and the development of low back pain as well. It can be very difficult to determine if pain is being referred from the hip or lumbar spine or a combination of both. Consequently both areas need to be examined.

Specific clinical conditions of the hip are detailed below.

FEMOROACETABULAR IMPINGEMENT (FAI) AND LABRAL TEARS

Femoroacetabular impingement (FAI) has been defined as the abutment of the proximal femur against the acetabular rim (Lavigne et al 2004). Although first described as a surgical entity in the 1930s, in relation to old slipped upper femoral epiphyses (Smith-Peterson 1936), it has only become a more widely diagnosed condition towards the end of the 20th century. The natural history of untreated femoroacetabular impingement is the development of premature osteoarthritis (Ganz et al 2008).

Figure 12.3.1 shows patterns of femoroacetabular impingement.

PATTERNS OF FEMOROACETABULAR IMPINGMENT

Pincer impingement

In this type of impingement, contact that occurs between the femoral head/neck junction and the acetabular rim leads to rim ossification and deepening of the acetabulum (Box 12.3.1). This typically occurs in individuals in their fourth or fifth decade and is more common in women.

In practice, most cases of femoroacetabular impingement are probably a combination of both cam and pincer impingement (Beck et al 2005).

Cam impingement

In this type of impingement, an aspherical portion of the femoral head abuts on the acetabular rim (Box 12.3.2). Characteristically, but not exclusively, this occurs in young male patients with high-impact contact sport a common risk factor (Philippon et al 2007).

Labral tears

The functional acetabular labrum is a fibrocartilaginous lip that attaches to the bony acetabulum. The anterior part of the labrum is the common site for isolated labral tears and damage here is also the central feature of painful femoroacetabular impingement (Tanzer & Noiseux 2004). Labral tears are also more commonly found in patients with hip dysplasia (Haene et al 2007).

Functional impingement

Even with normal anatomy, hypermobile patients may impinge due to their abnormal arc of movement. This, with time, may lead to anterior labral damage in the same way that a patient with normal movement and anatomical abnormality may

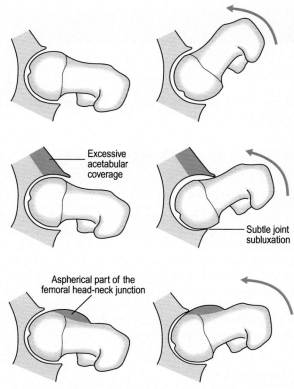

Excessive acetabular coverage

Subtle joint subluxation

Aspherical part of the femoral head-neck junction

Fig. 12.3.1 Patterns of femoroacetabular impingement

BOX 12.3.1 Causes of pincer impingement

Protrusio acetabula
Coxa profunda
Femoral retroversion
Post periacetabular osteotomy

BOX 12.3.2 Causes of cam impingement

Slipped upper femoral epiphysis
Perthes disease
Decreased femoral head neck offset
Epiphyseal dysplasia

---

develop damage to the labrum. Clearly, if a patient has both an increased range of movement and anatomical abnormality, then rim damage from impingement will be more likely to occur.

The clinical pictures of patients with labral tears, with or without femoroacetabular impingement,

share certain similarities and are considered together. Patients with labral tears may have a clear history of an injury, but often do not, particularly when there is an underlying structural bony abnormality. Characteristically, pain is felt in the groin, often following activity, and the patient describes the pain as deep in the hip, such that they 'can't get to it'. They may clasp the affected hip with their hand, placing the index finger in the groin and the thumb over the greater trochanter, in an attempt to localize the pain (the C-sign). Straight-line activity is less likely to cause pain than activities which involve twisting, particularly if associated with impact. Clicking, locking and catching are intermittent features, often occurring when getting up from a seated position. Constant pain, rest pain and night pain should raise suspicion of degenerate change, pain hypersensitivity or more serious pathology. Patients characteristically present with pain over many months and may have previously been treated for groin strains. On clinical examination, the routine Apley-style 'look, feel, move' examination may be entirely normal, but a subtle loss of internal rotation in flexion may be detected. The impingement sign is considered positive, if pain is elicited on internal rotation and adduction at 90 degrees of hip flexion (Klaue et al 1991), as shown in Figure 12.3.2. Whilst this test is sensitive, it is non-specific and may be positive in FAI, labral tears, degenerative disease or

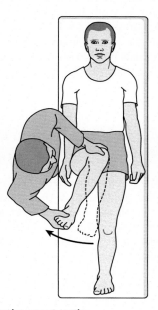

Fig. 12.3.2 Impingement testing

any other intra-articular pathology, and as such only serves to confirm the site of pain as the hip joint.

Treatment of labral tears and impingement

The treatment of labral tears in isolation has been effectively addressed by arthroscopic debridement or reattachment (Murphy et al 2006, Robertson et al 2007), but treatment of the underlying cause is also necessary. Cam femoroacetabular impingement requires removal of the neck bump causing the asphericity of the femoral head. Pincer impingement requires rim trimming, often in conjunction with labral detachment and refixation. Encouraging early and medium-term results have been achieved with both open surgery via safe surgical dislocation (Ganz et al 2001) and arthroscopic surgery (Philippon et al 2009), although there remains debate over which is most effective. Pincer impingement caused by retroversion may require treatment with a reverse periacetabular osteotomy.

HIP DYSPLASIA

There is a spectrum of severity in hip dysplasia, from the true congenital dislocated hip, detected at birth or infancy, to the subtle, shallow acetabulum that presents any time from adolescence onwards (Klaue et al 1991). Whilst adult dysplasia may manifest for the first time with end-stage arthritis, it usually shows with the clinical picture of a labral tear well before degeneration has occurred, in the second, third or fourth decade. Periacetabular osteotomy (PAO) to reorientate the acetabulum is highly effective at alleviating symptoms, by reducing forces on the labrum and acetabular cartilage (Murphy et al 1999, Peters et al 2006). PAO may also delay degenerative change for many years, and may even prevent it altogether (Fig. 12.3.3a, b).

LIGAMENTUM TERES RUPTURE

Whilst the ligamentum teres was long considered a vestigial blood supply to the femoral head (Kapandji 1978), the more widespread use of hip arthroscopy has led to renewed interest in the biomechanical function of the ligament. Rupture is reported in between 4% and 15% of hip

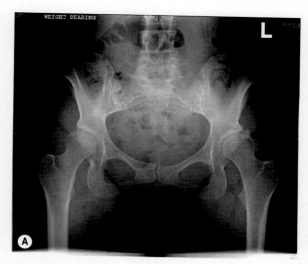

Fig. 12.3.3a Radiograph of hip dysplasia

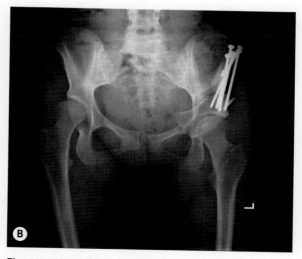

Fig. 12.3.3b Radiograph of same patient following periacetabular osteotomy

arthroscopies (Baber et al 1999, Rao et al 2001, Byrd & Jones 2004) and is the third most common diagnosis found at hip arthroscopy in athletes (Byrd & Jones 2001). The ligamentum teres is tightest in flexion, adduction and external rotation. Whilst one might expect the hypermobile patient to have a higher incidence of ligamentum teres rupture, it has not been our experience. Ligamentum teres rupture can be effectively treated with arthroscopic debridement (Bardarkos & Villar 2009).

SNAPPING HIP SYNDROME

Snapping of the iliopsoas tendon and iliotibial band (ITB) are sometimes grouped together as 'snapping hip syndrome', but these two entities are quite separate (Chapter 9).

ILIOPSOAS SNAPPING

The site of snapping has variously been described as the location where the iliopsoas tendon shifts from lateral to medial over the femoral head (Schaberg et al 1984, Allen et al 1995) catches on the iliopectineal eminence or even catches on a lesser trochanter exostosis (Staple et al 1988). Whatever the cause, the presentation is of a popping or snapping sensation in the groin, with or without pain. The snapping can usually be demonstrated by extending the hip from a flexed, abducted and externally rotated position to an extended and internally rotated position. It is often easiest to ask the patient to demonstrate the snapping themselves, in which case the patient will either reproduce a manoeuvre similar to the above while supine, or whilst standing by bringing the hip into extension.

Treatment of snapping ilopsoas

The snapping iliopsoas may require no treatment at all and simply giving the patient an explanation of the diagnosis may be all that is required. For others, it may be debilitating. Patients will often have learned avoidance tactics to prevent the tendon snapping and may have undertaken a course of physiotherapy. An ultrasound-guided local anaesthetic and steroid injection is helpful in confirming the diagnosis and may also be therapeutic. For cases for whom conservative measures have either been unsuccessful, or have had only a transient benefit, open surgical release can be considered. This is performed either at the pelvic brim, over the anterior capsule, or at the lesser trochanter (Jacobson & Allen 1990, Dobbs et al 2002). Arthroscopic extracapsular release via the peripheral compartment has also been described (Flanum et al 2007). It is the authors' practise to release the tendinous portion of the iliopsoas below the pelvic brim via a groin incision, with release at the lesser trochanter via a medial approach reserved for recalcitrant cases.

ILIOTIBIAL BAND SYNDROME

This is caused by the iliotibial band catching over the lateral aspect of the greater trochanter as it moves from a posterior position in extension to an anterior one with flexion. This leads to thickening of the posterior portion of the iliotibial band. The patient localizes the sensation laterally over the hip, which may or may not be painful. There is often a perception that the hip has dislocated, particularly in the hypermobile individual. The phenomenon is again often most easily demonstrated by the patient (usually in standing) and can be felt or even seen by the examiner. Localized tenderness may indicate an underlying trochanteric bursitis. The snapping is thought to be caused by a short or tight ITB which can be detected using the Ober test (Ober 1936). When examining hypermobile individuals it may be advisable to use the modified Ober test (Kendall et al 1993) as this produces less strain on the medial knee joint and less tension on the patella.

Treatment of iliotibial band syndrome

A simple explanation of the diagnosis and reassurance that the hip is not dislocating, combined with physiotherapy to lengthen the ITB and improve the balance of muscles around the hip, may be all that is required. Injection of local anaesthetic and steroid may be necessary and should certainly be tried before considering surgery. Surgical options described include z lengthening or excision of an ellipse of the iliotibial band. Alternatively, division of the ITB in conjunction with an anterior transposition of the lower fourth of the gluteus maximus muscle over the greater trochanter as a pad is highly effective (Brignall & Stainsby 1991, Provencher et al 2004).

IMAGING OF THE PAINFUL HIP JOINT

Plain radiographs may be normal, or at least reported as normal. An anteroposterior pelvis and lateral of the hip is the most useful initial imaging modality in any hip condition and will guide further imaging. If degeneration is seen, further imaging is unlikely to be helpful in establishing a diagnosis. Cam femoroacetabular impingement will be seen as a loss of the normal asphericity of the femoral head and a shoot through lateral in internal rotation will show the anterior femoral neck bump most clearly. Pincer impingement may be seen as a crossover sign on the AP pelvic radiograph (Reynolds et al 1999), although this will also be the case in true retroversion. If dysplasia is seen on the AP pelvis view, then supplementary dysplasia views, including false profile to assess the anterior uncovering of the femoral head, should be performed. If a bony anatomical abnormality is seen, fine cut CT scanning with 3D reconstructions gives the gold standard assessment of the bony hip (Klaue et al 1988) and may also detect degeneration not visible on plain X-ray imaging. Magnetic resonance imaging is extremely useful in excluding other pathology, such as avascular necrosis, transient osteoporosis, stress fractures or more distant pathology. It may also show inflammation associated with bursitis or tendonitis around the hip. In FAI, characteristic femoral neck cysts seen on MRI (Nokes et al 1989) can be helpful, particularly in the diagnosis of functional impingement, in cases where no bony abnormality is seen. In the diagnosis of labral tears, MRI has limited sensitivity (Edwards et al 2005), even with arthrography using intra-articular gadolinium (Toomayan 2006). The latter is often extremely unpleasant for the patient and not used routinely by the authors. The combination of plain radiography, CT and MRI will, in most cases, confirm a diagnosis. Rarely, bone scanning or SPECT CT may aid diagnosis.

GENERAL MANAGEMENT

Whilst the specific conditions discussed above will require treatment in their own right, this needs to be done in conjunction with overall treatment of the hypermobility syndrome. Patients identified as being hypermobile, but without a definitive diagnosis, should be referred to a hypermobility specialist for assessment and to allow, if necessary, for screening of associated conditions and genetic counselling. The overall treatment will also involve a physiotherapist, experienced in the management of hypermobility, for treatment aimed at controlling the patients' excessive movement, since it has been postulated that the increased femoral excursion, in isolation, may cause hip symptoms or exacerbate existing conditions (Chapter 9). In many cases, involvement of a chronic pain team is required, since pain hypersensitivity may lead to complex perioperative analgesic requirements.

HIP PAIN WITH NORMAL IMAGING

It is not uncommon, particularly in hypermobile patients, that all imaging is normal, but the hip is the localizing site of pain. If the site is in any doubt, a diagnostic local anaesthetic injection may be helpful in confirming the diagnosis, although failure of the injection may be due to resistance to local anaesthetic. Whilst the diagnosis in hypermobile cases is usually functional impingement, hip arthroscopy should be considered as the final diagnostic tool (Baber et al 1999), particularly as some small labral tears or labral inflammation may be invisible on imaging studies (Figs 12.3.4 and 12.3.5). However, confirming an absence of structural problems in hypermobile patients is extremely useful, since it allows

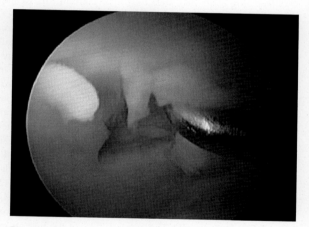

Fig. 12.3.4 Anterior chondral damage as seen at hip arthroscopy

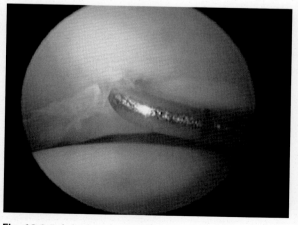

Fig. 12.3.5 Labral tear seen at hip arthroscopy

the patient and their health care professionals to concentrate on pain management. It must be borne in mind, however, that hip arthroscopy can be followed by a lengthy rehabilitation period and should not be undertaken without careful consideration.

SUMMARY

A variety of hip conditions are seen in hypermobile patients. These may be predisposed to by the excessive range of movement seen in this group of patients. Assessment and treatment requires a multidisciplinary and multimodal approach. It is important that those treating hip conditions in this group appreciate that hypermobility as a sole source of hip pain is a diagnosis that can only be reached after thorough assessment of underlying anatomical abnormalities. Likewise, assessment of joint hypermobility should be considered part of the assessment of the painful hip joint, particularly in young patients.

References

Allen WC, Cope R: Coxa Saltans: the snapping hip revisited, *J Am Acad Orthop Surg* 3:303–308, 1995.

Baber YF, Robinson AHF, Villar N: Is diagnostic arthroscopy of the hip worthwhile?: a prospective review of 328 adults investigated for hip pain, *Br J Bone Joint Surg* 81-B:600–603, 1999.

Bardakos NV, Villar RN: The ligamentum teres of the adult hip, *Br J Bone Joint Surg* 91-B:8–15, 2009.

Beck M, Kahlhor M, Leunig M, et al: Hip morphology influences the pattern of acetabular cartilage damage, *Br J Bone Joint Surg* 87-B:1012–1018, 2005.

Brignall CG, Stainsby GD: The snapping hip. Treatment by Z-plasty, *Br J Bone Joint Surg* 73:253–254, 1991.

Byrd JWT, Jones KS: Hip arthroscopy in athletes, *Clin Sports Med* 20:749–761, 2001.

Byrd JWT, Jones KS: Traumatic rupture of the ligamentum teres as a source of hip pain, *Arthroscopy* 20:385–391, 2004.

Dobbs MB, Gordon JE, Luhmann SJ, et al: Surgical Correction of the Snapping Iliopsoas Tendon in Adolescents, *Am J Bone Joint Surg* 84:420–424, 2002.

Edwards DJ, Lomas D, Villar RN: Diagnosis of the painful hip by magnetic resonance imaging and arthroscopy, *Br J Bone Joint Surg* 77-B:374–376, 1995.

Flanum ME, Keene JS, Blankenbaker DG, et al: Arthroscopic treatment of the painful 'internal' snapping hip: results of a new endoscopic technique and imaging protocol, *Am J Sports Med* 35:770–779, 2007.

Ganz R, Gill TJ, Gautier E, et al: Surgical dislocation of the adult hip: a technique with full access to the femoral head and acetabulum without the risk of avascular necrosis, *Br J Bone Joint Surg* 1(83-B):1119–1124, 2001.

Ganz R, Leunig M, Leunig-Ganz K, et al: The etiology of osteoarthritis of the hip: an integrated mechanical concept, *Clin Orthop Relat Res* 466:264–272, 2008.

Haene RA, Bradley M, Villar RN: Hip dysplasia and the torn acetabular labrum: an inexact relationship, *Br J Bone Joint Surg* 89-B: 1289–1292, 2007.

Jacobson T, Allen WC: Surgical correction of the snapping iliopsoas tendon, *Am J Sports Med* 18:470–474, 1990.

Kapandji IA: The physiology of the ligamentum teres. In *The physiology of the joints*, vol 2, ed 2, New York, 1978, Churchill Livingstone, p. 42.

Kendall FP, McCreary EK, Provance PG: *Muscles Testing and Function*, ed 4, Baltimore, 1993, Williams & Wilkins, p. 57.

Klaue K, Wallin A, Ganz R: CT evaluation of coverage and congruency of the hip prior to osteotomy, *Clin Orthop Relat Res* 232:15–25, 1988.

Klaue K, Durnin CW, Ganz R: The acetabular rim syndrome: a clinical presentation of dysplasia of the hip, *Br J Bone Joint Surg* 73-B:423–429, 1991.

Lavigne M, Parvizi J, Beck M, et al: Anterior femoroacetabular impingement. Part I: techniques of joint preserving surgery, *Clin Orthop Relat Res* 418:61–66, 2004.

Murphy SB, Millis MB, Hall JE: Surgical correction of acetabular dysplasia in the adult. A Boston experience, *Clin Orthop Relat Res* 363:38–44, 1999.

Murphy KP, Ross AE, Javernick MA, et al: Repair of the adult acetabular labrum, *Arthroscopy* 22:567, 2006.

Nokes SR, Vogler JB, Spritzer CE, et al: Herniation pits of the femoral neck: appearance at MR imaging, *Radiology* 172:231–234, 1989.

Ober FR: The role of the ilio-tibial band and fascia lata as a factor in the causation of low back disabilities and sciatica, *J Bone Joint Surg* 18:105–110, 1936.

Peters CL, Erickson JA, Hines JL: Early results of the Bernese periacetabular osteotomy: the learning curve at an academic medical center, *Am J Bone Joint Surg* 88:1920–1926, 2006.

Philippon MJ, Schenker M, Briggs K, et al: Femoroacetabular impingement in 45 professional athletes: associated pathologies and return to sport following arthroscopic decompression, *Knee Surg Sports Traumatol Arthrosc* 15:908–914, 2007.

Philippon MJ, Briggs KK, Yen YM, et al: Outcomes following hip arthroscopy for femoroacetabular impingement with associated chondrolabral dysfunction: minimum two-year follow-up, *Br J Bone Joint Surg* 91-B(1):16–23, 2009.

Provencher MT, Hofmeister EP, Muldoon MP: The surgical treatment of external coxa saltans (the snapping hip) by Z-plasty of the iliotibial band, *Am J Sports Med* 32:470–476, 2004.

Rao J, Zhou YX, Villar RN: Injury to the ligamentum teres: mechanism, findings, and results of treatment, *Clin Sports Med* 20:791–799, 2001.

Reynolds D, Lucas J, Klaue K: Retroversion of the acetabulum: a cause of hip pain, *Br J Bone Joint Surg* 81-B:281–288, 1999.

Robertson WJ, Kadrmas WR, Kelly BT: Arthroscopic management of labral tears in the hip: a systematic review of the literature, *Clin Orthop Relat Res* 455:88–92, 2007.

Schaberg JE, Harper MC, Allen WC: The snapping hip syndrome, *Am J Sports Med* 12:361–365, 1984.

Smith-Petersen MN: Treatment of malum coxae senilis, old slipped upper femoral epiphysis, intrapelvic protrusion of the acetabulum, and coxa plana by means of acetabuloplasty, *J Bone Joint Surg* 18:869–880, 1936.

Staple TW, Jung D, Mork A: Snapping tendon syndrome: hip tenography with fluoroscopic monitoring, *Radiology* 166:873–874, 1988.

Tanzer M, Noiseux N: Osseous abnormalities and early osteoarthritis: the role of hip impingement, *Clin Orthop Relat Res* 429:170–177, 2004.

Toomayan GA, Holman WR, Major NM, et al: Sensitivity of MR arthrography in the evaluation of acetabular labral tears, *Am J Roentgenol* 186:449–453, 2006.

12.4 The knee joint

Fares Haddad and Rohit Dhawan

INTRODUCTION

This chapter will discuss how hypermobility (JHM) and joint hypermobility syndrome (JHS) affect the knee joint making it more vulnerable to injury, instability and painful conditions. The most common conditions are described with suggestions for conservative and surgical management.

CHARACTERISTICS OF THE HYPERMOBILE KNEE

Clinical assessment of a hypermobile knee reveals laxity that would be considered pathological were it not symmetrical and physiological for that patient. Compared to the average patient, the hypermobile knee may be grossly lax and unstable. This renders them not only vulnerable to other injuries but also means that they have a lower physiological reserve and hence have more difficulty recovering from more minor injuries.

According to the 'Theory of Tissue Homeostasis' described by Dye (1996), the knee joint is more of an active complex system rather than just a mechanical structure. In this, the range of load that can be applied within a joint without causing structural failure is called the 'Envelope of Function' that covers the 'Zone of Homeostasis'. The boundaries of this zone are determined by four factors, namely – anatomical, kinematic, involving the biomechanics of the knee, physiological factors involving the cell function and repair and fourthly, the treatment modalities involved. The aim of any therapy should be to 'maximise the boundaries of the envelope of function' (Bridges et al 1992, Dye 1996). In patients with JHM we believe that the envelope of function is reduced and that these patients are therefore vulnerable to a whole range of knee problems.

Patients with JHM are at increased risk of 'standard' knee injuries that are suffered by non-JHM patients and have their own spectrum of specific problems such as genu recurvatum pain, patello-femoral pain and patellar instability that require specific attention. In the experience of the senior author, patients who are hypermobile are much more sensitive to even minor knee injuries and therefore have to be treated very carefully. A typical hypermobile patient takes twice as long to recover from a medial collateral ligament (MCL) strain or a minor contusion to the anterior aspect of the knee. Close liaison between carers is necessary in order to reinforce the need for patience and appropriate rehabilitation.

KNEE PROPRIOCEPTION AND POSTURE CONTROL

The only objective evidence of a pathology in JHS is the known fact of a proprioceptive deficit in the knee joints along with the proximal interphalangeal joints (Mallik et al 1994, Hall et al 1995). The imbalance of autonomic dysfunction has also been described as an extra-articular manifestation of the syndrome. There have been reports suggesting a delayed motor development in patients as well (Jaffe et al 1988, Tirosh et al 1991). Efficient postural control depends on proprioceptive feedback from the joints. In JHS patients, this feedback is reduced due to decreased proprioceptive acuity leading to an imbalance in posture maintenance (Chapter 6.4).

Current research based on histological, proprioceptive and nerve studies suggests that the generation of nerve impulses from the intra-articular components of the knee help in conscious perception of position of the knee in space (Barrack et al 1989, Barrett et al 1991, Biedert et al 1992, Clark et al 1979, Denti et al 1994, Dye et al 1998, Freeman & Wyke 1967, Gardner 1948, Grabiner et al 1994, Newton 1982, Pitman et al 1992, Proske et al 1988, Warren et al 1993). The study by Hall et al (1995) has shown that there is a reduction in the proprioceptive acuity in the knee joint in patients suffering from JHS resulting in a poor feedback from the joint. Such patients tend to have a higher threshold level for detection of the start of flexion of the knee joint as well. There is no increase in the acuity seen on extending the knee joint in JHS patients (Hall et al 1995). This is responsible for biomechanically inefficient positions adopted by the joints leading to an uneven distribution of force which can cause pain and possibly osteoarthritis in the long run (El Shahaly & El Sherif 1991, Bridges et al 1992).

An 8-week physiotherapy regimen consisting of closed kinetic chain (CKC) and static hamstring exercises has been shown to improve proprioception, balance and muscle strength as well as reduce pain and improve quality of life in patients with JHS (Ferrell et al 2004). In the study, the CKC exercises consisted of squats, pliés, front and lateral lunges, performed alongside exercises on the balance board and static hamstring exercises to strengthen the hamstrings. Compared to the traditional open kinetic chain exercises (OKC), CKC are considered safer, more specific and more functional. They are also thought to increase joint stability by facilitating co-contraction of the muscles of the knee joint and so help in recruitment of quadriceps, hamstrings and gastrocnemius (Lass et al 1991). The CKC exercises also put less strain on the ligaments (Henning et al 1985) than the OKC. The Ruffini nerve endings in the knee joint are sensitive to volume and pressure changes in the intra-articular fluid and CKC are thought to facilitate these receptors by increasing the pressure in the joints and thereby help in improving the proprioceptive acuity of the joint (Wood & Ferrell 1984). This, in turn, improves the posture of the joint and the body as a whole, and helps to reduce symptoms.

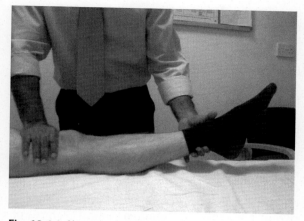

Fig. 12.4.1 Hyperextension at the knee

COMMON CONDITIONS IN THE HYPERMOBILE KNEE

GENU RECURVATUM

Excessive hyperextension, or genu recurvatum (Fig. 12.4.1), of the knee can lead to increased pressure and irritation of the infrapatellar fat pad due to the patella lying more inferiorly. This can present as pain and swelling around the inferior aspect of the patella. The pain is exacerbated by prolonged standing with the knee hyperextended. This can be clinically demonstrated by extension overpressure. The infrapatellar fat pad can also be compressed by maltracking of the patella which is common in hypermobility. As well as having an influence on the position of the patella, excessive hyperextension at the knee also changes the contact between the femur and tibia to a more anterior position potentially increasing the compression on the anterior

structures in the knee including the anterior horn of the medial meniscus.

Hyperextension of the knee in the hypermobile individual often occurs in combination with overpronation of the feet and internal rotation of the femurs and may result in postural bowlegs (genu varum) as the hyperextension occurs in a posterolateral direction. Less commonly, hyperextension occurs in combination with oversupination in the feet and lateral rotation of the femurs resulting in knock-knees (genu valgum), due to the hyperextension producing adduction at the knees (Kendall et al 1993).

The effects of hyperextension at the knee are felt above and below the knee and need to be considered in any planned treatment. Treatment is aimed at reducing the tendency of the hypermobile individual to stand or rest at end of range at their knees in order to prevent soft tissue strain. Treatment involves re-education of the hamstrings and quadriceps to co-contract during standing and hold the knee in full extension without going into hyperextension. It is essential that both hamstrings and quadriceps are trained together as the training of only one set of muscles would lead to an imbalance of forces acting on the knee. Attention also needs to be given to the muscles in the rest of the leg, to improve control of pronation in the foot and internal rotation at the hip as well as improving core/trunk stability.

ANTERIOR KNEE PAIN

The causes of anterior knee pain can be obscure or distinct (Jackson 2001). It is much easier to diagnose and treat the distinct causes that result from trauma, dysplasia, overuse, tumours or have an iatrogenic cause. These all tend to result in focal lesions that can be dealt with relatively easily. The unexplained anterior knee pain that results from hypermobility, subtle maltracking and/or subluxation of the patella, or where no cause is found, is more difficult to manage (Jackson 2001).

Underlying structural factors which may contribute to the development of pain include anteversion of the femur, patella alta, patella baja, increased Q angle, genu valgum, genu varum, excessive foot pronation and genu recurvatum (Malek & Mangine 1981) as they affect the balance of the soft tissues surrounding the patella. The last two in particular are common clinical features of JHS and make the individual more susceptible to anterior knee pain.

The patellofemoral joint (PFJ) is subject to a large amount of shear stress and compression forces when the knee is in motion. It has been shown that due to the small moment arm of the patellar tendon, the magnitude of forces in the PFJ can vary from 2–17.5 times bodyweight (Perry et al 1975, Zernicke et al 1977). In a hypermobile knee with lax ligaments and tendons, it is not surprising that symptoms occur in the patellofemoral joint, given the immense magnitude of the stresses incurred in the joint.

Movement of the patella is controlled by the balance of soft tissue structures around the knee joint as well as the thickness and shape of the patellofemoral chondral cartilage and surrounding musculature. The tracking of the patella – the movement of the patella within the trochlear groove of the femur – is also affected by an imbalance of forces on the patella. This leads to an uneven distribution of stresses on the infrapatellar surface resulting in articular damage. Being avascular in nature, hyaline cartilage has a poor healing capacity and its surface properties, including its shock absorption efficiency, deteriorate over time. Synovitis and pain may be caused at an early stage by irritation of the synovium due to degenerative changes in the superficial layer of cartilage (Fulkerson & Hungerford 1990). Ultimately, if patellar maltracking is not addressed, continued chondral damage leads to exposure of the underlying subchondral bone, and a direct transfer of force to the bones results in an increase in the intraosseous pressure and hence severe pain.

In a growing adolescent, the muscles and soft tissues become tight and less flexible. This reduction in flexibility of the hamstrings, quadriceps, gastrocnemius-soleus complex, tensor fascia lata and lateral retinaculum adversely affects patellar tracking and can initiate knee symptoms (Chapter 10). A short lateral retinaculum pulls on the patella as flexion is initiated and draws it into the trochlear groove. There is a further increase in the tension as the iliotibial band moves posterior to the lateral condyle of the femur and increases the tension on the already tense lateral retinaculum. These changes in the force distribution lead to a lateral tilting and lateral tracking of the patella (Dye 1996). A weakness of the vastus medialis obliquus (VMO) adds to the lateral tilt of the patella, as it is unable to pull the patella medially.

The typical characteristics of anterior knee pain include vague, non-specific pain on the anterior and anteromedial aspect of the knee. The pain is exacerbated on walking or running and particularly with stair climbing, and is sometimes accompanied by an effusion of the knee joint. The patient may also complain of a feeling of the knee 'giving way', due to subluxation of the patella or quadriceps inhibition. On examination quadriceps wasting may be seen along with crepitus on movement. VMO has been shown to develop reflex inhibition after a knee effusion (Spencer et al 1984) and when present, this leads to subsequent atrophy of the muscle so that abnormal tracking occurs.

Muscle imbalances around the hips and pelvis as well as abnormal gait patterns can also lead to patellofemoral problems. An appropriate rehabilitation programme to address the relevant imbalances is based on an in-depth assessment of the length, strength, timing and control of the muscles of the lower limbs and pelvis, with particular attention to the relative balance of the medial and lateral quadriceps and tensor fascia lata/ilio-tibial band (TFL/ITB). Treatment will frequently involve manual techniques to relax and lengthen short overactive tissues (TFL/ITB) in combination with facilitation and strengthening of VMO. Patellar taping can be an effective adjunct, having been shown to increase VMO activity (Christou 2004, Macgregor et al 2005), enhance proprioception (but only in those whose proprioception is poor) (Callaghan et al 2002, 2008) and produce a beneficial effect on dynamic postural control in patients with patellofemoral pain syndrome compared to healthy individuals (Aminaka and Gribble 2008) (Chapters 9 and 13).

PATELLOFEMORAL INSTABILITY

Patellofemoral instability is a variant of the patellofemoral pain syndromes. It is found to be more prevalent in females, people with generalized hypermobility and hyperextension of the knee, those having patella alta, a Q angle (the angle subtended by a line from the anterior superior iliac spine to the centre of the patella, and a line from the centre of the patella to the tibial tuberosity) of greater than 20 degrees and dysplasia of the trochlea and patella (Insall 1979, Hughston 1989). The patella is known to dislocate or sublux laterally. The patient shows apprehension on passive movement of the patella laterally and the patellar glide test shows a translation of more than 75% of the width of the patella. In a normal individual, the subluxation of the patella can cause damage to the articular cartilage but it has been shown that patients with JHS are less likely to sustain articular cartilage damage – this may be because the hypermobility leads to less articular pressure during subluxation/dislocation than it would in a tighter knee (Stanitski 1995).

Recent studies on unstable patellofemoral joints (PFJ) have focused more on passive restraints against 'mediolateral patellofemoral motion' (Fithian et al 2004). In such knees, although the muscle alignment is important, it still has only a secondary role to play in maintaining the stability, which is primarily controlled passively by the medial patellofemoral ligaments.

Physiotherapy aimed at improving the biomechanical alignment of the joint and also addressing the patellar soft tissue balance has been found to be successful (Crossley et al 2005, McConnell 2007) (Chapter 9). Exercises that involve strengthening programmes such as to the VMO and pelvic muscles are useful. Patients with hypermobility should be taught specific exercises aimed at improving their proprioceptive acuity and kinaesthesia (Chapter 6.4).

In a stable PFJ, the patella gets locked into the trochlea in early flexion, so the ligaments come to play only in full extension. But in an unstable PFJ, the medial patellofemoral ligaments have a bigger role to play in preventing lateral dislocation (Fithian et al 2004). Each individual must be assessed thoroughly with regards to the risk of dislocation, disability, pain and the anatomical structure of the joint before preparing a multidisciplinary treatment plan.

Surgical treatment is a last resort in these cases as the secondary muscle wasting that occurs after surgery often worsens the patient's symptoms. Moreover, any form of soft tissue plication is likely to stretch over time due to the basic nature of the tissue in these cases. In cases where a decision for surgical management has been made, simple operations involving repair of the retinacular structures are not as effective as more complex realignment procedures that also address patellofemoral dysplasia – these include trochleoplasty, tibial tuberosity transfer, medial plication and medial patellofemoral ligament reconstruction. Fithian et al (2004) have also appropriately argued that lateral release (which was frequently undertaken in the past for patellar tilt/subluxation) has very little role in treating a hyperlax PFJ as it in fact, adds laxity to an already unstable system.

ANTERIOR CRUCIATE LIGAMENT (ACL) INJURY

ACL injury is more common in individuals with joint laxity and hyperextension of the knee joint (Nicholas 1970, Ramesh et al 2005). There are numerous factors that predispose to the rupture of ACL. Among the extrinsic factors (potentially changeable) are strength, hamstring flexibility, proprioception, neuromuscular rhythm, poor co-ordination and footwear. Among the intrinsic factors (unchangeable) are limb alignment, physiological laxity, hyperextension of the knee, ACL size, femoral notch shape and size and hormonal influence (Arendt & Dick 1995, Rozzi et al 1999, Boden et al 2000, Griffin et al 2000, Ireland 2002, Ramesh et al 2005).

During movement of the knee joint, at the time of injury there is an attempt to rectify any flexion. This involves excessive contraction of the quadriceps leading to hyperextension of the knee and anterior translation of the tibia (Hirokawa et al 1992, Shoemaker et al 1993, Boden et al 2000, Griffin et al 2000). The anterior translation force is the highest when the quadriceps contract at high acceleration with the knee in a small flexion angle (Borsa et al 1997). In the presence of knee hyperextension, the knee moves further in its arc and the femoral notch impinges on the ACL resulting in it being guillotined. A simultaneous strong hamstring contraction would reduce this risk.

Attempts to prevent ACL injury in hypermobile individuals has increasingly come to the fore, particularly in the sporting population. The simplest method is the use of a knee brace which is a useful adjunct for sports such as skiing. Other preventative strategies involve improving neuromuscular control of the leg (Hewett et al 1999), proprioceptive training programmes (Caraffa et al 1996) and plyometric training programmes involving stretching before contraction of muscles (Hewett et al 1996).

Once they occur, ACL injuries can be treated non-operatively or surgically. In the hypermobile patient, a trial of non-operative treatment is attempted but if patients complain of insecurity/instability, the authors have a very low threshold for proceeding to a reconstruction. Operative treatment involves reconstruction of the ACL. There is controversy regarding the optimal graft type for such cases as loss of either hamstring or quadriceps strength and control can be very deleterious for hypermobile patients. The bone–tendon–bone grafts have been shown to be more successful in stabilization than four bundle hamstring grafts (Kim et al 2008). Others favour reconstruction using double bundle quadriceps tendon–bone graft which allows less translation than single bundle bone-patellar tendon–bone graft (Kim et al 2009). The senior author has seen very favourable

outcomes using allograft reconstruction in these cases as it removes the morbidity of donor site harvest. Regardless of the technique used, full recovery for hypermobile patients requires at least a year of committed rehabilitation.

OSTEOARTHRITIS

Hypermobile individuals develop knee osteoarthritis in the same way as other individuals do, either as part of their genetic fate or in relation to injuries sustained early in life (Chapter 1 and 2). The commonest presentation relates to patellofemoral osteoarthritis, in that chronic patellofemoral mal-alignment leads to progressive chondral damage and erosion of the patella and trochlear surfaces. The patient typically presents with increasing difficulty climbing stairs and pain with activity.

Ultimately, hypermobile patients are assessed and treated in the same way as non-hypermobile patients with osteoarthritis, but greater attention needs to be paid at the time of surgery to both patellofemoral and tibio-femoral stability. A large proportion of such patients have isolated patellofemoral osteoarthritis and benefit from

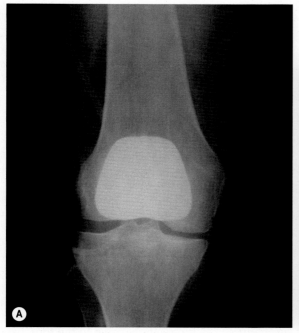
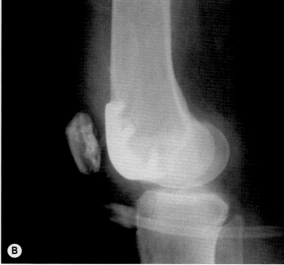

Fig. 12.4.2a, b Patello-femoral arthroplasty

isolated patello-femoral arthroplasty (Fig. 12.4.2). This is generally a successful procedure that allows the tibio-femoral joint to continue functioning in a kinematically normal way. A conversion to a total knee replacement, should this loosen or fail, is subsequently straightforward.

Where a total knee replacement is required, it is the author's experience that prehabilitation and strengthening prior to surgery is helpful. The patients cope with the subsequent trauma of surgery much better. In most cases, a standard condylar knee replacement can be used. It is unusual to have to resort to hinged or very constrained implants, as is the scenario in patients with polio or other neuromuscular conditions. It is critical, however, to obtain excellent alignment and soft tissue balance in these cases.

SUMMARY

The knee joint in individuals with JHS frequently demonstrates increased laxity and a deficit in proprioception. This produces an increased vulnerability to injury and a lower physiological reserve. The envelope of function is reduced and therefore even minor injuries to the knee can generate quite severe symptoms. The greatest problem for patients with hypermobility is patellofemoral mal-alignment and instability. Physiotherapy rehabilitation aimed at improving the biomechanical alignment and soft tissue balance is the treatment of choice. Although hypermobile patients develop similar symptoms as non-hypermobile patients, they require greater input in terms of rehabilitation and have less physiological reserve in terms of knee control.

References

Aminaka N, Gribble P: Patellar taping, patellofemoral pain syndrome, lower extremity kinematics and dynamic postural control, *Journal of Athletic Training* 43:21–28, 2008.

Arendt E, Dick R: Knee injury patterns among men and women in collegiate basketball and soccer. NCAA data and review of literature, *Am J Sports Med* 23:694–701, 1995.

Barrack RL, Skinner HB, Buckley SL: Proprioception in the anterior cruciate deficient knee, *Am J Sports Med* 17:1–6, 1989.

Barrett DS, Cobb AG, Bentley G: Joint proprioception in normal, osteoarthritic and replaced knees, *J Bone Joint Surg Br* 73:53–56, 1991.

Biedert RM, Stauffer E, Friederich NF: Occurrence of free nerve endings in the soft tissue of the knee joint. A histologic investigation, *Am J Sports Med* 20:430–433, 1992.

Boden BP, Dean GS, Feagin JA Jr, et al: Mechanisms of anterior cruciate ligament injury, *Orthopedics* 23:573–578, 2000.

Borsa PA, Lephart SM, Irrgang JJ, et al: The effects of joint position and direction of joint motion on proprioceptive sensibility in anterior cruciate ligament-deficient athletes, *Am J Sports Med* 25:336–340, 1997.

Bridges AJ, Smith E, Reid J: Joint hypermobility in adults referred to rheumatology clinics, *Annals of Rheumatic Disease* 51:793–796, 1992.

Callaghan MJ, Selfe J, Bagley PJ, et al: The effects of patellar taping on knee joint proprioception, *Journal of Athletic Training* 37:19–24, 2002.

Callaghan MJ, Selfe J, McHenry A, et al: Effects of patellar taping on knee joint proprioception in patients with patellofemoral pain syndrome, *Man Ther* 13:192–199, 2008.

Caraffa A, Cerulli G, Projetti M, et al: Prevention of anterior cruciate ligament injuries in soccer. A prospective controlled study of proprioceptive training, *Knee Surg Sports Traumatol Arthrosc* 4:19–21, 1996.

Christou EA: Patellar taping increases vastus medialis oblique activity in the presence of patellofemoral pain, *J Electromyogr Kinesiol* 14:495–504, 2004.

Clark FJ, Horch KW, Bach SM, et al: Contributions of cutaneous and joint receptors to static knee-position sense in man, *J Neurophysiol* 42:877–888, 1979.

Crossley KM, Cowan SM, McConnell J, et al: Physical therapy improves knee flexion during stair ambulation in patellofemoral pain, *Med Sci Sports Exerc* 37:176–183, 2005.

Denti M, Monteleone M, Berardi A, et al: Anterior cruciate ligament mechanoreceptors. Histologic studies on lesions and reconstruction, *Clin Orthop Relat Res* 308:29–32, 1994.

Dye SF: The knee as a biologic transmission with an envelope of function: a theory, *Clin Orthop Relat Res* 325:10–18, 1996.

Dye SF, Vaupel GL, Dye CC: Conscious neurosensory mapping of the internal structures of the human knee without intraarticular anesthesia, *Am J Sports Med* 26:773–777, 1998.

El Shahaly HA, El Sherif AK: Is the benign joint hypermobility syndrome benign? *Clin Rheumatol* 10:302–307, 1991.

Ferrell WR, Tennant N, Sturrock RD, et al: Amelioration of symptoms by enhancement of proprioception in patients with joint hypermobility syndrome, *Arthritis Rheum* 50:3323–3328, 2004.

Fithian DC, Paxton EW, Cohen AB: Indications in the treatment of patellar instability, *J Knee Surg* 17:47–56, 2004.

Freeman MA, Wyke B: The innervation of the knee joint. An anatomical and histological study in the cat, *J Anat* 101:505–532, 1967.

Fulkerson JP, Hungerford DS: *Disorders of the Patellofemoral Joint,* ed 2, Baltimore, 1990, Williams and Wilkins.

Gardner E: The innervation of the knee joint, *Anatomical Record* 101:109–130, 1948.

Grabiner MD, Koh TJ, Draganich LF: Neuromechanics of the patellofemoral joint, *Med Sci Sports Exerc* 26:10–21, 1994.

Griffin LY, Agel J, Albohm MJ, et al: Noncontact anterior cruciate ligament injuries: risk factors and prevention strategies, *J Am Acad Orthop Surg* 8:141–150, 2000.

Hall MG, Ferrell WR, Sturrock RD, et al: The effect of the hypermobility syndrome on knee joint proprioception, *Br J Rheumatol* 34:121–125, 1995.

Handler CE, Child A, Light ND, et al: Mitral valve prolapse, aortic compliance, and skin collagen in joint hypermobility syndrome, *Br Heart J* 54:501–508, 1985.

Henning CE, Lynch MA, Glick KR Jr: An in vivo strain gauge study of elongation of the anterior cruciate ligament, *Am J Sports Med* 13:22–26, 1985.

Hewett TE, Stroupe AL, Nance TA, et al: Plyometric training in female athletes. Decreased impact forces and increased hamstring torques, *Am J Sports Med* 24:765–773, 1996.

Hewett TE, Lindenfeld TN, Riccobene JV, et al: The effect of neuromuscular training on the incidence of knee injury in female athletes. A prospective study, *Am J Sports Med* 27:699–706, 1999.

Hirokawa S, Solomonow M, Lu Y, et al: Anterior-posterior and rotational displacement of the tibia elicited by quadriceps contraction, *Am J Sports Med* 20:299–306, 1992.

Hughston JC: Patellar subluxation. A recent history, *Clin Sports Med* 8:153–162, 1989.

Insall J: Chondromalacia patellae: patellar malalignment syndrome, *Orthop Clin North Am* 10:117–127, 1979.

Ireland ML: The female ACL: why is it more prone to injury? *Orthop Clin North Am* 33:637–651, 2002.

Jackson AM: Anterior knee pain, *J Bone Joint Surg Br* 83:937–948, 2001.

Jaffe M, Tirosh E, Cohen A, et al: Joint mobility and motor development, *Arch Dis Child* 63:159–161, 1988.

Kendall FP, McCreary EK, Provance PG: *Muscles: testing and function,* ed 4, Baltimore, 1993, Williams and Wilkins, p 97.

Kim SJ, Kim TE, Lee DH, et al: Anterior cruciate ligament reconstruction in patients who have excessive joint laxity, *J Bone Joint Surg Am* 90:735–741, 2008.

Kim SJ, Chang JH, Kim TW, et al: Anterior cruciate ligament reconstruction with use of a single or double-bundle technique in patients with generalized ligamentous laxity, *J Bone Joint Surg Am* 91:257–262, 2009.

Lass P, Kaalund S, leFevre S, et al: Muscle coordination following rupture of the anterior cruciate ligament. Electromyographic studies of 14 patients, *Acta Orthop Scand* 62:9–14, 1991.

McConnell J: Rehabilitation and nonoperative treatment of patellar instability, *Sports Med Arthrosc* 15:95–104, 2007.

Macgregor K, Gerlach S, Mellor R, et al: Cutaneous stimulation from patella tape causes a differential increase in vasti muscle activity in people with patellofemoral pain, *J Orthop Res* 23:351–358, 2005.

Malek MM, Mangine RE: Patellofemoral pain syndromes: a comprehensive and conservative approach, *J Orthop Sports Phys Ther* 2:108–116, 1981.

Mallik AK, Ferrell WR, McDonald AG, et al: Impaired proprioceptive acuity at the proximal interphalangeal joint in patients with the hypermobility syndrome, *Br J Rheumatol* 33:631–637, 1994.

Newton RA: Joint receptor contributions to reflexive and kinesthetic responses, *Phys Ther* 62:22–29, 1982.

Nicholas JA: Injuries to knee ligaments. Relationship to looseness and tightness in football players, *J Am Med Assoc* 212:2236–2239, 1970.

Perry JD, Antonelli D, Ford W: Analysis of knee-joint forces during flexed-knee stance, *J Bone Joint Surg Am* 57:961–967, 1975.

Pitman MI, Nainzadeh N, Menche D, et al: The intraoperative evaluation of the neurosensory function of the anterior cruciate ligament in humans using somatosensory evoked potentials, *Arthroscopy* 8:442–447, 1992.

Proske UH, Schaible G, Schmidt RF: Joint receptors and kinaesthesia, *Exp Brain Res* 72:219–224, 1988.

Ramesh R, Von Arx O, Azzopardi T, et al: The risk of anterior cruciate ligament rupture with generalised joint laxity, *J Bone Joint Surg Br* 87:800–803, 2005.

Rozzi SL, Lephart SM, Gear WS, et al: Knee joint laxity and neuromuscular characteristics of male and female soccer and basketball players, *Am J Sports Med* 27:312–319, 1999.

Shoemaker SC, Adams D, Daniel DM, et al: Quadriceps/anterior cruciate graft interaction. An in vitro study of joint kinematics and anterior cruciate ligament graft tension, *Clin Orthop Relat Res* 294:379–390, 1993.

Spencer JD, Hayes KC, Alexander IJ: Knee joint effusion and quadriceps reflex inhibition in man, *Arch Phys Med Rehabil* 65:171–177, 1984.

Stanitski CL: Articular hypermobility and chondral injury in patients with acute patellar dislocation, *Am J Sports Med* 23:146–150, 1995.

Tirosh E, Jaffe M, Marmur R, et al: Prognosis of motor development and joint hypermobility, *Arch Dis Child* 66:931–933, 1991.

Warren PJ, Olanlokun TK, Cobb AG, et al: Proprioception after knee arthroplasty. The influence of prosthetic design, *Clin Orthop Relat Res* 297:182–187, 1993.

Wood L, Ferrell WR: Response of slowly adapting articular mechanoreceptors in the cat knee joint to alterations in intra-articular volume, *Annals of Rheumatic Diseases* 43:327–332, 1984.

Zernicke RF, Garhammer J, Jobe FW: Human patellar-tendon rupture, *J Bone Joint Surg Am* 59:179–183, 1977.

12.5 The hypermobile foot

Ron S McCulloch and Anthony Redmond

With contribution from Rosemary Keer

INTRODUCTION

The foot is a complex structure containing 26 bones, more than 30 small joints, and more than 100 muscles, tendons and ligaments. These components are not only structurally complex but also depend on carefully coordinated timing of force and motion in order to produce normal foot function. The normal foot goes through a pronation/re-supination cycle in each stance phase, acting first as a mobile adapter during weight acceptance and later as a rigid lever in terminal stance. The coordination of this cycle is a product of bony architecture, active muscle control and also of soft tissue restraining mechanisms.

The loads on the foot are both repetitive and high compared with some other joints, such as, those in the upper limb. During normal walking, forces experienced by the foot can be up to 1.3 times those experienced during still standing, and during more strenuous activity the forces to which the foot is exposed can increase even further. Running results typically in forces equivalent to 3–4 times body weight and during extreme activity such as running downhill, forces can exceed 8 times body weight equivalent.

The cyclical mechanism above can become defective if external demands on the foot are too great or if the coupling mechanisms that control it are compromised by, for example, bony mal-alignment or ligament laxity.

Patients with joint hypermobility (JHM) are particularly susceptible to the effects of bio-mechanical osseous mal-alignments and ligamentous laxity. The presence of JHM should always be considered where any intervention on the foot is planned, as failure to do so can lead to disappointing outcomes and avoidable complications.

Assessment should include biomechanical morphology and function, through open and closed chain evaluation with both clinical and quantitative gait analysis.

FOOT PROBLEMS IN THE GENERAL POPULATION

Foot problems are relatively common in the general population with some 20–24% of all adults having had an episode of foot pain in the past month and some 60% in the past 6 months (Garrow et al 2004). The incidence and impact of foot problems increases with age, with a quarter of all people over 55 years reporting ongoing foot pain (Benvenuti et al 1995, Leveille et al 1998, Gorter et al 2001, Chen et al 2003, Thomas et al 2004). Foot pain is also five times more prevalent in females than males (Black & Hale 1987, Benvenuti et al 1995, Leveille et al 1998, Munro & Steele 1998, Dunn et al 2004, Garrow et al 2004).

It is generally assumed that foot problems associated with JHM are more common and more severe than in the rest of the population. Pathologies are largely mechanical in origin, with sites in the heel, midfoot and forefoot all affected.

THE FOOT AND HYPERMOBILITY

The Beighton hypermobility scale does not assess foot JHM (Chapter 1). Furthermore, a high positive score will not always coincide with pedal joint laxity (see later). Significantly, patients can present with marked pedal laxity without further joint involvement.

As noted above foot pain of mechanical origin is relatively common. People with JHM appear to develop similar sorts of 'overuse'-type symptoms as the rest of the population (tenosynovitis, arthralgia) but do so more frequently, and possibly more severely.

Joint-specific presentations around the lower leg include: ankle pain, instability and impingement syndromes, midfoot joint pain and symptoms across the forefoot (Finsterbush & Pogrund 1982). More common are soft tissue disorders resulting from instability of structure and function, with the resulting increase in stress on surrounding tissues. Common soft tissue presentations will include tendo-Achilles pain and other posterior heel presentations, plantar heel pain (plantar fasciitis), tendonitis around the medial malleolus (tibialis posterior tenosynovitis) or lateral malleolus (peroneal tenosynovitis), flexor/extensor tendonopathy and bursitis. Long-term changes occurring in the presence of altered foot function such as the development of bunions at the 1st metatarsophalangeal (MTP) joint or clawed lesser toes can also cause their own specific symptoms.

Marfan syndrome is associated with JHM although interestingly, the presenting foot type is often highly arched, rather than flattened, reflecting processes other than local JHM. Joint hypermobility can be associated with some unusual presentations in the feet including a 'skewfoot'-type presentation often seen in Marfan syndrome, and talipes equinovarus type features (Agnew 1997).

THE FOOT AND JOINT HYPERMOBILITY SYNDROME

Joint hypermobility syndrome (JHS) has been cited as a potential cause for a number of foot conditions including digital deformities, hallux valgus and flexible collapsed pes plano valgus (Ross et al 1988, Harris & Beeson 1998, Murray 2006). There is an increased incidence of soft tissue injury, including tendinopathy in individuals with JHS. This is particularly well documented in music, dance and sport (Nicholas 1970, McCormack et al 2004, Stewart & Burden 2004). Pain in the lower limb is also considered to be as common as spinal and upper limb pain in these patients (Ainsworth & Aulicino 1993, Hudson et al 1995, Sacheti et al 1997). This is not surprising given ankle and foot JHM has been reported to affect as many as 60% to 94% of adults with JHS (Bulbena et al 1992, Riano et al 2001).

Hypermobility of foot joints is thought to predispose the individual to a more pronated or flat-footed presentation (pes planus). Certain types of hypermobility (e.g. classical EDS (Chapter 1)) may be more closely associated with pes planus.

Whatever the relationship with JHM, people with JHS undoubtedly experience a significantly greater degree of pain and impairment. In a large prevalence study of the effects of JHS on joint pain and health status Redmond et al (2006a) found that individuals with JHS reported significantly worse general health, as measured by the EQ-5D, a widely used 100-point rating scale for overall health status (Kind et al 2005). In this study, the JHS group rated

their health status at a median of only 65/100, compared with 90/100 for age- and gender-matched controls. Much of this impaired health status was associated with foot problems. The JHS group reported far higher levels of foot pain on a 100-mm visual analogue scale (34 mm vs 0.4 mm for the controls) and far greater degrees of resulting impairment (16/33 vs 0/33) using the Manchester Foot Pain and Disability Questionnaire (MFPDQ) (Garrow et al 2000). Most sites in the lower limb were affected, with 77% of the JHS group reporting hip symptoms, 87% reporting knee problems, 74% ankle problems and 72% foot problems. In summary, compared with age- and gender-matched controls people with JHS reported:

- Poorer general health and quality of life
- Worse lower limb pain
- Greater lower limb disability
- A propensity for lower limb joint involvement.

Little scientific data exist to explain any link between the mechanical factors assumed to be influential in JHS and associated pain and health status. An attempt has been made to explore associations between overall hypermobility, mechanical features in the lower limb, and resulting pain and health status (Redmond et al 2006b). In 75 people with a rheumatologist diagnosis of JHM (Beighton score current or confirmed historical of ≥5/9) and musculoskeletal foot symptoms, the study examined a range of self-reported outcomes including measures of general health status (EQ-5D), foot health status (MFPDQ) and foot pain using the pain subscale of the Foot Function Index (Budiman-Mak et al 1991). These were analysed for associations with clinician-derived data from a range of clinical variables including general joint mobility (Beighton score), standing foot posture (Foot Posture Index (Keenan et al 2007, Redmond et al 2006c)) (see below), and dynamic foot function during normal walking. There was a significant linear relationship between the degree of hypermobility and poorer general health and even more so with poorer foot health status and with worse foot pain. Interestingly though, there was no evidence of any direct link between the Beighton score and severity of flat-foot in quiet standing, and no evidence of any link between the Beighton score and abnormal pronation of the ankle/subtalar joint complex during gait. Despite the absence of any association within these classic models of foot function, a moderate association was found to exist between the Beighton score and magnitudes of midfoot joint excursion during walking. A further link was found between larger magnitudes of midfoot motion during gait and impaired foot health status.

Rather than the traditional assumption of generalized hypermobility being associated simply with flat feet, it may therefore be that excessive movement in the joints of the midfoot leads to poor coupled movement with neighbouring joints and a breakdown of the normal pronation/supination cycle when walking. This would seem a plausible explanation for some of the foot pain experienced by hypermobile individuals where static foot anatomy appears normal.

ASSESSMENT OF THE FOOT

HISTORY

The history should include those areas of general health pertinent to JHS such as questions related to a personal and familial predisposition to fractures, osteoarthrosis, compromised healing, excessive bruising, vaso-vagal incidents (faints), heart valve disease and abnormal scarring. A history of previous surgical complications must be noted (Tompkins & Bellacosa 1997). The presence of an excessively thin, papyraceous scarring is a feature of JHS. In addition, thought should be given to secondary skin manifestations including symptomatic hyperkeratoses, digital lesions and ulcerations (Port et al 1980). A positive family history for local anaesthetic resistance is also more common (Hakim et al 2005).

Environmental factors such as type or extent of weight-bearing/non-weight-bearing activity, or diurnal variation and footwear worn can help to identify whether local mechanical factors might be driving the pathology. In particular the clinician should also be aware of activities such as ballet and gymnastics, as the pathologies associated with these activities can be uniquely challenging.

Previous treatments employed should be explored in detail, both as a pointer to the disease process and to avoid duplication of effort.

BIOMECHANICS

The hypermobile patient is more likely to develop deformity and symptoms if biomechanical asymmetries and imbalances co-exist. A detailed mechanical assessment assists with planning therapy and in particular informs more realistic expectations as to the outcome of surgery.

Formal examination of the many components of the foot is complex and can be time-consuming to perform. Specific examples are discussed below. An in-depth description of examination of the foot is beyond the scope of this book. The reader is referred to two resources by Redmond & Helliwell (2005) and Redmond (2008) detailing assessment of the foot and lower limb respectively.

Many of the deforming forces which may lead to the development of conditions such as flexible pes planus, hallux valgus and digital deformity do not derive from the foot itself and failure to recognize and consider these will often lead to disappointing outcomes. An abducted foot position, for example, may derive from the ankle, mid tarsal and sub talar joints or from the hip. With the last, the deforming forces are likely to continue regardless of the treatment applied to the foot. Similarly, an in-toe gait, genu varum and valgum can profoundly compromise foot function.

The standing examination

The assessment may begin with the patient standing. These observations provide valuable information which can be cross-referenced against the non-weight-bearing examination.

It is often helpful to start from the head down. Unequal shoulder height may indicate a scoliosis or limb length discrepancy. A limb length discrepancy is supported by downward frontal plane pelvic tilt on the shorter side. Excessive anterior pelvic tilt may also lead to an overall compromise in foot and lower limb function.

Starting proximally in the lower limb the position and alignment of the hip, upper leg, knee, lower leg, and ankle should be assessed for rotation, varus/valgus, fixed flexion deformities and joint/soft tissue swelling.

Internally rotated patellae, often referred to as 'squinting patellae', would indicate either a primary internal neutral hip position or a secondary internal rotation from an abnormally pronated foot. The underlying cause can be determined by asking the patient to invert their feet to neutral whilst standing. The relaxed stance position is shown in Figure 12.5.1. If the patellar position corrects, then the internal rotation is most likely to derive from the foot. The reverse may be true

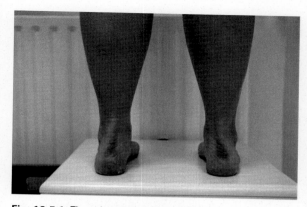

Fig. 12.5.1 The relaxed stance position

of an external neutral hip position, although this more commonly derives from the hip joint itself. The presence of genu valgum can be assessed in a similar way. Tibia or genu varum may result in varus heels during stance which would increase the patient's predisposition to lateral instability. Internal tibial torsion can markedly increase abnormal pronation. Figure 12.5.2 shows hindfoot pronation and midfoot eversion.

The presence of ankle equinus can be determined by asking the patient to stand on a 15 degree incline (commercial incline boards being readily available). A rectus posture without compensation through abnormal pronation or postural change suggests normal calf flexibility. Compensations such as forward lean, foot abduction, and knee flexion and knee hyperextension suggest a lack of ankle dorsiflexion; similar compensations may occur during gait.

Particular attention should be paid to the midfoot arch during transition from weight-bearing to non-weight-bearing. Feet that appear high arched while non-weight-bearing can look normal on weight-bearing, while perfectly normal-looking non-weight-bearing feet can become significantly flattened when under load. The easiest way to test that a flat-footed posture is reducible is to ask the patient to stand on tip-toes.

Most of the traditional methods of quantifying variation in foot posture are of limited reliability or require complex techniques or instrumentation. The Foot Posture Index (FPI) is a recently developed and validated tool (Redmond et al 2006c, Keenan et al 2007). It is a simple classification system, scoring six observations against set criteria (Box 12.5.1) applying a common rating system to the observations with positive scores for signs associated with pronated/planus postures and negative scores for signs associated with supinated/cavus postures. The FPI predicts about 60% of the true variance in standing posture relative to other forms of laboratory testing and about 40% of the variance observed by laboratory analysis of walking; this is about twice as much as traditional measures such as calcaneal position and navicular height. Further information, manuals and normative datasheets are obtainable free of charge from www.leeds.ac.uk/medicine/FASTER/FPI (Redmond et al 2008). Whilst these data cannot be directly interpreted as pedal joint laxity they form a valuable part of the assessment process and results should be cross-referenced against some of the more specific hypermobility tests outlined below.

One subjective test that may be helpful is the 'standing eversion stress test'. This will often highlight increased degrees of hindfoot laxity. Whilst individuals without hindfoot laxity are generally unable to evert their heels beyond their relaxed position, the hypermobile patient can often achieve much greater levels of eversion.

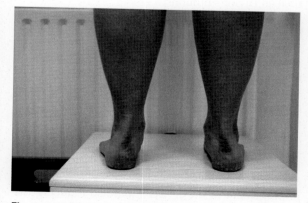

Fig. 12.5.2 Hindfoot pronation and midfoot eversion

BOX 12.5.1 The six criteria which make up the FPI rating scale

1. Talar head palpation
2. Supra- and infralateral malleolar curvature
3. Calcaneal frontal plane position
4. Prominence in the region of the talonavicular joint
5. Congruence of the medial longitudinal arch
6. Abduction/adduction of the forefoot on the rearfoot

The non-weight-bearing examination

The non-weight-bearing assessment can help to crystallize some of the conclusions from the standing examination. The presence of a length discrepancy will be supported by unequal malleolar level in the presence of parallel superior and posterior iliac spines. The patient should be assessed for an internal or external neutral hip position with the hip joint extended and flexed. Gastrocnemius flexibility should be assessed with the hindfoot held close to neutral and the knee extended. Soleus involvement can be assessed by repeating this test with the knee flexed.

Further non-pedal manifestations of lower limb JHM are characterized by a loss of inherent stability with reduced joint 'end feel' and greater ranges of motion. This can typically be appreciated when examining hip joint rotation, abduction and adduction and whilst performing routine ligamentous tests of the knee such as the anterior drawer test.

Examination of the hindfoot

Laxity within the ankle joint can often be appreciated from simply observing the relaxed position of the foot whilst the patient lies supine on the examination couch (Fig. 12.5.3). The hypermobile ankle typically rests with exaggerated plantarflexion. The head of the talus is often prominent and the extensor tendons may be bowed. This leads to digital retraction which can over time result in weight-bearing deformities of the toes, such as varus and claw digits.

The posterior and anterior drawer test will often reveal increased laxity of the ankle joint. Greater motion and loss of 'end feel' is often noted

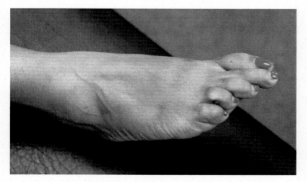

Fig. 12.5.3 Laxity within the ankle joint can often be appreciated from simply observing the relaxed position of the foot whilst the patient lies supine on the examination couch

with inversion, particularly where there is a history of symptomatic or asymptomatic inversion sprains. Radiological stress tests are less useful in evaluating the hypermobile ankle unless a comparison is sought with the asymptomatic side.

One of the most important clues for hindfoot laxity is a predisposition to lateral ankle instability. Practitioners should avoid using the term ankle sprain, as repetitive 'giving way' of the ankle may be considered as incidental to the patient, causing no apparent ill effect. Whilst bruising or pain is often not reported there are likely to be long-term implications, including worsening instability with lateral collateral ankle ligament attenuation, ankle impingement syndromes and osteoarthrosis (Mangwani et al 2001).

Examination of the midfoot

Frontal plane motion can best be assessed by rotating the forefoot in varus and valgus whilst stabilizing the hindfoot with the other hand. Excessive frontal plane motion will be noted in the hypermobile midfoot.

The term anterior equinus is used to express a sagittal mal-alignment whereby the forefoot is excessively plantarflexed in relation to the hindfoot. Excessive forefoot laxity in the sagittal plane can be assessed by holding the hindfoot stable with one hand and dorsiflexing and plantarflexing the entire forefoot. The experienced examiner will note a lack of resistance and excessive motion with this test. Patients with an anterior equinus and a hypermobile forefoot will often stand with increased levels of forefoot abduction, creating the appearance of a lateral 'C'-shaped border. Here the foot may be more predisposed to lateral column deformity, such as Taylor's bunions.

Lisfranc's JHM and instability can be appreciated by mobilizing the metatarsals in dorsiflexion and plantarflexion against the tarsus. The 2nd and 3rd metatarsals have limited range of motion in relation to the medial column (1st metatarsal) and lateral column (4th and 5th metatarsals). Palpable osteophytosis is an indicator of abnormal compression and compromised function. Radiographs are invaluable in supporting these clinical observations.

Hallux dorsiflexion may be excessive in the hypermobile foot (Fig. 12.5.4) but concomitant abnormal pronation can also result in functional impingement of the 1st MTP joint, so reducing the reliability of this test.

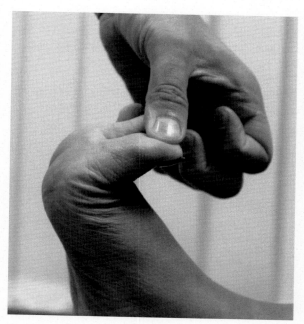

Fig. 12.5.4 The hypermobile hallux

Examination of the medial column

Hypermobility of the medial column has been discussed extensively in the literature (Roukis & Landsman 2003, Blitz 2009, Rush & Jordan 2009). Particular emphasis has been placed on the presence of hypermobility at the 1st metatarso-cuneiform (MC) joint. This is regularly cited as significant in the development of 1st MTP joint pathology, including hallux valgus and rigidus and must be considered during surgical planning. A definitive link between hypermobility of the 1st MC joint and the development of hallux valgus has not yet been established.

Clinical diagnosis of isolated hypermobility of the 1st MC joint can be challenging and potentially difficult to distinguish from laxity at other joints of the medial column. Radiographs are often useful as a means of identifying the level at which instability occurs.

Instability of the medial column should be assessed in all three planes. An apparent increase in transverse plane abduction of the 1st metatarsal in relation to the 2nd can be appreciated by compressing the hallux against the lateral border of the 1st metatarsal head. Appreciable movement often suggests instability between the medial and intermediate cuneiforms.

Excessive sagittal plane dorsiflexion and plantarflexion of the 1st ray can be appreciated by mobilizing this segment whilst stabilizing the midfoot with the other hand. An experienced examiner will readily appreciate excessive motion not seen in the 'normal' foot. A simple clinical method for assessing 1st ray dorsiflexion has been described whereby relative dorsiflexion of the first metatarsal head is measured against the second, with an increase of 8–10 mm being deemed abnormal (Voellmicke & Deland 2002).

Frontal plane rotation of the medial column can also occur so that the 1st metatarsal will appear inverted in relation to the hallux. Rotational deformity is most likely to derive from the 1st MC and/or 1st MTP joint. The surgeon should ensure that surgery to correct rotational mal-alignment of the medial column is undertaken at the origin of the deformity.

The significance of hypermobility at the interphalangeal (IP) joint of the hallux must not be underestimated. Its presence compromises the great toe's ability to act as a stable propulsive lever. In the author's experience, hyperextension at the IP joint is sometimes associated with a plantar accessory ossicle. A painful hyperkeratotic lesion (e.g. corn) may form inferior to the 1st IP joint where such an accessory ossicle is present, often resulting in an antalgic gait pattern. Hallux IP joint hyperextension is frequently associated with deformity and instability at the 1st MTP joint, such as hallux limitus and rigidus. Whilst hyperextension at the IP joint of the hallux could logically derive from a sagittal plane compensation for hallux limitus or rigidus, it is entirely feasible that hallux hyperextension acts as the primary deforming force leading to secondary changes at the 1st MTP joint (Banks et al 2001).

Examination of the lateral column

The 5th metatarsal may be assessed in the same manner as the first with an evaluation of its transverse, frontal and sagittal plane motion. Hypermobility with excessive transverse plane abduction of the 5th metatarsal may lead to deformities such as Tailor's bunions. As previously discussed, the presence of a mobile anterior equinus can increase lateral pressures.

Examination of the lesser digits

Digital deformities are commonly seen in the hypermobile foot. A drawer test is one of the most useful methods for assessing inherent digital laxity (Thomas et al 2009). This test is executed by gliding the base of the digit against the metatarsal head in a dorsal and plantar direction, with little to no motion being apparent in the normal foot.

Increased degrees of digital dorsiflexion and retraction are seen in many types of foot dysfunction and are not necessarily an indicator of increased laxity.

GAIT ANALYSIS

The patient needs to walk a few metres to and from the observer several times to get a genuine representation of their normal gait. The aim is to determine whether segments accelerate and decelerate noticeably. From the head down an assessment of gait should include observation of:

- Carriage of the head and the levels of the shoulders
- Curvature of the spine (scoliosis, kyphosis, lordosis), either primary to spinal deformity or secondary to external factors
- Upper limb carriage and determine whether there is evidence of flexion at the elbows or of asymmetry in arm carriage
- Pelvic tilt, both in the frontal plane (left to right side tilt) and also in the sagittal plane (anteroposterior)
- The knees, noting if they are fully extending, hyperextending or permanently flexed and if any rotation is present
- Signs of knee valgus/varus
- Placement of the foot
- The foot in general, noting overall posture and whether the posture changes during the walking cycle (e.g. dynamic flattening of the arch or adductory/abductory twists).

Gait analysis is particularly useful in JHS because it is not uncommon for patients with pedal laxity to stand normally only to show marked instability and abnormal pronation during gait. Hypermobile dancers for example, often display good postural awareness and are hence particularly adept at masking their instability during the non-dynamic examination. They may nevertheless go on to show marked gait asymmetry and dysfunction during walking.

Gait analysis provides a wealth of additional information which can prove invaluable in planning and evaluating therapy. An improvement in

symptoms does not necessarily indicate better function; the introduction of post-operative gait analysis for example empowers the surgeon to objectively measure the dynamic effects of their operation.

Gait analysis can be divided into three broad categories:

- Simple video analysis: This type of observational analysis may highlight obvious asymmetries including early heel lift, excessive Trendelenburg and differences in transverse plane foot position. Systems can be relatively inexpensive.

- Kinetic analysis: The use of force platforms, pressures mats, and in shoe pressure systems have greatly added to our understanding of foot function. The hypermobile patient may present with various kinetic deficits, including:

(a) An asymmetrical irregular force–time curve (Fig. 12.5.5)

(b) Medial deviation of the centre of force trajectory, suggesting an inability to re-supinate the foot during the propulsive phase of gait

(c) Under utilization of the 1st MTP joint with high focal pressures inferior to the 2nd MTP joint and hallux. This pressure distribution

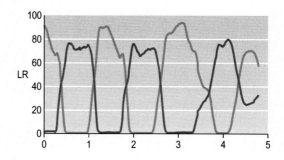

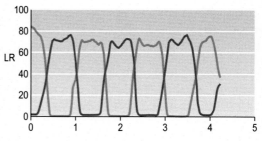

Fig. 12.5.5 An asymmetrical irregular force–time curve

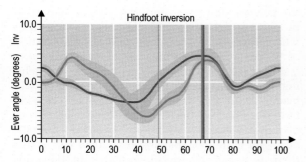

Fig. 12.5.6 Kinematic models such as the 'Oxford Foot Model' (McCahill et al 2008) are dramatically improving our understanding of foot function

may suggest a form of lateral weight transfer referred to as low gear propulsion.

(d) Excessive 1st metatarsal head pressures: Paradoxically, some hypermobile patients are unable to adopt a low gear propulsive gait pattern to compensate for functional restriction of their great toe joint. These patients often display marked abnormal pronation and instability

● Quantitative 3-dimensional (3D) analysis: Advancement in 3D technology has allowed for more detailed analysis of kinematic foot and lower limb function. Kinematic models such as the 'Oxford Foot Model' (McCahill et al 2008) are dramatically improving our understanding of foot function (Fig. 12.5.6).

RADIOGRAPHIC EVALUATION IN THE HYPERMOBILE FOOT

A number of the clinical tests that have been previously described can be investigated further radiologically.

Radiographs are a valuable imaging modality in the assessment of the hypermobile foot and weight-bearing anterior-posterior (AP), lateral and oblique views should generally be requested. Specific AP views of the ankle are indicated where there is suspected ankle pathology.

Radiological charting can be useful when assessing for pedal hypermobility. A decreased calcaneal pitch angle, increased 1st MTP angle and reduced talo-metatarsal angle have been shown to occur more frequently in hypermobile individuals (Kamanli et al 2004).

Medial column instability and ptosis can best be appreciated from weight-bearing lateral radiography.

The location of a hypermobile segment may be shown radiologically by joint sag at various points along the medial column. Splay between the medial and intermediate cuneiforms, which can best be appreciated from the AP view, suggests intercuneiform instability. Subluxation and instability at the talo-navicular and calcaneo-cuboid joints can best be appreciated from the AP views.

Magnetic resonance imaging (MRI) has greatly advanced diagnostic capabilities in the foot. In the ankle, however, a number of studies have questioned the reliability of MRI in certain pathologies and ankle arthroscopy is still often considered to be the gold standard (Kumar et al 2007, Joshy et al 2010).

TREATMENT

The four staple approaches used are:

● Strengthening/joint protection
● Improvement of proprioception
● Footwear and orthoses
● Surgery.

STRENGTHENING

The benefits of improving joint stability generally are well recognized in the management of hypermobility – typically a Pilates-type approach combined with specific exercises. Foot exercises can be limited in their effectiveness because the large forces involved in altering foot function during weight-bearing conditions are beyond the capacity of most muscle function. Nevertheless, a regimen that includes conditioning of muscles under natural loads may help to a degree. Barefoot walking is encouraged where safe and comfortable, and exercises involving repeated rising onto tip-toe may help strengthen intrinsic musculature and improve proprioception (see next section). It is helpful to instruct the patient to 'lift the heels' to improve muscle recruitment; rising onto tip-toe can be achieved by merely shifting body weight forwards with little muscle activation. Attention also needs to be given to control of the ankle during the lift, as hypermobile individuals frequently lose contact through the 1st MTP joint which leads to poor load transference through the foot during push-off, as well as encouraging a slow controlled descent to strengthen eccentric muscle activity.

Kulig et al (2009) found the inclusion of resistive exercises, and particularly eccentric muscle work produced additional benefits in terms of decreased pain and improved perceived function in treatment of tibialis posterior tendinopathy.

Paradoxically, hypermobile joints may lead to undue tightness of surrounding muscles and tendons and so gentle, controlled stretching may be useful. A combination of weight-bearing, strengthening exercises with calf stretches (either against the wall or on a step) and non-weight-bearing flexibility exercises (e.g. circling of feet, splaying of toes) are beneficial. Care should be taken when prescribing and teaching calf stretches because the midfoot, if hypermobile, can 'give' and become stressed while attempting to produce a stretch in the calf unless there is close attention to good technique.

PROPRIOCEPTION

Joint position sense is known to be reduced in people with hypermobility syndrome (Chapter 6.4) and techniques aimed at addressing this deficiency can have a positive impact on instability in joints such as the ankle. Tip-toe standing, or raising the heels, is a simple form with the patient starting with short-duration, low-repetition exercise, bearing weight on both feet simultaneously. If safe and appropriate they can, over time, progress to larger numbers of repetitions and single limb support for maximum effect. The non-weight-bearing flexibility exercises described above may also have some benefit to proprioception.

FOOTWEAR AND ORTHOSES

Sensible footwear choices are extremely important and simple changes here can make a significant difference in many people with JHM. Unstable ankles and overly flexible feet can benefit from greater control provided by the shoe, and the impact of overloaded joints and soft tissues can be offset to a significant degree through the judicious use of shock-absorbing and cushioning materials. In essence, the characteristics of the ideal shoe are seen in the more solid types of trainers readily available in the high street. A strong heel counter for stability, with robust strong fastenings for midfoot support, and a cushioned midsole are all ideal. Many trainer-type shoes now come in colours easier to reconcile with the workplace. They are excellent

for general daily use and can reduce abnormal pronation in the hypermobile patient. In settings where trainers are not appropriate, consideration of any of the above features will likely be helpful.

If exercises and footwear changes are not helping then some people with hypermobility will benefit from functional foot insoles or orthoses. Orthoses can be effective in treating many types of musculoskeletal condition (Scherer et al 2007, Springett et al 2007, Barrios et al 2009) and whilst there is a lack of specific research in JHS, this approach should always be considered prior to invasive treatment.

The introduction of kinetic technology, including pressure mats and in-shoe pressure systems have empowered practitioners to evaluate the effects of both surgical and orthotic intervention.

Most functional orthoses combine three key characteristics:

- contoured shell
- heel cup
- one or more wedges to influence joint positions.

Standard foot orthoses can be obtained over the counter and may suit many people. Depending on the severity of the instability and associated symptoms, more tailored devices may be required. Low-profile plastic composite semi-rigid foot orthoses which offer good stability, resilience and longevity are generally recommended (Woodburn et al 2002). Very soft EVA-type devices may distort rapidly whilst their increased bulk often creates issues with shoe fit and compliance.

Ankle supports can be considered an effective tool in the management of the hypermobile, unstable ankle (Dizon & Reyes 2009).

PHYSIOTHERAPY

Physiotherapy can be a valuable adjunct to the use of orthotics in improving pain and dysfunction in the hypermobile foot and occurs in the context of a global approach which includes evaluation and treatment of the entire lower extremity and pelvis (Wadsworth & Eadie 2005) as described in Chapters 9, 10, 11 and 13. In the hypermobile individual control of the hyperextending knee is of particular importance in improving function in the foot (Chapter 12.4).

Acute injuries, either through trauma or overuse, such as tenosynovitis, can be helped by ice and electrotherapy to reduce swelling and support to rest the injured tissues and allow graded movement and function. More chronic conditions, such as hallux rigidus/hallux valgus, can benefit from joint mobilization to improve mobility in combination with gait training and exercises to improve load transfer through the foot.

Functional stability can be improved in individuals with ankle instability through a rehabilitation programme involving exercises to address range of movement, strength, neuromuscular control and functional tasks (Hale et al 2007). Challenging balance and postural control through one-leg stand exercises and the use of unstable surfaces, such as balance boards, is thought to be particularly helpful.

Physiotherapy is important in the peri-operative management of the hypermobile patient. A pre-operative strengthening regimen will potentially help with recovery, especially in cases where the un-operated side will be favoured for a period of weeks or months, with obvious postural implications. It is advisable to allow patients time to 'practise' with their crutches for several weeks before their operation. Crutches should have ergonomically designed hand grips and casting materials should be as light as possible. When a redistributive post-operative 'heel walker' shoe is used, a heel lift should be placed in the shoe on the contralateral side to keep leg length relatively equal. Post-operative physiotherapy is particularly important for patients with JHS and long periods of inactivity should be counteracted by appropriate flexibility, proprioceptive and strengthening regimens. Post-operative soft tissue techniques including massage to optimize scar tissue formation and mobilizations to regain normal mobility are important.

SURGERY

Foot surgery in patients who exhibit pedal joint laxity should be considered with caution and only when conservative treatment options have been exhausted.

Re-alignment osteotomies of the hindfoot can be used in the treatment of the hypermobile flat foot and are often preferable over isolated soft tissue procedures. Equinus limitation of the ankle may present in the hypermobile flat foot and this must be considered as part of surgical management.

In cases of lateral ankle instability, an isolated ligamentous and capsular repair (e.g. Bröstrom Procedure) may prove less successful and tendon transfer or grafting procedures should be considered more readily. Concomitant pathology, including impingement syndromes, syndesmotic instability and peroneal tendinopathy must be investigated. In instances where there is calcaneal varus, a trans-positional or closing wedge osteotomy of the calcaneum can be undertaken.

When surgical arthrodesis is considered, weight-bearing radiographs should first be undertaken to identify areas of osteoarthrosis and/or deformity. Whilst certain joints in the foot may be considered 'less essential' than others, the pathological effects of arthrodesis on neighbouring joints is likely to be greater in the hypermobile foot.

The correction of 1st MTP joint deformity, such as hallux limitus and valgus can be managed with a variety of operations (Easley & Trnka 2007). Procedures of the 1st metatarsal and hallux may be associated with an increased risk of recurrence in the hypermobile foot, because varying levels of medial column and hindfoot instability are likely to persist post-surgically. A 1st MC joint arthrodesis may prove preferable, particularly where the majority of laxity and instability derives from this joint.

Arthrodesis of the 1st MC joint may be considered for a myriad of different conditions affecting the medial column. A hypermobile or unstable MC joint can be arthrodesed with concomitant correction of large 1st–2nd intermetatarsal angles, rotational changes and sagittal deviation of the 1st metatarsal, so managing such deformities as hallux valgus and hallux limitus. Where inter-cuneiform splay is present the fixation technique can be modified to stabilize this segment.

Hyperextension deformities of the hallux should include removal of an accessory ossicle when present. Hyperextension can also be managed with a closing elliptical plantar capsulotomy or interphalangeal arthrodesis of the hallux. Where de-rotation of a valgus hallux cannot be achieved through 1st metatarsal correction, a through and through de-rotational osteomy of the hallux can be considered.

In cases of digital deformity, interphalangeal joint arthrodesis may prove preferable over digital arthroplasty, particularly when significant degrees of extensor bowing are present. Tendon lengthening or tendon transfer surgery should also be considered.

Special consideration should be given to cutaneous surgery in the hypermobile foot (Whitaker et al 2009). Wound closure should achieve little to no tension on the skin edges. Techniques such as the running sub-cuticular suture can prove more challenging because of thin skin type and a smaller 5.0 suture can be helpful. Reinforcement sutures can be used to pre-empt possible dehiscence and tearing of the skin. The author generally removes sutures after 20 rather than the more usual 10–14 days. Where the surgeon wishes to use absorbable sutures, the author has found some of the new monofilament sutures to be less reactive, e.g. Monocryl®.

The use of non-adherent post-operative dressings is particularly important because of increased skin fragility. Paraffin-impregnated gauze is satisfactory, with Mepitel® being an excellent alternative. The author has found post-operative silicone dressings such as CICA – CARE® very helpful in the management of abnormal scar formation and these can be used for several weeks or months after surgery.

LOCAL ANAESTHETIC RESISTANCE

Patients with JHS may present with resistance to local anaesthetic (Chapter 1). Where resistance is suspected, cases can be scheduled under local anaesthesia with general anaesthesia on standby. This will avoid the need for rescheduling, should local anaesthesia fail.

The benefit of administering local anaesthetic post-operatively for pain relief will be lost or diminished in cases of resistance, and additional post-operative oral analgesia should be considered.

SUMMARY

Managing the hypermobile foot is both challenging and, in relation to surgery, potentially unforgiving. Results of surgery are generally less predictable than when compared to the non-hypermobile population, leading to a need to explore all the alternative conservative options highlighted above whenever possible.

Thorough understanding of the global implications of JHS and meticulous assessment of foot anatomy maximizes the chances of a successful outcome.

References

Agnew P: Evaluation of the child with ligamentous laxity, *Clin Podiatr Med Surg* 14(1):117–130, 1997.

Ainsworth SR, Aulicino PL: A survey of patients with Ehlers-Danlos syndrome, *Clin Orthop Relat Res* 286:250–256, 1993.

Banks AS, Downey MS, Martin DE, et al: *Comprehensive Textbook of Foot and Ankle Surgery*, ed 3, UK, 2001, Lippincott Williams and Wilkins.

Barrios JA, Crenshaw JR, Royer TD, et al: Walking shoes and laterally wedged orthoses in the clinical management of medial tibiofemoral osteoarthritis: A one-year prospective controlled trial, *Knee* 16(2):136–142, 2009.

Benvenuti F, Ferrucci L, Guralnik JM, et al: Foot pain and disability in older persons: an epidemiologic survey, *J Am Geriatr Soc* 43(5):479–484, 1995.

Black JR, Hale WE: Prevalence of foot complaints in the elderly, *J Am Podiatr Med Assoc* 77(6):308–311, 1987.

Blitz NM: The Versatility of the Lapidus Arthrodesis, *Clin Podiatr Med Surg* 26:427–441, 2009.

Budiman-Mak E, Conrad KJ, Roach KE: The Foot Function Index: a measure of foot pain and disability, *J Clin Epidemiol* 44(6):561–570, 1991.

Bulbena A, Duro JC, Porta M, et al: Clinical assessment of hypermobility of joints: assembling criteria, *J Rheumatol* 19(1):115–122, 1992.

Chen J, Devine A, Dick IM, et al: Prevalence of lower extremity pain and its association with functionality and quality of life in elderly women in Australia, *J Rheumatol* 30(12):2689–2693, 2003.

Dizon JM, Reyes JJ: A systematic review on the effectiveness of external ankle supports in the prevention of inversion ankle sprains among elite and recreational players, *J Sci Med Sport* Jul 7, 2009, (Epub ahead of print).

Dunn JE, Link CL, Felson DT, et al: Prevalence of foot and ankle conditions in a multiethnic community sample of older adults, *Am J Epidemiol* 159(5):491–498, 2004.

Easley ME, Trnka HJ: Current Concepts Review: Hallux Valgus Part II: Operative Treatment, *Foot Ankle Int* 28(6):748–758, 2007.

Finsterbush A, Pogrund H: The hypermobility syndrome. Musculoskeletal complaints in 100 consecutive cases of generalized joint hypermobility, *Clin Orthop Relat Res* 168:124–127, 1982.

Garrow AP, Papageorgiou AC, Silman AJ, et al: Development and validation of a questionnaire to assess disabling foot pain, *Pain* 85:107–113, 2000.

Garrow AP, Silman AJ, Macfarlane GJ: The Cheshire Foot Pain and Disability Survey: a population survey assessing prevalence and associations, *Pain* 110(1-2):378–384, 2004.

Gorter K, Kuyvenhoven M, de Melker R: Health care utilisation by older people with non-traumatic foot complaints. What makes the difference, *Scand J Prim Health Care* 19(3):191–193, 2001.

Hakim AJ, Grahame R, Norris P, et al: Local anaesthetic failure in joint hypermobility syndrome, *J R Soc Med* 98(2):84–85, 2005.

Hale SA, Hertel J, Olmsted-Kramer LC: The effect of a 4-week comprehensive rehabilitation program on postural control and lower extremity function in individuals with chronic ankle instability, *Journal of Orthopaedics and Sports Physical Therapy* 37(6): 303–311, 2007.

Harris M-CR, Beeson P: Generalized hypermobility: is it a predisposing factor towards the development of juvenile hallux abducto valgus? *The Foot* 8(12):203–209, 1998.

Hudson N, Starr MR, Esdaile JM, et al: Diagnostic associations with hypermobility in rheumatology patients, *Br J Rheumatol* 34(12): 1157–1161, 1995.

Joshy S, Abdulkadir U, Chaganti S, et al: Accuracy of MRI scan in the diagnosis of ligamentous and chondral pathology in the ankle, *J Bone Joint Surg Br* 92-B:243, 2010.

Kamanli A, Sahin S, Ozgocmen S, et al: Relationship Between Foot Angles and Hypermobility Scores and Assessment of Foot Types in Hypermobile Individuals, *Foot Ankle Int* 25:101–106, 2004.

Keenan AM, Redmond AC, Horton M, et al: The Foot Posture Index: Rasch analysis of a novel, foot-specific outcome measure, *Arch Phys Med Rehabil* 88(1):88–93, 2007.

Kind P, Brooks R, Rabin R, editors: *EQ-5D concepts and methods: a developmental history*, Rotterdam, The Netherlands, 2005, EuroQol Group Business Management, Springer.

Kulig K, Reischl SF, Pomrantz AB, et al: Nonsurgical management of posterior tibial tendon dysfunction with orthoses and resistive exercise: a randomized controlled trial, *Phys Ther* 89(1): 26–37, 2009.

Kumar V, Triantafyllopoulos I, Panagopoulos A, et al: Deficiencies of MRI in the diagnosis of chronic symptomatic lateral ankle ligament injuries, *J Foot Ankle Surg* 13(4):171–176, 2007.

Leveille SG, Guralnik JM, Ferrucci L, et al: Foot pain and disability in older women, *Am J Epidemiol* 148(7):657–665, 1998.

Mangwani J, Hakmi MA, Smith TWD: Chronic lateral ankle instability: review of anatomy, biomechanics, pathology, diagnosis and treatment, *The Foot* 11(2):76–84, 2001.

McCahill J, Stebbins J, Theologis T: Use of the Oxford Foot Model in clinical practice, *J Foot Ankle Res*, Sept 1 (Suppl 1):O28, 2008.

McCormack M, Briggs J, Hakim AJ, et al: Joint laxity and the benign joint hypermobility syndrome in student and professional ballet dancers, *J Rheumatol* 3:173–178, 2004.

Munro BJ, Steele JR: Foot-care awareness. A survey of persons aged 65 years and older, *J Am Podiatr Med Assoc* 88(5):242–248, 1998.

Murray K: Hypermobility disorders in children and adolescents, *Best Pract Res Clin Rheumatol* 20(2): 329–351, 2006.

Nicholas JA: Injuries to knee ligaments: relationship to looseness and tightness in football players, *J Am Med Assoc* 212:2236–2239, 1970.

Port M, McCarthy DJ, Chu S: The foot and systemic disease in the Veterans Administration: a quantitation of the relationship between systemic disease and

pedal problems, *J Am Podiatry Assoc* 70(8):397–404, 1980.

Redmond AC, Helliwell PS: Musculoskeletal Disorders. In Lorimer D, French G, West SG, editors: *Neale's Disorders of the Foot*, ed 7, Edinburgh, UK, 2005, Churchill Livingstone.

Redmond A, Hain J, Bird H: The distribution and prevalence of symptoms associated with hypermobility syndrome, *Ann Rheum Dis* 65(sII): 241, 2006a.

Redmond AC, Helliwell PS, Bird HA, et al: Pain and health status in people with hypermobility syndrome are associated with overall joint mobility and selected local mechanical factors, *Rheumatology* 45(1):108, 2006b.

Redmond AC, Crosbie J, Ouvrier RA: Development and validation of a novel rating system for scoring standing foot posture: the Foot Posture Index, *Clin Biomech* 21(1):89–98, 2006c.

Redmond AC: Functional Assessment. In Yates B, editor: *Assessment and Diagnosis of the Lower Limb*, Edinburgh, UK, 2008, Churchill Livingstone.

Redmond AC, Crane YZ, Menz HB: Normative values for the foot posture index. BioMed Central, *J Foot Ankle Res* 1(6):1–9, 2008.

Riano F, Sanchez O, Pena N, et al: Joint hypermobility syndrome: A prospective study of articular and non-rheumatic manifestation in a Venezuelan population, *Ann Rheum Dis* 60(Suppl 1):Thu 0217, 2001.

Ross CA, Evanski S, Waugh T: Hypermobility in hallux valgus, *Foot Ankle* 8:264–270, 1988.

Roukis TS, Landsman AS: Hypermobility of the first ray: a critical review of the literature, *J Foot Ankle Surg* 42(6):377–390, 2003.

Rush SM, Jordan T: Naviculocuneiform Arthrodesis for treatment of Medial Column

Instability, *Clin Podiatr Med Surg* 26(3):373–384, 2009.

Sacheti A, Szemere J, Bernstein B, et al: Chronic pain is a manifestation of the Ehlers-Danlos syndrome, *J Pain Symptom Manage* 14(2):88–93, 1997.

Scherer PR, Waters LL, Choate CS, et al: Is There Proof in the Evidence-Based Literature that Custom Orthoses Work? *Orthotics and Biomechanics* 9:109–122, 2007.

Springett KP, Otter S, Barry A: A clinical longitudinal evaluation of pre-fabricated, semi-rigid foot orthoses prescribed to improve foot function, *The Foot* 17 (12):184–189, 2007.

Stewart DR, Burden SB: Does generalised ligamentous laxity increase seasonal incidence of injuries in male first division club rugby players? *Br J Sports Med* 38:457–460, 2004.

Thomas E, Peat G, Harris L, et al: The prevalence of pain and pain interference in a general population of older adults: cross-sectional findings from the North Staffordshire Osteoarthritis Project (NorStOP), *Pain* 110:361–368, 2004.

Thomas JL, Blitch EL, Chaney DM, et al: Diagnosis and Treatment of Forefoot Disorders, *J Foot Ankle Surg* 48:230–250, 2009.

Tompkins MH, Bellacosa RA: Podiatric surgical considerations in the ehlers-danlos patient, *J Foot Ankle Surg* 36(5):381–387, 1997.

Voellmicke KV, Deland JT: Manual Examination Technique to Assess Dorsal Instability of the First Ray, *Foot Ankle Int* 23(11):1040–1041, 2002.

Wadsworth DJ, Eadie NT: Conservative Management of subtle Lisfranc injury: a case report, *J Orthop Sports Phys Ther* 35(3):154–164, 2005.

Whitaker IS, Rozen WM, Cairns SA, et al: Molecular genetic and clinical review of Ehlers Danlos Type VIIA: implications for management by the plastic surgeon in a multidisciplinary setting, *J Plast Reconstr Aesthet Surg* 62(5):589–594, 2009.

Woodburn J, Barker S, Helliwell PS: A randomised controlled trial of foot orthoses in rheumatoid arthritis, *J Rheumatology* 29:1377–1383, 2002.

12.6 Pregnancy and the pelvis

Rodney Grahame and Rosemary Keer

INTRODUCTION

Pregnancy is a time of massive change for the female reproductive organs. The weight of the uterus, normally 30–100 g can rise to 1 kg in pregnancy, during which time there is an 800% rise in its collagen content (Morrione 1962), a process that is rapidly reversed during the post-partum period. It is not surprising therefore, that pregnancy is a time of concern and anxiety for patients with hereditary disorders of connective tissue, their carers and health professionals. In the hypermobility clinic more questions are posed regarding pregnancy and childbirth than about any other single health issue. It behoves all those who are responsible for the care of women in pregnancy to be aware of these conditions (Chapter 1) and alert to their occurrence so that risks to mother and child may be minimized.

ISSUES IN PREGNANCY RELATED TO THE GENERAL POPULATION

JOINT LAXITY IN PREGNANCY

There is good evidence that peripheral joint laxity increases during pregnancy, but these changes do not correlate well with levels of maternal oestradiol, progesterone or relaxin (Marnach et al 2003). In one study, 54% of 46 women showed an increase of 10% or more in the mobility in either wrist joint (flexion/extension and abduction/adduction) from the first to the third trimester. Although levels of the three hormones rose generally in pregnancy, there was no difference between those who became lax during pregnancy and those who did not. Linear regression analysis of wrist joint laxity and levels of serum oestradiol, progesterone and relaxin demonstrated no significant correlation. Wrist flexion–extension laxity did, however, show some correlation with the level of maternal cortisol ($r = 0.18$, P value = 0.03). Subjective joint pain developed in 57% of women during pregnancy, which was not associated with increased joint laxity, but was associated with significantly increased levels of oestradiol and progesterone. There is some

evidence to suggest that laxity of the anterior cruciate ligament may correlate positively with blood oestradiol levels seen to be rising during the last trimester of pregnancy and falling after delivery (Charlton et al 2001). In this study high serum oestradiol levels during the third trimester of pregnancy correlated with increased anterior tibial translation, which decreased in parallel with the return of serum oestradiol to non-pregnant levels.

Thus, the relationships between the occurrence of joint pain, increased laxity and hormonal variations in pregnancy have yet to be clarified.

LOW BACK AND PELVIC PAIN IN PREGNANCY

Low back and pelvic pain is a common symptom in pregnancy. In one cross-sectional study 891 women giving birth in two hospitals in Sweden in 2002 completed a questionnaire designed to assess the prevalence of low back and pelvic pain (LBPP) in pregnancy and to identify risk factors. The overall prevalence of LBPP in this series was 72%. A history of hypermobility (HM) was one of several factors that were statistically significantly associated with the pain; others being multiparity, higher pre-pregnancy and end-pregnancy weight, high body mass index and reported periods of amenorrhoea. Factors not associated with LBPP were age at menarche and the use of contraceptives (Mogren & Pohjanen 2005).

A distinction is often made between back pain (lumbar spine) and peripartum pelvic pain (PPPP) (pain in the pelvic region) (Mens et al 1996). The PPPP group includes women with pain from the pubic symphysis as well as women with combined pain (back and pelvic pain). PPPP is more common than back pain during pregnancy and although fitness prior to pregnancy reduces the incidence of back pain it makes no difference to PPPP (Ostgaard et al 1994). The severity of pelvic pain has been shown to be related to the prevailing serum relaxin level (MacLennan 1991). Serum relaxin immunoreactivity was measured by means of a porcine relaxin radioimmunoassay in 35 patients with severe pelvic pain and pelvic joint instability during late pregnancy. The results were compared with a control group of 368 samples obtained throughout pregnancy from normal primagravidae. Most of the relaxin concentrations in the study group were above the 95% confidence limits of the median for the corresponding gestational age in the control group. The difference in relaxin levels between the study and control groups in the third trimester was highly significant. Relaxin levels in patients with pelvic pain were close to normal non-pregnant levels by the third postnatal day. The highest relaxin levels during pregnancy were found in the patients who were the most incapacitated clinically. The results suggest that there may be an association between high serum relaxin levels and pelvic pain and joint laxity during late pregnancy.

However, a study was undertaken to explore the association between HM with peri-partum pelvic pain (PPPP) among a South African Cape Coloured pregnant population of 509 patients. In this cross-sectional study joint mobility was measured using the Beighton score; using a rather severe cut-off point of $\geq 5/9$ (Chapter 1). In the event only 4.9% of the 509 pregnant women displayed HM by these criteria. No correlation between HM with the occurrence of PPPP was apparent and in fact only 20 very mild cases of PPPP were encountered. The incidence of back pain, by contrast, did increase significantly during pregnancy to a mean of 38% (van Dongen et al 1999).

SACROILIAC JOINT LAXITY IN PREGNANCY

There is evidence that increased instability of the sacroiliac joints may be responsible for pelvic pain in pregnancy.

In a prospective cohort study, the object was to determine the prognostic value of asymmetric laxity of the sacroiliac joints (SIJs) during pregnancy on pregnancy-related postpartum pelvic pain. The authors had previously found a correlation between asymmetric laxity of the SIJs and moderate to severe pelvic pain during pregnancy. In their latest study 123 women were prospectively questioned and examined, and SIJ laxity was measured by means of Doppler imaging at 36 weeks' gestation and at 8 weeks' postpartum. A left to right difference in SIJ laxity ≥ 3 threshold units was considered to indicate asymmetric laxity of the SIJs. In subjects with moderate to severe pelvic pain during pregnancy, SIJ asymmetric laxity

was predictive of moderate to severe pregnancy-related pelvic pain persisting into the postpartum period in 77% of the subjects. The sensitivity, specificity and positive predictive value of SIJ asymmetric laxity during pregnancy for pregnancy-related pelvic pain persisting postpartum were 65%, 83% and 77%, respectively. Subjects with moderate to severe pregnancy-related pelvic pain and asymmetric laxity of the sacroiliac joints during pregnancy have a threefold higher risk of continuing to experience pain postpartum than subjects with symmetric laxity. This would indicate that in women with moderate to severe complaints of pelvic pain during pregnancy, sacroiliac joint asymmetric laxity during pregnancy is predictive of pelvic pain persisting into the postpartum period (Damen et al 2001).

PUBIC SYMPHYSIS DYSFUNCTION IN PREGNANCY

Pubic symphysis dysfunction is a commonly encountered symptom in the hypermobility clinic and the onset usually occurs in the perinatal period. When it occurs, pubic symphysis diastasis is a cause of instability in the pubic synostosis and a potential source of pain and disability in postpartum women. Because the pubic symphysis is part of the pelvic ring, any instability here will also involve instability at one or both of the sacroiliac joints (Ostgaard 1998).

CLINICAL PRESENTATION

Hypermobile women often report a considerable change in their wellbeing during pregnancy. For some asymptomatic individuals it seems that pregnancy can be the start of their problems, while others report that they feel the best they have ever felt, or even become symptom-free for the first time in years, only to have their symptoms return soon after delivery.

Back pain is often considered inevitable during pregnancy and tends to consist of a localized ache in the lumbar spine. Pelvic pain is usually more intense and associated with pain around the sacroiliac joints, symphysis pubis and buttocks with radiation into the upper legs. Pain is time-dependent; increasing with time spent weight-bearing, such that standing and walking become progressively more difficult. Many women with PPPP show a characteristic waddling gait (Mens et al 1996), with or without a marked limp. Twisting and asymmetric loading of the pelvis, as in vacuum cleaning, is most provocative in the PPPP group (Ostgaard 1998).

The posterior pelvic pain provocation test (Fig. 12.6.1) was developed to differentiate women with back pain from pelvic pain (Ostgaard 1998). The test consists of a gentle longitudinal force applied along the length of the femur with the hip in 90 degrees of flexion (Fig. 12.6.1). It is considered positive if pain is reproduced in the posterior pelvis on the same side and has been shown to differentiate pain from the lumbar spine with sensitivity of 0.88 and specificity of 0.89 (Gutke 2009). The intensity of pain produced correlates with increased disability and can detect women with significant physical impairment (Ando & Osashi 2009).

Pubic symphysis instability is best detected by means of alternating single-stance (flamingo) plain radiography of the pelvis. A pubic translation of 5 mm or more is deemed to be abnormal (Garras et al 2008).

MANAGEMENT OF SYMPTOMS ASSOCIATED WITH PREGNANCY

Pregnant women presenting with lumbar spine pain should be treated in the same way as non-pregnant individuals as far as their pregnancy allows (Ostgaard 1998) (Chapters 9 and 12.8). The increased weight of the developing uterus and fetus may be a contributing factor in the development of pain and this may be eased by a prenatal cradle (Fig. 12.6.2). While there is limited scientific evidence to support the effectiveness of maternity supports (Ho 2009), anecdotal evidence in the hypermobile population suggests that if pain is eased by lifting and supporting the abdomen from underneath using the hands, then a maternity support can be helpful.

It is thought that increased mobility in the SIJs, in response to hormonal changes, is responsible for PPPP. But it is not known if hypermobile women are more at risk, although clinical experience suggests that many hypermobile women do have problems with SIJ pain during pregnancy (Keer et al 2003).

Accurate measurement of mobility at the SIJ is difficult in the clinic. However, it is thought to be the difference in mobility between the two SIJs that is important in the production of pain (Pool-Goudzwaard et al 1999) and this has been, to some

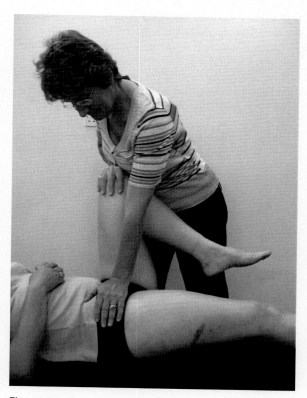

Fig. 12.6.1 Posterior pelvic pain provocation test

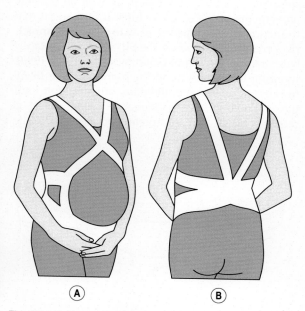

Fig. 12.6.2 Prenatal cradle

extent, confirmed in the study by Damen et al (2001). It would appear that the pelvis is similar to other areas of the body in which relative *hypomobility* produces increased stress on the hypermobile joint(s). Treatment should be directed at the *hypomobile* joint to restore mobility. Gentle mobilizing techniques applied to the joint in combination with soft tissue release can be effective in relieving pain and restoring mobility. Effective recruitment of the stability muscles (transversus abdominus, pelvic floor, multifidus) and gluteal muscles helps to compensate for the instability in the pelvis by increasing the muscle force. This only works for a short time (Vleeming et al 1995) and external force, via a non-elastic belt, is frequently necessary to increase force closure and provide some stability (Fig. 12.6.3). Mens et al (1996) found that PPPP was relieved by wearing such a belt in 50% of women while pregnant and in about two-thirds of women after delivery. Damen et al (2002) also draw attention to the benefits of a pelvic belt, particularly when used in a high position. Severe cases of SIJ instability may need the support of a stick or crutches to decrease the load through the pelvis.

Educating the patient about the condition is important to encourage a change of lifestyle, where possible, to accommodate the insufficiency of the pelvis. Activities which stress the pelvis should be avoided, such as climbing stairs, one-leg standing, stepping up onto a high step, as well as extreme movements of the spine or hips. It is thought that the action of the iliopsoas leads to a large asymmetric force being placed on the SIJ, which can exacerbate symptoms (Pool-Goudzwaard et al 1999). Ignoring the pain will not help and is more likely to cause an increase in the pain, often not felt until the following day (Ostgaard 1998). Rest is recommended, but complete bed rest is to be avoided due to the deleterious effect on muscle strength and endurance.

Posterior pelvic pain disappears in the majority of women within 3 months after delivery (Ostgaard 1998, Elden et al 2008). Once the posterior pelvic pain provocation test is negative, showing that the pelvis has regained its stability, specific training of the pelvic floor, back and abdominal muscles should be started. Rehabilitation is slow lasting, between 6–12 months and normally contains periods of relapse (Ostgaard 1998), probably due to the extra physical work involved in looking after a new baby. Ostgaard (1998) also emphasizes that strenuous work should be avoided for 6 months after delivery even if the pain has disappeared, in order to avoid a relapse.

Hypermobile patients are invariably concerned about other factors, such as looking after the child, breastfeeding, whether the child will have problems and the effect of another pregnancy as well as about the labour. Generally, caesarean operations are not recommended in cases of low back pain or PPPP (Ostgaard 1998), although they may be appropriate in the case of hypermobility type III Ehlers-Danlos syndrome (Charvet et al 1991). Problem-solving and advice, as well as speaking to the consultant obstetrician or midwife, can relieve some of the patient's anxiety. It is not known which is the best position for delivery but it would seem advisable to support the patient's legs and back and prevent excessive unsupported hip abduction.

SURGERY

Pelvic pain which does not respond to treatment and becomes chronic can continue to cause considerable disability. When a pubic symphysis diastasis >3 cm is present, surgical intervention may be needed to preserve the integrity of the pubic symphysis joint. Surgical procedures for reduction of pubic symphysis diastasis have usually been via internal fixation with plates and screws on the superior pubic rami. External fixation is an alternative method of treatment for those patients with severe postpartum pubic symphysis diastasis with reproductive organ damage (Chang & Wu 2008). Stabilization surgery has a place in the treatment of chronic pelvic pain, but a minority of patients experience a worsening of their symptoms or the development of new ones (Vercellini et al 2009) and no significant difference in outcome was found between surgically treated

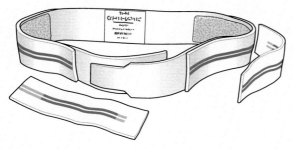

Fig. 12.6.3 Sacroiliac (non-elastic) belt

patients and the non-operatively treated patients in a study by Weil et al (2008). It would seem sensible therefore as far as possible to follow a more conservative approach, focusing on stabilization through more effective muscle function, which has been shown to be more effective than physical therapy without stabilizing exercises (Stuge et al 2004).

COMPLICATIONS OF PREGNANCY RELATED TO JOINT HYPERMOBILITY SYNDROME

Both cervical incompetence and premature rupture of the membranes have been reported in patients with the hypermobility type of EDS (Chapter 2). In one report the patient had the misfortune to suffer both complications in successive pregnancies (De Vos et al 1999). Successful prophylactic use of the McDonald cerclage allowed the second pregnancy to go to 23 weeks, whereupon premature spontaneous rupture of the membranes occurred. A female infant was delivered at 26 weeks but died shortly after birth. Electron microscopical examination of fetal skin revealed abnormalities in the collagen fibres compatible with EDS. These authors urge their obstetric colleagues to be on the lookout for connective tissue disorders in their pregnant patients and to work closely with geneticist colleagues. A less invasive alternative approach is the use of the Smith-Hodge pessary, which can be equally effective (Leduc & Wasserstrum 1992).

Anecdotally, many patients with joint hypermobility syndrome (JHS) fail to develop striae gravidarum (stretch marks) during pregnancy. This either passes unobserved or is attributed to skin creams that may have been applied or, even less plausibly, to their good luck. The more likely explanation, is the fact that mature EDS/JHS skin is inherently stretchy and thereby totally capable of encompassing the shape and size of the pregnant uterus without undergoing the process of viscous slip when its degree of stretch has reached the elastic limit (Tregear 1966). By the same mechanism many pregnant EDS/JHS patients are spared perineal tears or the need for an episiotomy during delivery of the baby. The question of skin change is taken up further in Chapter 2. The author is aware that the clinical picture in EDS/JHS is full of paradoxes! Notwithstanding what has been written here, a minority of patients manifest the direct opposite effect, producing the most extreme forms of striae gravidarum and suffering severe tears and damage to the perineum during childbirth.

PREMATURE RUPTURE OF THE MEMBRANES

Human amnion is a five-layer structure including a compact sheet of connective tissue mainly composed of types I and III collagen fibrils. Premature rupture of the fetal membranes is a major cause of preterm birth and its associated infant morbidity and mortality. The first report of a family with JHS showing obstetric complications was a report in 1988 (Thornton et al 1988). In the family described, four generations were affected by 'benign familial joint hyperlaxity' and, in the two generations for which obstetric data were available, pregnancies were complicated by unexplained mid-trimester vaginal bleeding. This prompted a study to determine whether unexplained antepartum haemorrhage (APH) and premature rupture of the membranes (PROM), both of which might reflect the structure of fetal membrane collagen, were associated with joint hyperlaxity in the offspring. The joint hyperlaxity of children born from such pregnancies was slightly greater than that found in age-matched children born from uncomplicated pregnancies.

Recently, it has become clear that rupture of the fetal membranes, either term or preterm, is not merely the result of the stretch and shear forces of uterine contractions, but is, in significant part, the consequence of a programmed weakening process. Work in the rat model has demonstrated that collagen remodelling, with activation of matrix metalloproteinases (MMPs), and apoptosis increase markedly in the amnion at end of gestation, suggesting that these processes are involved in fetal membrane weakening. Fetal membrane strength testing equipment and a systematic tissue sampling methodology have demonstrated that term, non-laboured, fetal membranes have a zone of weakness overlying the cervix, which contains biochemical markers of both collagen remodelling and apoptosis. These findings provide strong support for the concept of programmed fetal membrane weakening prior to labour (Morrione 1962). A model has also been used to establish the physical properties of individual fetal membrane components (amnion, chorion), determine the sequence of events during the fetal membrane rupture process, and demonstrate that treatment of fetal membranes with TNF or IL-1beta, in vitro, induces weakness and the identical biochemical markers of collagen remodelling and apoptosis seen in the physiological weak zone. The ability to simultaneously correlate macroscopic physical properties with histological and biochemical fetal membrane characteristics, presents a unique perspective on the physiology of fetal membrane rupture.

In one Belgian study skin biopsies were taken from 42 women aged from 21 to 41 years presenting with recurrent pre-term premature rupture of the membranes (PPROM) and miscarriages and compared with controls. Many of the women suffering from PPROM showed subtle dermal changes consistent with those found in EDS. However, there is no obvious clinical expression of these alterations other than the occurrence of PPROM (Hermanns-Le et al 2005).

LABOUR AND DELIVERY

There is evidence, albeit anecdotal, that the duration of labour in mothers with JHS is significantly shortened, almost, in some cases, to the point of precipitate labour! As an example of this phenomenon, in one of the present author's patients, in seven out of nine successive births the total duration of labour was one hour or less!

COMPLICATIONS IN LATER LIFE

To assess the relation between joint mobility and genital prolapse, joint mobility in 76 women with genital prolapse was compared with that in an age- and parity-matched control group without prolapse. Mobility was scored on a scale of 0–9. The number of patients with hypermobile joints and the total mobility scores were higher in the genital prolapse group ($P < 0.005$), which also had more joint complaints and twice the prevalence of backache when compared with the control group (Al-Rawi & Al-Rawi 1982).

UTERINE PROLAPSE, URINARY INCONTINENCE AND HYPERMOBILITY

The original observation linking uterine prolapse and HM is attributed to Al-Rawi (Al-Rawi & Al-Rawi 1982). Later studies broadened the relevance to include other manifestations of pelvic floor weakness such as rectocele and cystocele (Norton

et al 1995) and the complaint of stress incontinence (after coughing, sneezing, laughing, exercise and straining at stool). In a study in 1995 the frequencies of prolapse (29.3%), incontinence complaints (59%), endometriosis (27%), dyspareunia (57%), and previous hysterectomy (44%) among 41 EDS women with a mean age of 41 years were all higher than expected (McIntosh et al 1995). However, there was no significant relationship between prolapse and HM, but wrist dorsiflexion ($P < 0.05$) and palmar flexion ($P = 0.05$) alone among 18 joint measures correlated with incontinence (McIntosh et al 1996). Tincello et al (2002) found that elbow hyperextension was associated with an increased incidence of post-natal urinary incontinence.

A larger recent Russian study of 208 women with genital prolapse found that over a half (52.4%) of females with HM developed severe prolapse within 3 years of delivery (Smol'nova et al 2004). Pelvic organ prolapse with urinary incontinence has also been identified in a study of patients with Marfan syndrome and EDS giving more credence to the notion that connective tissue weakness provides the important pathogenetic link in these patients (Carley et al 2000).

In a group of fit, nulliparous women, Bo et al (1994) found 38% reported symptoms of stress urinary incontinence (SUI), with evidence of increased incidence of urethral sphincteric incompetence and JHS when compared to the control group. Karan et al (2004) found joint hypermobility (measured as > 3 on Beighton scale) featured more frequently in a group of patients with SUI compared to a control group. There appears therefore to be a tenuous association between SUI and JH. Whereas hypermobility of the bladder base is a predictor of SUI and this is strongly associated with vaginal childbirth (particularly the first delivery) and vaginal operative deliveries (Meyer et al 1998, Dietz et al 2002, Shek & Dietz 2008). These findings suggest alteration in urethral support and therefore development of SUI is due to increased fascial compliance (Dietz et al 2003) which may be particularly relevant for hypermobile individuals.

MANAGEMENT

Post-partum pelvic floor exercises are of particular importance in patients who have lax tissues such as those with JHS and EDS. It has been shown that supervised pelvic floor exercises can decrease the incidence of SUI post-partum (Reilly et al 2002,

Harvey 2003, Hay-Smith et al 2008). In the study by Reilly et al (2002), 268 at-risk primigravidae, with ultrasonically proven bladder neck mobility, took part in a single-blind randomized control trial based in the UK. Patients randomly allocated to the active group attended a physiotherapist monthly from 20 weeks until delivery for supervised pelvic floor exercises. Both the active group and the control group received verbal advice on pelvic floor exercises from midwives antenatally. Subjective stress incontinence improved in the treated group but pelvic floor strength and bladder neck mobility were unchanged (Reilly et al 2002). On the basis of a review of 16 trials Hay-Smith et al (2008) concluded that there was evidence that pelvic floor muscle training can prevent urinary incontinence in late pregnancy and postpartum and that the more intensive the programme the greater the treatment effect.

Urinary continence depends on both tonic and phasic pelvic floor muscle activity (Sapsford 2004). Examination of the pelvic floor can be performed by digital vaginal palpation by experienced physiotherapists or through external hand contact over the perineum. It is important that the perineum is felt to move up and in rather than bulging, as the latter indicates an increase in intra-abdominal pressure which can force the pelvic organs and vagina down. This frequently occurs with breath-holding and may necessitate breathing re-education as part of the pelvic floor muscle retraining programme. There is often over-recruitment of the abdominal muscles leading to a bracing strategy.

Co-activation of the pelvic floor muscles with transversus abdominus (TrA) is desirable and should occur without global abdominal muscle activity. Real-time ultrasound imaging of the pelvic floor and TrA can be helpful in identifying aberrant activation and correcting it through biofeedback (Fig. 12.6.4). A delay in the timing of activation of the pelvic floor muscles with arm movement has been identified in incontinent women compared to continent women despite a greater amplitude of contraction (Smith et al 2007). Furthermore, pelvic floor activity decreased and abdominal and erector spinae muscle activity increased when the bladder was moderately full, which would be expected to have negative consequences for continence and lumbopelvic stability in women with incontinence.

Training often starts in lying because it is easier to relax the abdominal muscles. The patient is taught to gently activate the pelvic floor muscles, in isolation from surrounding muscles such as the buttocks or adductors but in conjunction with a gentle TrA contraction while maintaining a relaxed diaphragmatic breathing pattern with lateral rib expansion. Tonic activity is improved through repetition of gentle holds with the hold time progressively increased, while phasic muscle activity is improved by fast repetitions over a short period of time. Pelvic floor muscles fatigue easily and it is important to rest and relax the muscle fully in between repetitions and after exercising. Hypertonic pelvic floor muscles are also thought to contribute to urinary incontinence in some individuals. Once the patient is confident about

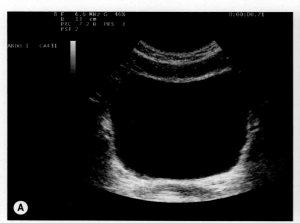 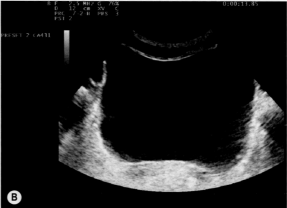

Fig. 12.6.4 Real-time ultrasound imaging of the bladder to assess the efficiency of pelvic floor contractions. (a) Ideal transverse bladder view of a relaxed pelvic floor. (b) Transverse bladder view with pelvic floor and TrA contraction. Note slight asymmetrical lift of bladder

exercising in lying the exercises can be progressed to more functional positions such as sitting, standing and walking and during functional activities.

PREGNANCY AND DELIVERY IN THE RARER FORMS OF EHLERS–DANLOS SYNDROME

EDS – HYPERMOBILITY TYPE (EDS TYPE III)

Turning from symptoms in HM to EDS, in a recent extensive review of the EDS literature, surprisingly, only 39 cases of EDS hypermobility type could be identified (Volkov et al 2007), which considering the relatively high prevalence, is perplexing. Of these, 32 women (82%) delivered live-born infants while 18% suffered either first or second trimester pregnancy loss. Two-thirds of the pregnancies were carried to term, and 30 (77%) patients had a vaginal delivery. Intra-partum and post-partum haemorrhage occurred in 10% and 5% respectively. In the view of these authors, severe and significant complications in this type of EDS have never been reported. This may be a somewhat misleading statement and presumably refers to the absence of the major life-threatening complications seen in the vascular type, described below.

EDS – CLASSICAL TYPE (EDS TYPES I/II)

There is a dearth of published case-reports relating to pregnancy and childbirth in the classic type. A handful of individual case-reports only are available. The overarching impression is that pregnancy in the classic form of EDS is uncommon and that the complications, such as premature rupture of the membranes when they occur are similar to those seen in the hypermobility type. The possible exception is the occasional occurrence of extensive vaginal lacerations or dehiscence of an episiotomy. With foresight these complications may be prevented by appropriate adaptations of the surgical technique. The prognosis is generally very good provided close obstetric supervision is available and results of caesarean section when required have been uncomplicated.

EDS – VASCULAR TYPE (TYPE IV)

The situation is quite the contrary in the vascular type of EDS. In their seminal study Pepin et al (2000) describe 81 women with EDS type IV who had had a total of 183 pregnancies, with 167 deliveries of live-born infants at term. There were three stillbirths, ten spontaneous abortions, and three elective terminations. Twelve women died during the peripartum period or within 2 weeks of delivery (five from uterine rupture during labour, two of vessel rupture at delivery, and five in the post-partum period after vessel rupture). There were five pregnancy-related deaths among the 81 women who had been pregnant once, three among the 53 who had been pregnant twice, two among the 24 who had been pregnant three times, two among the 13 who had been pregnant four times, and no deaths among the six women who had been pregnant five times, the two who had been pregnant six times, or the one who had been pregnant seven times. The overall mortality rate was 11.5%. These figures leave no doubt as to the high risks of pregnancy in vascular EDS.

On the basis of their findings, these authors recommended that women with the vascular type of EDS undergo preconception counselling and be advised against pregnancy. If such women do become pregnant, they should be advised against continuing with the pregnancy. Elective termination of pregnancy before 16 weeks has been successfully accomplished without significant sequelae. However, it is not without risk and in at least one case emergency hysterectomy was required. If the woman chooses to continue the pregnancy, close follow-up is mandatory and elective hospitalization is recommended during the third trimester with restriction of physical activity. Consideration should be given to delivery by planned caesarean section, before the onset of labour, approximately at 32 weeks (after steroid administration). Although there are inadequate data to support this management, it might theoretically be beneficial for the following reasons:

(a) The majority of spontaneous deliveries in EDS patients occur between 32 and 35 weeks gestation.

(b) Maternal plasma volume peaks at or before 32 weeks, and plasma volume might have a role in the severity of vascular complications.

(c) Caesarean delivery may minimize the fluctuations in maternal cardiac output and blood pressure associated with labour, a factor that may augment the risk for arterial rupture.

(d) It may reduce the risk for significant perineal trauma.

Arguing against caesarean delivery is the fact that it may be associated with increased risk of perioperative haemorrhage. In addition, wound healing may be impaired, and there is an increased likelihood of wound dehiscence. Before delivery the woman should be counselled against subsequent pregnancy and tubal ligation should be offered.

SUMMARY

It is important that all patients with JHS or EDS who become pregnant ensure that their obstetrician or midwife is made aware of their condition so that appropriate arrangements can be made for their antenatal and postnatal care as well, of course, for the conduct and mode of delivery.

Unlike the vascular form of the Ehlers-Danlos syndrome (EDS), formerly EDS type IV, the joint hypermobility syndrome (JHS), which is equivalent to EDS hypermobility type (formerly EDS III) is not associated with heart disease or major hazards during pregnancy and labour. However there are a number of considerations that are worthy of highlighting:

- There is a tendency for joint and spinal pains to increase temporarily during the course of the pregnancy.
- Because they rely on the tensile strength afforded by their collagen content, the membranes may rupture prematurely, resulting in premature labour and birth.
- Anecdotally, there is a tendency for labour to be unusually rapid.
- There is an apparent resistance to the effects of local anaesthetics seen in about two thirds of patients with JHS and this can cause problems during epidural anaesthesia or infiltration of the tissues prior to the repair of a tear or episiotomy.
- Healing of either a perineal tear or an episiotomy may be slow and extra sutures may be required and the time they are retained may need to be extended to allow full healing.
- Lactation and care of the newborn baby may be more taxing than with other mothers.
- Pelvic floor problems (uterine prolapse etc.) are more likely to occur in later life so that the practice of postnatal exercises is doubly important.
- Since JHS follows a dominant pattern of inheritance there is a 50% chance that any offspring will carry the gene, although this does not mean that he/she will necessarily develop symptoms of tissue laxity subsequently.

References

Al-Rawi ZS, Al-Rawi ZT: Joint hypermobility in women with genital prolapse, Lancet 1 (8287):1439–1441, 1982.

Ando F, Osashi K: Using the posterior pelvic pain provocation test in pregnant Japanese women, Nursing Health Science 11:3–9, 2009.

Bo K, Stien R, Kulseng-Hanssen S, et al: Clinical and urodynamic assessment of nulliparous young women with and without stress incontinence symptoms: a case-control study, Obstet Gynecol 84:1028–1032, 1994.

Carley ME, Schaffer J, Carley ME: Urinary incontinence and pelvic organ prolapse in women with Marfan or Ehlers Danlos syndrome, Am J Obstet Gynecol 182(5):1021–1023, 2000.

Chang JL, Wu V: External fixation of pubic symphysis diastasis from postpartum trauma, Orthopedics 31(5):493, 2008.

Charlton WP, Coslett-Charlton LM, Ciccotti MG: Correlation of estradiol in pregnancy and anterior cruciate ligament laxity, Clin Orthop Relat Res 387:165–170, 2001.

Charvet PY, Sale B, Rebaud P, et al: Ehlers-Danlos syndrome and pregnancy. A proposal of a case (Abstract – article in French), Journal of Gynaecology Biology and Reproduction (Paris) 20:75–78, 1991.

Damen L, Buyruk HM, Guler-Uysal F, et al: Pelvic pain during pregnancy is associated with asymmetric laxity of the sacroiliac joints, Acta Obstet Gynecol Scand 80(11):1019–1024, 2001.

Damen L, Spoor CW, Snijders CJ, et al: Does a pelvic belt influence sacroiliac joint laxity? Clin Biomech (Bristol, Avon) 17(7):495–498, 2002.

De Vos M, Nuytinck L, Verellen C, et al: Preterm premature rupture of membranes in a patient with the hypermobility type of the Ehlers-Danlos syndrome. A case report, Fetal Diagn Ther 14 (4):244–247, 1999.

Dietz HP, Clarke B, Vancaillie TG: Vaginal childbirth and bladder neck mobility, Aust N Z J Obstet Gynecol 42:522–552, 2002.

Dietz HP, Steensma AB, Hastings R: Three-dimensional ultrasound imaging of the pelvic floor: the effect of parturition on paravaginal structures, Ultrasound Obstet Gynecol 21:589–595, 2003.

Dumoulin C, Hay-Smith J: Pelvic floor muscle training versus no treatment for urinary incontinence in women. A Cochrane systematic review, *European Journal of Rehabilitation Medicine* 44:47–63, 2008.

Elden H, Hagberg H, Olsen MF: Regression of pelvic pain after delivery: follow-up of a randomised single blind controlled trial with different modalities, *Acta Obstet Gynecol Scand* 87:201–208, 2008.

Garras DN, Carothers JT, Olson SA: Single-leg-stance (flamingo) radiographs to assess pelvic instability: how much motion is normal? *J Bone Joint Surg Am* 90(10):2114–2118, 2008.

Gutke A, Ostgaard HC, Oberg B: Association between muscle function and low back pain in relation to pregnancy, *J Rehabil Med* 40:304–311, 2008.

Gutke A, Hansson ER, Zetherstrom G, et al: Posterior pelvic pain provocation test is negative in patients with lumbar herniated discs, *Eur Spine J* Apr 24, 2009. (Epub ahead of print).

Harvey MA: Pelvic floor exercises during and after pregnancy: a systematic review of their role in preventing pelvic floor dysfunction, *J Obstet Gynaecol Can* 25:487–498, 2003.

Hay-Smith J, Morkved S, Fairbrother KA: Pelvic floor muscle training for prevention and treatment of urinary and faecal incontinence in antenatal and postnatal women, *Cochrane Database Syst Rev* Oct 8(4): CD007471, 2008.

Hermanns-Le T, Pierard G, Quatresooz P: Ehlers-Danlos-like dermal abnormalities in women with recurrent preterm premature rupture of fetal membranes, *Am J Dermatopathol* 27(5):407–410, 2005.

Ho SS, Yu WW, Lao TT: Effectiveness of maternity support belts in reducing low back pain during pregnancy: a review, *J Clin Nurs* 18:1523–1532, 2009.

Jarrell JF, Vilos GA, Allaire C: Consensus guidelines for the management of chronic pelvic pain, *J Obstet Gynaecol Can* 27:781–826, 2005.

Karan A, Isikoglu M, Aksac B, et al: Hypermobility Syndrome in 105 women with pure urinary stress incontinence and in 105 controls, *Arch Gynecol Obstet* 269:89–90, 2004.

Keer R, Edwards-Fowler A, Mansi E: Management of the hypermobile adult. In Keer R, Grahame R, editors: *Hypermobility Syndrome, Recognition and Management for Physiotherapists*, Edinburgh, 2003, Butterworth Heinemann, pp 94–95.

Leduc L, Wasserstrum N: Successful treatment with the Smith-Hodge pessary of cervical incompetence due to defective connective tissue in Ehlers-Danlos syndrome, *Am J Perinatol* 9(1):25–27, 1992.

MacLennan AH: The role of the hormone relaxin in human reproduction and pelvic girdle relaxation, *Scand J Rheumatol Suppl* 88:7–15, 1991.

Marnach ML, Ramin KD, Ramsey PS, et al: Characterization of the relationship between joint laxity and maternal hormones in pregnancy, *Obstet Gynecol* 101(2): 331–335, 2003.

McIntosh LJ, Mallett VT, Frahm JD, et al: Gynecologic disorders in women with Ehlers-Danlos syndrome, *J Soc Gynecol Investig* 2(3):559–564, 1995.

McIntosh LJ, Stanitski DF, Mallett VT, et al: Ehlers-Danlos syndrome: relationship between joint hypermobility, urinary incontinence and pelvic floor prolapse, *Gynecol Obstet Invest* 41(2):135–139, 1996.

Mens JMA, Vleeming A, Stoeckart R, et al: Understanding peripartum pelvic pain. Implications of a patient survey, *Spine* 21:1363–1370, 1996.

Meyer S, Schreyer A, De Grandi P, et al: The effects of birth on urinary continence mechanisms and other pelvic-floor characteristics, *Obstet Gynecol* 92:613–618, 1998.

Mogren IM, Pohjanen AI: Low back pain and pelvic pain during pregnancy: prevalence and risk factors, *Spine* 30(8):983–991, 2005.

Morrione TG, Seifter S: Alteration in the collagen content of the human uterus during pregnancy and post-partum involution, *J Exp Med* 115:357–365, 1962.

Norton PA, Baker JE, Sharp HC, et al: Genitourinary prolapse and joint hypermobility in women, *Obstet Gynecol* 85(2):225–228, 1995.

Ostgaard HC, Zetherstrom G, Roos-Hansson E: Reduction of back and posterior pelvic pain in pregnancy, *Spine* 19:894–900, 1994.

Ostgaard HC: Back pain in relation to pregnancy: state of the art. Where are we now? In Vleeming A, Mooney V, Tilscher H, et al, editors: *Proceedings of the Third Interdisciplinary World Congress on Low Back Pain and Pelvic Pain*, Vienna, Austria, 1998a, pp 158–160.

Ostgaard HC: Assessment and treatment of low back pain in the working pregnant woman. In Vleeming A, Mooney V, Tilscher H, et al, editors: *Proceedings of the Third Interdisciplinary World Congress on Low Back Pain and Pelvic Pain*, Vienna, Austria, 1998b, pp 161–171.

Pepin M, Schwarze U, Superti-Furga A, et al: Clinical and genetic features of Ehlers-Danlos syndrome type IV the vascular type, [see comment] [erratum appears in *N Engl J Med* 344 (5):392, 2001] *N Engl J Med* 342 (10):673–680, 2000.

Pool-Goudzwaard AL, Vleeming A, Stoeckart R, et al: Insufficient lumbo-pelvic stability: a clinical, anatomical and biomechanical approach to 'aspecific' low back pain, *Man Ther* 3:12–20, 1998.

Reilly ET, Freeman RM, Waterfield MR, et al: Prevention of postpartum stress incontinence in primigravidae with increased bladder neck mobility: a randomised controlled trial of antenatal pelvic floor exercises, *Br J Obstet Gynaecol* 109(1):68–76, 2002.

Sapsford R: Rehabilitation of pelvic floor muscles utilizing trunk stabilization, *Man Ther* 9:3–12, 2004.

Shek KL, Dietz HP: The urethral motion profile: a novel method to evaluate urethral support and mobility, *Aust N Z J Obstet Gynaecol* 48:337–342, 2008.

Smith MD, Coppieters MW, Hodges PW: Postural activity of the pelvic floor muscles is delayed during rapid arm movements in women with stress urinary incontinence, *Int Urogynecol J Pelvic Floor Dysfunct* 18:901–911, 2007.

Smol'nova TI, Savel'ev SV, Grishin VL, et al: [Genital prolapse in women and articular hypermobility syndrome in connective tissue dysplasia], [Russian] *Ter Arkh* 76(11):83–88, 2004.

Stuge B, Laerum E, Kirkesola G, et al: The efficacy of a treatment program focusing on specific stabilising exercises for pelvic girdle pain after pregnancy: a randomised controlled trial, *Spine* 29:351–359, 2004a.

Stuge B, Veierod MB, Laerum E, et al: The efficacy of a treatment program focusing on specific stabilising exercises for pelvic girdle pain after pregnancy: a two year follow-up of a randomised clinical trial, *Spine* 29:E197–E203, 2004b.

Thornton JG, Hill J, Bird HA: Complications of pregnancy and benign familial joint hyperlaxity, *Annals of Rheumatic Diseases* 47 (3):228–231, 1988.

Tincello DG, Adams EJ, Richmond DH: Antenatal screening for postpartum urinary incontinence in nulliparous women: a pilot study, *Eur J Obstet Gynecol Reprod Biol* 101:70–73, 2002.

Tregear RT: Force between molecules. Mechanics of skin. In Tragear RT, editor: *Physical Functions of the Skin*, ed 1, London, 1966, Academic Press, pp 73–95.

van Dongen PW, de Boer M, Lemmens WA, et al: Hypermobility and peripartum pelvic pain syndrome in pregnant South African women, *Eur J Obstet Gynecol Reprod Biol* 84(1):77–82, 1999.

Vercellini P, Vigano P, Somigliana E, et al: Medical, Surgical and alternative treatment for chronic pelvic pain in women; a descriptive review, *Gynecol Endocrinol* 25:208–221, 2009.

Vleeming A, Pool-Goudzwaard AL, Stoeckart R: The posterior layer of thoracolumbar fascia. Its function in load transfer from spine to legs, *Spine* 20:753–758, 1995.

Volkov N, Nisenblat V, Ohel G, et al: Ehlers-Danlos syndrome: insights on obstetric aspects, [Review] [37 refs] *Obstet Gynecol Surv* 62(1):51–57, 2007.

Weil YA, Hierholzer C, Sama D: Management of persistent postpartum pelvic pain, *Am J Orthop* 37:621–626, 2008.

12.7 The cervical spine and jaw – (a) The cervical spine

Rosemary Keer

INTRODUCTION

The cervical spine has been described as 'a triumph of packaging' (Grieve 1988) because while being the most mobile part of the spinal column, it also protects and transports many vital tissues as well as supporting the weight of the head. Stability has been sacrificed for mobility, making the cervical spine more vulnerable to injury (Magee 2008). It is no surprise then, that it can be responsible for some unpleasant symptoms, ranging from pain in the head, neck and face to symptoms affecting the vascular, auditory, visual and equilibrium systems.

Because of the close anatomical association between the cervical spine and the temporomandibular joints, this chapter is divided into sections which address each area in its own right as well as discussing their relationship.

UPPER CERVICAL SPINE (C0–2)

The craniovertebral area is particularly important for regulating body posture, both static and dynamic, via afferent impulses from the connective tissue structures and muscles associated with the upper synovial joints. Stability of the area relies on bony integrity and associated muscles, with an important part played by the craniovertebral ligaments. Any damage through trauma or disease can cause neurological complications, with rare but potentially serious consequences (MacKenzie & Rankin 2003).

There are no discs between the occipitoatlantal and the atlantoaxial joints. The principal movement at C0/1 is flexion/extension or nodding of the head, while rotation is the principal movement at C1/2, the most mobile articulation of the spine.

The head weighs approximately 11 lb (5 kg) in a 150 lb (68 kg) individual (Grieve 1988, p. 22) and poor postural habits can lead to 'a poking chin' posture, with the head being held forward (Fig. 12.7a.1). This can produce adaptive shortening of the sub-occipital muscles and weakness of the deep neck flexors, changing the alignment of the cervical spine resulting in increased joint compression.

The upper cervical spine is closely linked to the temporomandibular joint (TMJ). In particular, the forward head posture (Gonzalez & Manns 1996, D'Attilio et al 2004), as well as segmental stiffness at C0/3 and tender points in sternocleidomastoid and trapezius muscles (De Laat 1998), are thought to contribute to temporomandibular disorders (TMD), which are discussed in more detail below.

MID/LOWER CERVICAL SPINE (C2–7)

The plane of the facet joints, together with lax capsules, facilitates movement into flexion and extension, with the largest range of movement at C5/6. The neutral or resting position of the cervical spine is in slight extension, producing a cervical lordosis. This, along with the other curves in the spine, provides a shock-absorbing mechanism. The common forward head posture (Fig. 12.7a.1) can lead to increased flexion at the lower cervical spine with increased stress on the posterior elements of the vertebrae.

NECK PAIN

Neck pain is a common symptom in the population, with prevalence rates varying from 17% to 75%. It is generally reported more often in women than men, after injury, and in association with other chronic co-morbidities (Cote et al 2000, Fejer et al 2006).

Changes in segmental mobility can be associated with symptoms. The chronic pain of whiplash is thought to be due to *hypermobility* at C3/4 and C5/6 as a result of unphysiological movements during the accident (Dvorak 1993, Kristjansson et al 2003).

Conversely, motion studies have found *hypomobility*, most significantly at C6/7, associated with degenerative change and radicular symptoms (Dvorak 1993) and clinically it is common to find *hypomobility* in the cervico-thoracic junctional area.

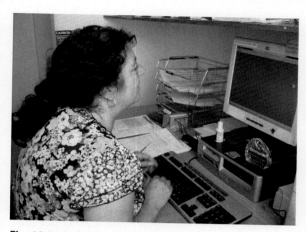

Fig. 12.7a.1 'Poking chin' or forward head posture

There is evidence that this is linked to neck–shoulder pain, particularly if there is less mobility in the C7/T1 segment compared to the T1/T2 segment (Norlander et al 1997, 1998). In addition, Norlander et al (1996) found *hypermobility* at C7/T1 in older subjects to have a protective influence.

HEADACHE

Headache can be considered one of the most prevalent pain conditions in the world (Stovner et al 2007). Although different forms of headache can co-exist, it is important that a correct diagnosis is established to ensure successful treatment. This is particularly true for physiotherapy intervention, because cervicogenic headache with a prevalence of 4% (Sjaastad & Bakketeij 2007) is currently the only headache form with evidence to support manual treatment (Hall et al 2008). Examination is very important and should include the articular, neural, muscle and fascial structures innervated by the upper three cervical nerves as a potential source for the headache.

Consideration should be given to the spinal nucleus of the trigeminal (fifth cranial) nerve as a cause of pain in the head and upper neck. The nucleus of the nerve descends from the pons to the 3rd or 4th cervical segment receiving nociceptive inputs from the V, VII, IX and X cranial nerves as well as C1–3 dorsal nerve roots. Furthermore the trigeminal nerve is accompanied by both sympathetic and parasympathetic neurons. It is thought that nociceptive traffic from the upper cervical joints may produce excitation of neurons in the associated cord segments, which are close to where afferents innervating tissues of the face and head synapse. This close relationship can initiate symptoms of pain and paraesthesiae to be felt in tissues of the face and jaw some distance from the articular irritation. In addition, the nucleus occupies a watershed area in the upper cervical cord and may be subject to ischaemic changes (Grieve 1988).

Cervical spine joint hypermobility has been suggested as a predisposing factor in the development of new daily persistent headache (Rozen et al 2006), a recently recognized form of the chronic daily headache, which has a prevalence of 3% (IHS 2004). Other rather more rare causes of headache associated with hypermobility which have been reported are spontaneous cerebrospinal fluid (CSF) leaks in two sisters with joint hypermobility (Mokri 2008).

INSTABILITY

Panjabi et al (1998) found, with an in vitro experimental model, that the osteoligamentous elements of the cervical spine support only 20–25% of the weight of the head. Therefore the surrounding musculature plays a significant role in mechanical stability. In addition, Panjabi et al (1994) in their study found support for the hypothesis that the neutral zone is more closely related to instability than range of motion (Chapter 12.8, 'neutral zone').

Six clinical features have been identified as important in the diagnosis of minor clinical instability (MCI) (Niere & Torney 2004). They are: a history of major trauma, reports of the neck catching, or locking, or giving way, poor muscular control, signs of hypermobility on X-ray, excessively free end-feel on passive movement testing and unpredictability of symptoms. MCI should be considered in any hypermobile patient with neck pain, even if there is no major trauma reported. Instability can be confirmed through functional X-ray and MRI scans into flexion and extension.

A syndrome of occipitoatlantoaxial hypermobility, cranial settling and Chiari malformation type I (CM-I) has been described recently in patients with Hereditary Disorders of Connective Tissue (HDCT) (Milhorat et al 2007). CM-I is defined as tonsillar herniation of 5 mm or more below the foramen magnum. The authors report that the impetus for the study was the observation that in a group of patients referred for failure of CM-I surgery, there was a subset of patients with HDCT with varying degrees of craniovertebral instability. In a study population of 2813, 12.7% were found to meet the criteria for HDCT and this group appeared to experience a greater incidence of lower brainstem symptoms including nausea, dysphagia, throat tightness, sleep apnoea, shortness of breath, palpitations, facial pain, double vision and syncope ($P < 0.001$). There was also an increased incidence of Raynaud phenomenon, dizziness, POTS, orthostatic hypotension, mitral valve prolapse and regurgitation ($P < 0.001$). Imaging distinctions included an increased incidence of retro-odontoid pannus, cervical disc disease, cervical joint subluxation and TMD ($P < 0.001$). In addition, hypermobile patients demonstrated hypermobility of the occipitoatlantoaxial complex (posterior gliding of occipital condyles) and cranial settling (a reduction in the distance between basion and odontoid) that occurs in the upright position but not caused by bone or cartilage destruction and which resolves on resumption of the supine position or with traction. The authors cite reports of fusion resolving the pannus formation which provides indirect evidence of hypermobility as the cause. The increased motion may be due to damage or disruption of the ligaments or laxity as a result of hypermobility.

In addition, there is evidence of an increased prevalence of atlantoaxial hypermobility in Marfan syndrome (Hobbs et al 1997, Herzka et al 2000, MacKenzie & Rankin 2003). It is recommended that rotatory subluxation should be included in the differential diagnosis of Marfan syndrome patients presenting with neck pain after injury (Herzka et al 2000) and that sport with risks of high-impact loading of the cervical spine should be avoided (Hobbs et al 1997).

There is considerable overlap between symptoms diagnosed as fibromyalgia and cervical myelopathy, although Heffez et al (2004) remark that a detailed neurological evaluation is not routine. In their study, 270 patients (87% female) diagnosed with fibromyalgia underwent clinical neurological and neuroradiological evaluation. The predominant reported symptoms were: neck/back pain (95%), fatigue (95%), cognitive impairment (92%), instability of gait (82%), parasthesiae (80%), dizziness (71%) and numbness (69%). Symptom exacerbation was reported in 88% on neck extension and the neurological examination was consistent with cervical myelopathy. In addition, MRI and contrast-enhanced CT imaging of the cervical spine revealed

spinal stenosis, with 46% of patients demonstrating a clinically significant spinal canal stenosis at C5/6 with the neck positioned in mild extension. MRI of the brain revealed a Chiari I malformation (tonsillar ectopia > 5mm) in 20% of patients. Similar findings are reported by Holman (2008) with a prevalence of 71% (Chapter 5) in patients with FM demonstrating cervical cord compression. While there is no mention of hypermobility or JHS in either study, it is acknowledged that there is considerable overlap between symptoms of fibromyalgia and JHS and it is possible that instability and poor segmental movement control during extension may be producing the functional cord compression. C5–6 is the most mobile segment of the cervical spine and poor posture and weak musculature may make the hypermobile individual more susceptible.

There is considerable overlap between symptoms of JHS and fibromyalgia. Sahin et al (2008) describe a group of 94 patients presenting to an out-patient clinic with cervical myofascial pain syndrome, in whom 88% were female, 58% suffered cervical trauma, 53% had trigger points in the trapezius muscle with associated autonomic phenomena, 40% also had fibromyalgia and 18% had JHS.

CERVICAL ARTERIAL DYSFUNCTION

The arterial supply to the head and neck, which comprises the vertebrobasilar system, internal carotid arteries and the circle of Willis, can be subject to trauma with injury to the neck, in particular from road traffic accidents. This is considered a rare occurrence, but one which may be more common than previously reported (Biffl et al 2000). Injury can result in dissection or aneurysm which can produce ischaemia in the brain.

There are reports of spontaneous dissection (Brandt et al 2005, Sasaki et al 2009) and dissection with trivial trauma (Haneline & Lewkovich 2007) in otherwise healthy individuals. Brandt et al (2005) investigated the morphology of the connective tissue in the carotid vessel walls and skin of individuals with spontaneous cervical artery dissection (sCAD). Results showed that while the skin was essentially normal, there were mild ultrastructural connective tissue alterations similar to EDS III – hypermobility type, or EDS IV, with collagen fibres containing fibrils with highly variable diameters, or the abnormalities were restricted to the elastic fibres. Interestingly, similar connective tissue findings were detected in some first-degree relatives and <5% of the patients with sCAD and connective tissue abnormalities had clinical manifestations of skin, joint or skeletal abnormalities of a defined HDCT. This suggests a weakening of the vessel wall may make it more susceptible to tearing as a result of minor trauma. This is particularly important for therapists treating the hypermobile cervical spine with manual therapy.

Head and neck pain are commonly reported symptoms of sCAD, therefore therapists must be vigilant to the fact that patients may present with an existing arterial dissection and that manual therapy may cause further damage (Kerry et al 2008). Manipulative (thrust) techniques, particularly in the upper cervical spine, are thought to be most hazardous because of the tortuous path of the vertebral artery between C2 and the occiput. However, flow studies show that gentler, repeated movement also has the potential to produce a dissecting force (Kerry et al 2008) and, in addition, the low/mid cervical spine cannot be considered safe because internal carotid artery plaques are most prevalent around the bifurcation of the internal/external vessels, which is level with this area (Kerry et al 2008). Functional pre-treatment screening tests have been recommended by Physiotherapy Associations in Australia (AJP 2001) and the UK, but there is no evidence to support the validity of these tests to identify patients at risk and the testing procedures can be provocative because end-range extension and rotation are sustained. The argument to stop pre-treatment screening tests is compelling (Thiel & Rix 2005), particularly in those with hypermobility, JHS or other connective tissue disorders.

EXAMINATION

It is not the remit of this chapter to describe in detail the examination of the cervical spine and readers are recommended to consult Magee (2008) for details on comprehensive assessment of the cervical spine. There are, however, some aspects of the examination which are particularly important in the hypermobile patient, which are highlighted below.

POSTURE

As previously mentioned (Chapter 9), observation of postural alignment of the whole body, in addition to head and neck posture, is particularly valuable. Ideally, assessment should be performed in both standing and sitting, with any deviation from an ideal alignment noted. If the habitual 'poking chin' or forward head posture is apparent it is useful to correct it and assess any change in symptoms and also to check if it is related to poor eyesight, bifocals or temporomandibular joint problems. It may be necessary to sustain the sitting position to test the endurance capability of the postural muscles. Patients with neck pain have demonstrated a reduced ability to maintain an upright posture during a computer task, showing a subtle forward drift of the head and increase in thoracic flexion curve (Falla et al 2007).

Problems originating in the neck can refer symptoms into the head, jaw, shoulders, upper back and arms, therefore an examination is not complete until all areas related to the symptoms are assessed.

RANGE OF MOVEMENT

Upper cervical spine

Movement of the upper cervical spine can be distinguished from the lower cervical spine. Movement between the first two cervical vertebrae can occur without involving the other levels, and amounts to a nodding action (flexion) and lifting the chin up (extension) without moving the rest of the neck. Upper cervical extension can be provocative and produce symptoms of dizziness, loss of balance or parasthesiae if there is an element of cord compression or vertebrobasilar dysfunction, secondary to hypermobility. Overpressure should be applied with extreme care in a hypermobile individual even if no symptoms are produced.

Lower cervical spine

In a hypermobile individual with no movement restriction it is not uncommon to find that the chin reaches the plane of the shoulder in rotation, the ear reaches very close to the shoulder in side flexion and in extension the occiput rests on the upper back (Fig. 12.7a.2). It can be very difficult to bring the head back from this latter position without poking the chin out, demonstrating muscular weakness of the deep neck flexors, with the sternocleidomastoid muscle initiating and dominating the movement. The quality of the movement (as in other areas) is

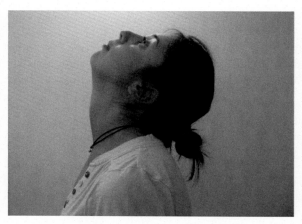

Fig. 12.7a.2 Cervical extension in a hypermobile individual. Note the increased mobility or 'hinging' in the mid-low (C5/6) cervical spine

of the utmost importance with extension frequently revealing a 'hinging' or 'buckling' in the mid-low cervical spine as movement occurs more readily at the most mobile segments compared to the lower cervical spine which is stiffer (Fig. 12.7a.2).

Passive movement testing in supine will reveal an increased range of movement because the muscles which hold the head up when sitting will be relaxed. Palpating the joints while testing passive movements, as in passive physiological intervertebral movement testing (PPIVM) and passive accessory intervertebral movement (PAIVM), can identify hyper/hypomobility at individual joints as well as give information regarding endfeel.

SPECIAL TESTS

There are special tests that can be performed, if indicated, such as the vertebral artery test and upper cervical ligament tests. These are generally recommended if treatment is to be given to the upper cervical spine and particularly if end-range techniques or manipulations are contemplated. However, they are provocative and should be applied with extreme caution in the hypermobile individual. Any suggestion of instability or obstruction in blood supply to the brain will contraindicate the use of such techniques.

PROPRIOCEPTION

The cervical spine is very important for balance and postural control and studies have shown a reduction in balance control following whiplash injuries (Dehner et al 2008), osteoarthritis of the cervical spine (Boucher et al 2008), cervical myelopathy (Yoshikawa 2008) and reduced cervical proprioceptive acuity in non-traumatic neck pain patients (Pinsault et al 2008). Clinically, it may be appropriate to test balance stability with the Romberg test as discussed in Chapter 6.3 and head and neck position sense using the cervicocephalic relocation test (Pinsault et al 2008) or similar. As yet there has been no research looking specifically at hypermobility and proprioception in the cervical spine, although anecdotal evidence suggests hypermobility can adversely affect proprioceptive acuity as has been shown in knee and finger joints.

MUSCLE STRENGTH AND CONTROL

Segmental stability is primarily achieved through co-contraction of the deep flexors (longus capitis and colli) and extensors (multifidus) of the neck. The craniocervical flexion test (CCFT) is a clinical test of the action and endurance of the deep neck flexors (DNF) (Jull et al 2008). Research has shown that patients with chronic neck pain have altered neuromotor control during the test, with decreased activity in the DNF and increased activity in the superficial flexors (sternocleidomastoid, hyoid and anterior scalene muscles). The test and subsequent training take place in a supine position with an air-filled pressure sensor (Chattanooga Stabilizer – Fig. 12.7a.3) to monitor the subtle flattening of the cervical lordosis as the patient gently performs upper cervical flexion without substitution from the superficial flexors (Jull et al 2004).

Strength of the neck flexors can be tested by asking the patient to lift and move their head through a full range of movement into flexion and back while in a supine position. Muscles which produce rotation and side flexion can be tested in a similar way. Multifidus can be tested by isometric neck/head extension with the cranio-cervical spine maintained in a flexed position (Lee et al 2007). It is important to observe the quality of the movement and the repetitions or hold time to highlight weakness and fatigue. It is the author's experience that hypermobile individuals have difficulty lifting the weight of the head off the bed in a smooth and controlled way and fatigue quickly.

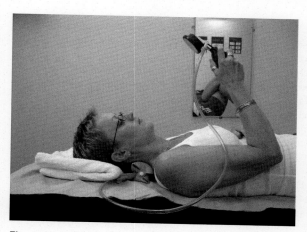

Fig. 12.7a.3 Craniocervical flexion test (CCFT) with pressure biofeedback

TREATMENT

Treatment for symptoms attributed to the cervical spine should follow the principles outlined in Chapter 9, and address abnormalities found on examination. The main aim of intervention will be to restore a full range of motion, improve posture and movement control, muscle strength and endurance.

One of the most important aspects of treatment in the hypermobile patient will be to improve or restore an effective stability mechanism. While proprioceptive exercise has played a large part in the rehabilitation of injuries in the lower limbs, it has featured much less prominently in the cervical spine (Armstrong et al 2008). It is thought that receptors in the muscle spindles of the deep cervical muscles play a key role, therefore muscle co-contraction exercise along with eye and neck coordination exercises have been advocated, although there is as yet little research confirming their efficacy (Armstrong et al 2008).

While there is evidence that the CCFT and neck flexor endurance strength training can significantly reduce neck pain and perceived disability, and improve ability to maintain an upright cervical and thoracic spine posture during a functional computer task (Falla et al 2007), the benefits may not automatically result in better muscle activation during functional activity (Falla et al 2008). Clinical experience suggests that while it may be appropriate to start initially with specific muscle retraining, to improve movement patterns, this should be progressed to more functional exercises involving, in the case of the neck, the rest of the spine and upper limbs. Improving strength and stability around the shoulder girdle can be particularly important in the hypermobile patient to ensure that the weight of the upper limb is supported evenly across the shoulder girdle and upper back, rather than predominantly by passive tension in the upper trapezius muscles, causing chronic strain and spasm.

SURGERY

Cervical spondylosis, a common cause of radiculopathy and myelopathy, is often treated by discectomy and interbody fusion, performed most often at C5–7 (Park et al 2007). However, there is a risk of increasing motion at segmental levels above and below the fusion which can accelerate degenerative disease at these levels (Eck et al 2002, Seo & Choi 2008). These clinical findings have been confirmed in cadaveric studies (Schwab et al 2006, Park et al 2007). This has lead to a change in operation techniques away from fusing procedures to motion preserving technologies, such as arthroplasty, and minimally invasive techniques (Korinth 2008), but it is too early to say whether the use of artificial disc replacements will decrease the incidence of adjacent segment disease.

References

Armstrong B, McNair P, Taylor D: Head and neck position, *Sports Med* 38:101–117, 2008.

Australian Journal of Physiotherapy Pre-manipulative testing of the cervical spine; Forum:*Aust J Physiother* 47:163–168, 2001.

Biffl WL, Moore EE, Elliott JP, et al: The devastating potential of blunt vertebral arterial injuries, *Ann Surg (US)* 231:672–681, 2000.

Boucher P, Descarreaux M, Normand MC: Postural control in people with osteoarthritis of the cervical spine, *J Manipulative Physiol Ther* 31:184–190, 2008.

Brandt T, Morcher M, Hausser I: Association of cervical artery dissection with connective tissue abnormalities in skin and arteries, *Front Neurol Neurosci* 20:16–29, 2005.

Cote P, Cassidy JD, Carroll L: The factors associated with neck pain and its related disability in the Saskatchewan population, *Spine* 25:1109–1117, 2000.

D'Attilio M, Epifania E, Ciuffolo F, et al: Cervical lordosis angle measured on lateral cephalograms; findings in skeletal class II female subjects with and without TMD: a cross sectional study, *Cranio* 22:27–44, 2004.

Dehner C, Heym B, Maier D, et al: Postural control deficit in acute QTF grade II whiplash injuries, *Gait Posture* 28:113–119, 2008.

De Laat A, Meuleman H, Stevens A, et al: Correlation between cervical spine and temporomandibular disorders, *Clin Oral Investig* 2:54–57, 1998.

Dvorak J, Panjabi MM, Grob D, et al: Clinical validation of functional flexio/extension radiographs of the cervical spine, *Spine* 18:120–127, 1993.

Eck JC, Humphreys SC, Lim TH, et al: Biomechanical study on the effect of cervical fusion on adjacent – level intradiscal pressure and segmental motion, *Spine* 27:2431–2434, 2002.

Falla D, Jull G, Russell T, et al: Effect of neck exercise on sitting posture in patients with chronic neck pain, *Phys Ther* 87(4):408–417, 2007.

Falla D, Jull G, Hodges P: Training the cervical muscles with prescribed motor tasks does not change muscle activation during a functional activity, *Man Ther* 13:507–512, 2008.

Fejer R, Kyvik KO, Hartvigsen J: The prevalence of neck pain in the world population: a systemic critical review of the literature, *Eur Spine J* 15:834–848, 2006.

Gonzalez HE, Manns A: Forward head posture: its structural and functional influence on the stomatognathic system, a conceptual study, *Cranio* 14:71–80, 1996.

Grieve GP: *Common Vertebral Joint Problems*, ed 2, Edinburgh, 1988, Churchill Livingstone, p 325.

Hall T, Briffa K, Hopper D: Clinical evaluation of cervicogenic headache: a clinical perspective, *Journal of Manual & Manipulative Therapy* 16:73–80, 2008.

Haneline M, Lewkovich GN: A narrative review of pathophysiological mechanisms with cervical artery dissection, *Journal of the Canadian Chiropractic Association* 51:146–157, 2007.

Heffez DS, Ross RE, Shade-Zeldow Y, et al: Clinical evidence for cervical myelopathy due to Chiari malformation and spinal stenosis in a non-randomized group of patients with the diagnosis of fibromyalgia, *Eur Spine J* 13:516–523, 2004.

Herzka A, Sponseller PD, Pyeritz RE: Atlantoaxial rotatory subluxation in patients with Marfan syndrome. A report of three cases, *Spine* 25:524–526, 2000.

Hobbs WR, Sponseller PD, Weiss AP, et al: The cervical spine in Marfan syndrome, *Spine* 22:983–989, 1997.

Holman AJ: Positional cervical spinal cord compression and fibromyalgia: a novel comorbidity with important diagnostic and treatment implications, *J Pain* 9:613–622, 2008.

International Headache Society: The International Classification of Headache Disorders, ed 2. *Cephalalgia* 24(Suppl 1):9–160, 2004.

Jull G, Falla D, Treleaven J, et al: A therapeutic exercise approach for cervical disorders. In Boyling JD, Jull G, editors: *Grieve's Modern Manual Therapy: The Vertebral Column*, ed 3, Edinburgh, 2004, Elsevier.

Jull GA, O'Leary SP, Falla DL: Clinical assessment of the deep neck flexor muscles: the craniocervical test, *J Manipulative Physiol Ther* 31:525–533, 2008.

Kerry R, Taylor AJ, Mitchell J, et al: Manual therapy and cervical arterial dysfunction, directions for the future: a clinical perspective, *Journal of Manual & Manipulative Therapy* 16:39–48, 2008.

Korinth MC: Treatment of cervical degenerative disc disease – current status and trends, *Zentralbl Neurochir* 69:113–124, 2008.

Kristjansson E, Leivseth G, Brinckmann P, et al: Increased sagittal plane segmental motion in the lower cervical spine in women with chronic whiplash-associated disorders, grades I & II: a case-control study using a new measurement protocol, *Spine* 28:2215–2221, 2003.

Lee JP, Tseng WY, Shau YW, et al: Measurement of segmental cervical multifidus contraction by ultrasonography in asymptomatic adults, *Man Ther* 12:286–294, 2007.

MacKenzie JM, Rankin R: Sudden death due to atlantoaxial subluxation in Marfan syndrome, *American Journal of Forensic Medical Pathology* 24:369–370, 2003.

Magee DJ: Cervical Spine. In *Orthopedic Physical Assessment*, ed 5, St Louis, 2008, Saunders, p 130.

Milhorat TH, Bolognese PA, Nishikawa M, et al: Syndrome of occipitoatlantoaxial hypermobility, cranial settling and Chiari malformation Type I in patients with hereditary disorders of connective tissue, *J Neurosurg Spine* 7:601–609, 2007.

Mokri B: Familial occurrence of spontaneous spinal CSF leaks: underlying connective tissue disorder, *Headache* 48:146–149, 2008.

Niere KR, Torney SK: Clinicians' perceptions of minor cervical instability, *Man Ther* 9:144–150, 2004.

Norlander S, Aste-Norlander U, Nordgren B, et al: Mobility in the cervico-thoracic motion segment: an indicative factor of musculoskeletal neck-shoulder pain, *Scand J Rehabil Med* 28:183–192, 1996.

Norlander S, Gustavsson BA, Lindell J, et al: Reduced mobility in the cervico-thoracic motion segment – a risk factor for musculoskeletal neck-shoulder pain: a two-year prospective follow-up study, *Scand J Rehabil Med* 29:167–174, 1997.

Norlander S, Nordgren B: Clinical symptoms related to musculoskeletal neck-shoulder pain and mobility in the cervico-thoracic spine, *Scand J Rehabil Med* 30:243–251, 1998.

Panjabi MM, Lydon C, Vasavada A, et al: On the understanding of clinical instability, *Spine* 19:2642–2650, 1994.

Panjabi MM, Cholewicki J, Nibu K, et al: Critical load of the human cervical spine: an in vitro experimental study, *Clinical Biomechnics (Bristol, Avon)* 13:11–17, 1998.

Park DH, Ramakrishnan P, Cho TH, et al: Effect of lower two-level anterior cervical fusion on the superior adjacent level, *J Neurosurg Spine* 7:336–340, 2007.

Pinsault N, Vuillerme N, Pavan P: Cervicocephalic relocation test to the neutral head position: assessment in bilateral labyrinthe-defective and chronic, nontraumatic neck pain patients, *Arch Phys Med Rehabil* 89:2375–2378, 2008.

Rozen TD, Roth JM, Denenberg N: Cervical spine joint hypermobility: a possible predisposing factor for new daily persistent headache, *Cephalalgia* 26:1182–1185, 2006.

Sahin N, Karatas O, Ozkaya M, et al: Demographics features, clinical findings and functional status in a group of subjects with cervical myofascial pain syndrome, *Agri: The Journal of the Turkish Society of Algology* 20:14–19, 2008.

Sasaki M, Makajima M, Hirano T, et al: A young patient with ischaemic stroke due to carotid artery dissection in whom a number of microembolic signals was followed up (article in Japanese), *Rinsho Shinkeigaku* 49:127–129, 2009.

Schwab JS, Diangelo DJ, Foley KT: Motion compensation associated with single-level cervical fusion: where does the lost motion go? *Spine* 31:2439–2448, 2006.

Seo M, Choi D: Adjacent segment disease after fusion for cervical spondylosis; myth or reality? *Br J Neurosurg* 22:195–199, 2008.

Sjaastad O: Cervicogenic headache: comparison with migraine without aura; vågå study, *Cephalalgia* 28(Suppl 1):18–20, 2008.

Stovner LJ, Hagen K, Jensen R, et al: The global burden of headache: a documentation of headache prevalence and disability worldwide, *Cephalalgia* 27:193–210, 2007.

Thiel H, Rix G: Is it time to stop functional pre-manipulation testing of the cervical spine? *Man Ther* 10:154–158, 2005.

Yoshikawa M, Doita M, Okamoto K: Impaired postural stability in patients with cervical myelopathy: evaluation by computerised static stabilometry, *Spine* 33:E460–E464, 2008.

12.7   The cervical spine and jaw – (b) Temporomandibular joint – physiotherapy management

Lynn Bryden

INTRODUCTION

Physiotherapy management of patients with temporomandibular dysfunction (TMD), as with other musculoskeletal problems, involves careful subjective and objective examination of the individual patient. In this section the association between generalized joint hypermobility (JHM), joint hypermobility syndrome (JHS) and TMD is explored and the relevance of this relationship in the physiotherapeutic management of TMD is discussed.

HYPERMOBILITY AND TMD

There is evidence to support a relationship between JHM and the presence of TMD (Buckingham et al 1991, Westling 1992, Adair & Hecht 1993, Westling & Mattiasson 1992, Kavuncu et al 2004, Hirsch et al 2008), although evidence for a relationship between JHS and TMD is harder to find.

Hypermobility of the TMJ is said to occur when the mandibular condyle translates anteriorly and inferiorly beyond the articular eminence of the temporal bone (Kavuncu et al 2006). Westling (1992) found that in a group of patients with craniomandibular dysfunction (CMD) those patients with TMD had significantly more hypermobile joints than other CMD patients. Similarly, Buckingham et al (1991) in a study of patients with temperomandibular (TMJ) dysfunction found 54% to be hypermobile. Interestingly, radiographs in this study showed TMJ hyperextensibility in only four of these hypermobile patients.

In a study of 20 children aged 4–19 years with JHS 75% exhibited some signs and symptoms of TMD in comparison to 50% of the control group (Adair & Hecht 1993) and in a further study of 17-year-olds by Westling and Mattiasson (1992), 22% of girls and 3% of boys, scoring five or more on the Beighton scale, showed a higher prevalence of signs and symptoms of TMD.

Hirsch et al (2008), in a larger study of 895 subjects aged 20–60, found that hypermobile subjects (with a score of >4 on the Beighton scale) had a higher risk of reciprocal TMJ clicking (as an indicator of disc displacement) and a lower risk for limited mouth opening (<35 mm). Generalized joint hypermobility was found to be associated with non-painful presentations of TMD.

Kavuncu et al (2006) screened 64 patients aged 15–60 years attending a hospital outpatient clinic for different reasons for TMD based on the Research Diagnostic Criteria for Temporo-mandibular Disorders (RDC/TMD). Systemic joint hypermobility (SJH) was evaluated using the Beighton score, and local condylar hypermobility (LCH) was also measured radiographically. A combination of SJH and LCH correlated most highly with TMD. It is important to note that excess range of mouth opening did not correlate with LCH, since the main cause of condylar subluxation is early translation, rather than rotation, of the mandible, suggesting that measurement of intra-incisal opening alone will not identify LCH. It should also be remembered that muscle spasm may mask any excess translation in TMD patients with LCH.

De Coster et al (2004) assessed oral health in 31 subjects with Ehlers-Danlos syndromes. In addition to other parameters, signs and symptoms of TMD were assessed, based on the RDC for TMD. Subjects with a history of whiplash, facial trauma, rheumatic disease and/or arthritis of the neck/shoulder complex were excluded as these may mimic orofacial pain. Four indicators were evaluated for TMD diagnosis: orofacial pain, joint sounds, range of mandibular opening and radiographic evaluation of joint surfaces. TMD diagnoses were divided into three groups: muscle disorders, disc disorders and joint disorders. Oral parafunctions, psychosocial factors, and frequency of dislocation (open lock or subluxation) were also recorded. Dislocation can describe either jamming of the disc–condyle complex beyond the articular eminence, or true hypertranslation of this complex beyond the articular eminence. The results showed that 100% of subjects were symptomatic in some way for TMD, though only 22% of these were seeking treatment. Eighty-three per cent of subjects were assigned unilateral myofascial pain diagnosis, 78% had bilateral disc displacement with reduction, and 51% had bilateral TMJ arthralgia. Recurrent TMJ dislocation was reported in 100% of cases, with higher frequency in those with a high chronic pain score.

However, other authors have reported inconclusive evidence for a link between TMD and generalized joint hypermobility (GJH) (Conti et al 2000, Winocur et al 2000, Dijkstra et al 2002). Conti et al (2000) evaluated 60 TMD subjects and 60 non-symptomatics looking at both the Beighton scale and lateral X-rays of the TMJ, taken in mouth open and mouth closed positions. No association was found between intra-articular disorders of the TMJ and systemic hypermobility or between systemic and TMJ hypermobility (condyle hypertranslation).

Dijkstra et al (2002) also struggled to find an association in a bibliographic search of 14 papers. Only three studies met the methodological criteria and had data available for analysis. Of 113 cases and 95 controls, 26 cases and five controls were hypermobile. However, they concluded that it was unclear whether GJH is associated with TMD but suggested that the clinician should consider that patients presenting with signs and symptoms of TMD may also have a background of GJH.

Winocur et al (2000) examined 248 girls aged 15–16 for signs and symptoms of TMD, TMJ hypermobility and GJH. The prevalence of GJH was 43% and TMJ hypermobility was 27% with a significant though weak correlation between the two. The presence of joint clicks was negatively associated with GJH. Their conclusions were that 'GJH did not seem to jeopardize the health of the stomatognathic system as expressed in the signs and symptoms of TMD'.

There is certainly evidence of an association between JHM and TMD, although very little work has been done looking at JHS and TMD. Nevertheless, this has implications both for physiotherapists involved in the treatment of patients with JHS, who report symptoms associated with the TMJ, and for physiotherapists who are involved in the management of patients presenting with signs and symptoms of TMD.

ANATOMICAL AND PATHOLOGICAL CONSIDERATIONS

The ligaments, fibrocartilage structure, disc and the retrodiscal tissues of the TMJ are composed mainly of collagen (Fig. 12.7b.1). In the presence of a genetic

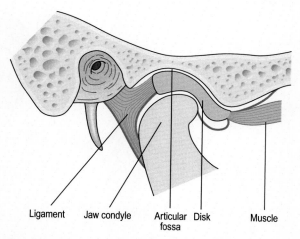

Ligament   Jaw condyle   Articular   Disk   Muscle
                            fossa

Fig. 12.7b.1 Cross-section of TMJ showing retrodiscal tissue, disc and superior head of lateral pterygoid muscle. *From McDevitt (1989, p. 80) with permission*

defect in the synthesis of collagen there may be an increased likelihood of developing dysfunction related to increased joint movement (Fig. 12.7b.2).

The percentage of the general population with signs of TMD is reported to be between 50–75% (Gray et al 1995), while the percentage with symptoms is reported to be between 20–25%, and those who seek treatment 3–4%. The peak age range for myofascial pain symptoms is between 15–30 years and over 40 years for degenerative joint disease. Internal derangement of the joint is reported at any age. Although the prevalence of symptoms is reported equal for both sexes, more females than males present for treatment, in a ratio of 5:1, with pain being the most common reason for seeking treatment. The indications from the literature are that in known JHS patients there is a high incidence of TMD. In light of this the physiotherapist should be aware that patients presenting with signs and symptoms of TMD may have underlying JHS which may not have been previously identified.

When examining a patient with signs and symptoms of TMD, it is always important to consider the influence of the cervical spine, which is a significant source of referred symptoms to the area of the TMJ, head and masticatory system. The structural and neurophysiological links between the TMJ and the cervical spine have been explored by many authors (Clark & Wyke 1974, Mohl 1976, Daly et al 1982, Darling et al 1984, Rocabado 1984, Frumker & Kyle 1985).

Common postural alterations, such as forward head posture, increase the elastic tension on the

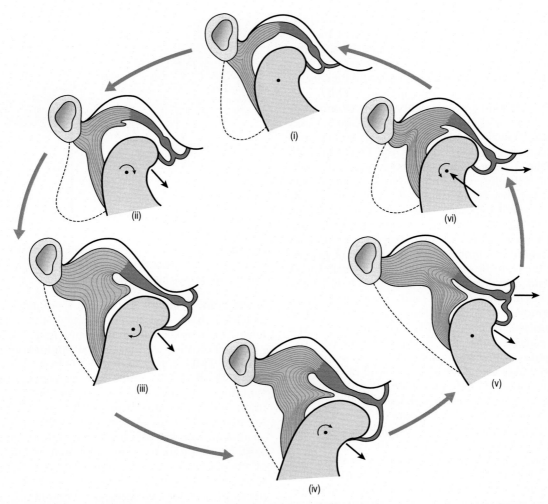

Fig. 12.7b.2 Structural relationships of the craniomandibular joint during functional jaw movement. In hypermobility of the joint the disc–condyle complex continues to translate beyond the articular eminence. *From McDevitt (1989, p. 103) with permission*

supra- and infrahyoid muscles, and via their thoracic attachments produce a downward and backward force on the mandible (Rocabado 1984).

The changes involved in forward head posture include:

- extension of the cervical spine at C0–1 and C1–2
- a decrease in cervical lordosis and an increase in thoracic kyphosis
- protraction and elevation of the shoulder girdle
- a downward and backward movement of the mandible
- adoption of 'mouth-breathing'.

This in turn may lead to:

- an increase in compressive forces on cervical apophyseal joints

- lengthening of the short neck flexors and infrahyoid muscles
- elevation of the hyoid bone
- shortening of the suprahyoids and neck extensors.

ASSESSMENT

Examination of the cervical spine is an important element in assessment of the TMJ (see above).

The subjective examination should include a detailed history and description of the symptoms and signs. Suggestions of particular questions to ask are given in Box 12.7b.1.

It should also be acknowledged that psychosocial factors often feature in the presentation of

BOX 12.7b.1 **Typical histories associated with TMJ pathology**

- Joint noises on mandibular movement such as clicking (which may indicate the recapture of an anteriorly dislocated disc, particularly if the click is reciprocal on opening and closing)
- Reports of locking and difficulty in opening the mouth
- Clenching or grinding of teeth (often during sleep)
- Pain associated with chewing food
- Pain or difficulty in opening the mouth (e.g. biting an apple, yawning)
- A sensation of fullness or tinnitus in the ear
- Oral parafunction – e.g. gum chewing, pen chewing, repetitive jaw clicking

head and neck pain (as with other musculoskeletal presentations). This is particularly so in TMD patients presenting with myofascial pain dysfunction syndrome. Therefore, assessment should include open questions regarding possible life stresses that may have contributed to the development of symptoms. People are known to respond to stress physiologically and this is often with a particular system. Patients with head and neck pain may be 'oral responders' and generate increased muscle tension in the stomatognathic system. Studies have shown an increased level of anxiety among TMD patients as well as hypermobile individuals (Bulbena et al 1993, 2006, Martin-Santos et al 1998) (Chapter 4).

The physiotherapist may need to refer the patient for assessment by a dental practitioner with expertise in the field of TMD management if this has not already occurred, for example, if the assessment indicates there is significant contribution to the symptoms from the occlusal position, or disc derangement where corrective splinting may be employed.

PHYSICAL EXAMINATION

It is not the purpose of this chapter to present detail of a comprehensive examination of the TMJ and the reader is directed to Kraus (1994) for further information. However, points of particular relevance to hypermobility will be highlighted.

The examination will provide information as to the type of dysfunction. TMD, as stated above, can be broadly divided into three main groups:

myofascial pain dysfunction syndrome, internal joint derangement/disc disorders, and degenerative joint disease. It is of course possible and not uncommon for a patient to present with a combination of two or more of the above.

The physical examination should include observation of facial symmetry and simple assessment of dental occlusion.

The range of mouth opening should be recorded by measurement of the inter-incisal distance (allowing for depth of overbite) and noting any deviation or deflection that occurs during movement. Likewise, the range of lateral glide is measured, using the incisors as markers and noting any discrepancy in range between sides.

Palpation of the lateral and posterior aspects of the TMJ during movement provides information on the point at which forward translation occurs, and the range of excursion of the disc–condyle complex along the articular eminence. Any discrepancy between sides should be noted. Clicking or crepitus should also be evaluated and it may be useful to load the joint to gain more information regarding pain, quality and regularity of clicks.

Muscles surrounding the TMJ, such as temporalis, masseter and medial pterygoid, are palpated to assess their involvement. The lateral pterygoid can be palpated intraorally, although this may be uncomfortable for the patient. Palpation of further masticatory and cervical spine muscles will be determined by the presenting symptoms and history.

TREATMENT

Hypermobile patients may present with a range of TMD signs and symptoms. Treatment should be directed empirically as with any other musculoskeletal presentation. While it is beyond the scope of this text to describe the many treatment methods that may be employed in the management of a patient with TMD, treatment of particular problems associated with hypermobility of the TMJ is discussed.

HYPOMOBILITY

It is not always the case that an individual with JHS will present with hypermobility of the TMJ. The history may reveal repetitive subluxation in the past that has now developed into a loss of range due to a repeatedly traumatized disc. Treatment should be directed at improving range of movement through joint mobilization and muscle relaxation techniques. If the restriction of movement is related to internal derangement of the disc then treatment is often in combination with appropriate splinting or other dental management.

HYPERMOBILITY

However, a significant number of JHS patients will present with local hypermobility of the TMJ. The clinician will feel hypertranslation of the mandibular condyle along the articular eminence by palpating over the lateral pole on mouth opening. If this movement is associated with pain and/or there is a history of 'open locking', which has to be manually reduced, then treatment is indicated.

Inflammation may be present from the repetitive trauma associated with the hypertranslation and can be reduced with low-dose ultrasound, gentle heat and, on occasions, ice. It is also important to educate the patient to reduce joint loading by avoiding parafunctional activity (such as gum chewing) and eating a soft-food diet. If there is evidence of clenching or grinding (often occurring during sleep) a splint may be helpful for night-time and teaching the patient the rest position of the tongue allows a decrease in masticatory muscle activity. In the rest position the anterosuperior tip of the tongue rests against the palate just posterior to the upper central incisors.

A further useful exercise is to perform repetitive condylar rotation with the tongue maintained in the rest position. This avoids the translation that tends to cause inflammation but helps to prevent any stiffness that may develop as a result of the patient avoiding painful translation.

The hypermobile patient should be instructed to avoid opening wide, for example, when yawning. Again, maintaining a tongue-up position will largely limit movement to condylar rotation with minimal translation.

Isometric exercises of the mandibular muscles can be helpful to improve proprioception and thereby movement control. The easiest way for the patient to do this is to hold the mandible still while applying pressure with the index finger in a variety of directions. It may be appropriate to do this with the head supported against a backrest or similar initially, and then progress to an unsupported head position.

It is advisable to avoid long periods with the mouth open. During dental treatment the patient should be allowed to take breaks to allow the mouth to close for a while. Similarly, during intubation, the anaesthetist should be alerted to avoid a wide open position if possible and take extra care with positioning of the cervical spine.

SUMMARY

It should be stressed that not all hypermobile TM joints are symptomatic and that there are many factors that may contribute to the development of signs and symptoms of TMD. There is, however, evidence of an association between hypermobility and TMD, and therefore the assessment and treatment of TMD should be performed in the context of possible generalized hypermobility or JHS. Conservative management of TMD is the treatment of choice, but this can often be lengthy, requiring good patient compliance to regular exercising.

References

Adair SM, Hecht C: Association of generalized joint hypermobility with history, signs and symptoms of temporomandibular joint dysfunction in children, *Pediatric Dental* 15(5):323–326, 1993.

Buckingham RB, Braun T, Harinstein DA, et al: Temporomandibular joint dysfunction syndrome: A close association with systemic joint laxity (the hypermobile joint syndrome), *Oral Surg Oral Med Oral Pathol* 72(5):514–519, 1991.

Bulbena A, Duro JC, Porta M: Anxiety disorders in the joint hypermobility syndrome, *Psychiatry Res* 46:59–68, 1993.

Bulbena A, Sperry L, Pailhez G, et al: Anxiety, temporomandibular disorders and joint hypermobility syndrome. Response to 'Psychological assessment of patients with temporomandibular disorders: confirmatory analysis of the dimensional structure of the Brief Symptoms Inventory 18, Journal of Psychosomatic Research 60: 365–370'. *J Psychosom Res* 61:851, 2006.

Clark RKF, Wyke BD: Contributions of temporomandibular mechanoreceptors to the control of mandibular posture: an experimental study, *J Dent* 2:121, 1974.

Conti PC, Miranda JE, Araujo CR: Relationship between systemic joint laxity, TMJ hypertranslation and intra-articular disorders, *Cranio* 18(3):192–197, 2000.

Daly P, Preston CB, Evans WG: Postural response of the head to bite opening in adult males, *Am J Orthod* 82:157–160, 1982.

Darling D, Krause S, Glasheen-Wray M: Relationship of head posture and the rest position of the mandible, *J Prosthet Dent* 52(1): III, 1984.

De Coster PJ, Martens LC, De Paepe A: Oral health in prevalent types of Ehlers-Danlos syndromes, *J Oral Pathol Med* 34:298–307, 2005.

Dijkstra PU, Kropmans TJ, Stegenga B: The association between generalised joint hypermobility and temporomandibular joint disorders: a systematic review, *J Dent Res* 81:158–163, 2002.

Frumker SC, Kyle MA: The dentist's contribution to rehabilitation of

cervical posture and function: Orthopaedic and neurological considerations in the treatment of craniomandibular disorders, *Basal Facts* 9(3):105–109, 1985.

Gray RJ, Davies SJ, Quayle AA: *Temporomandibular Disorders: a clinical approach*, London, 1995, British Dental Association, p 2.

Hirsh C, John MT, Stang A: Association between generalised joint hypermobility and signs and diagnoses of temporomandibular disorders, *Eur J Oral Sci* 116:525–530, 2008.

Kavuncu V, Sezai S, Ayhan K, et al: The role of systemic hypermobility and condylar hypermobility in temporomandibular joint dysfunction syndrome, *Rheumatol Int* 26:257–260, 2006.

Kraus SL: Physical therapy management of TMD. In *Temporomandibular Disorders. Clinics in Physical Therapy*, ed 2, New York, 1994, Churchill Livingstone, Chapter 7.

Martin-Santos R, Bulbena A, Porta M: Association between joint hypermobility syndrome and

panic disorder, *Am J Psychiatry* 155:1578–1583, 1998.

McDevitt WE: *Functional anatomy of the masticatory system*, London, 1989, Butterworth and Company.

Mohl N: Head posture and its role in occlusion, *NY Dental J* 42:17–23, 1976.

Rocabado M: Diagnosis and Treatment of Abnormal Craniocervical and Craniomandibular Mechanics. In Solberg WK, Clark GE, editors: *Abnormal jaw mechanics diagnosis and treatment*, Chicago, 1984, Quintessence.

Westling L: Temporomandibular joint dysfunction and systemic joint laxity, *Swedish Dental Journal: Supplement* 81:1–79, 1992.

Westling L, Mattiasson A: General joint hypermobility and temporomandibular joint derangement in adolescents, *Ann Rheum Dis* 51:87–90, 1992.

Winocur E, Gavish A, Halachmi M, et al: Generalized joint laxity and its relation with oral habits and temporomandibular disorders in adolescent girls, *J Oral Rehabil* 27:614–622, 2000.

12.7 The cervical spine and jaw – (c) Temporomandibular joint – surgical intervention

Waseem Jerjes and Colin Hopper

INTRODUCTION

Pathology of the temporomandibular joint (TMJ) and its associated muscles of mastication are termed temporomandibular disorders (TMDs). TMDs present with a variety of symptoms which include pain in the joint and the surrounding musculature, jaw clicking, limited mouth opening and headaches. They encompass the most common non-infective pain conditions of the orofacial region (Jerjes et al 2008).

ASSOCIATION BETWEEN TMD AND HYPERMOBILITY

It has been suggested that a close association exists between TMDs and joint hypermobility syndrome (JHS). This was initially studied in a group of 40 patients; 18 were found to have symptomatic joint hypermobility (JHM) and three had Ehlers-Danlos syndrome (EDS) (Harinstein et al 1988). The same group, but this time increased to 70 patients with severe, end-stage degenerative changes of the TMJ was reported by Buckingham et al (1991). The study suggested that 38 (54%) of these patients met criteria for symptomatic JHM. Five patients had classical EDS, and an additional two cases were described as 'Marfanoid' with possible EDS – akin to JHS by the later 1998 Brighton criteria (Chapter 1).

Patients with TMJ dysfunction are known to have higher prevalence of JHM when compared to craniomandibular dysfunction patients. Lower values of total collagen and a higher ratio of collagen type III to III + I have also been noticed in hypermobile patients (Westling 1992).

The dysfunction is believed to be associated with TMJ disc and capsular ligamentous attachment abnormalities (Goodman & Allison 1969, Fridrich et al 1990). This results in chronic subluxation or dislocation (Sacks et al 1990), with resultant pain crises refractory to most treatment modalities (Rossi & Kappel 2006).

MANAGING TMJ DYSFUNCTION

Management of disorders related to TMD in JHS and EDS can be very challenging. There is little doubt that conservative management should be considered in the first instance (Chapter 12.7b). Splint therapy is often tried but is of little long-term value and other physical therapies such as ultrasound, low-intensity laser, exercises and biofeedback are also of little use. Acupuncture, transcutaneous electrical nerve stimulation (TENS), cognitive behavioural therapy (CBT) (Chapter 8) and medical management with tricyclic antidepressants (Chapter 7) may have a role but responses are often disappointing.

SURGERY

Underlying collagen abnormalities can complicate joint surgery as it can result in poor wound healing and unpredictable surgical outcome (McDonald & Pogrel 1996). Associated with EDS is the problem of vascularity and bleeding disorders (Arneson et al 1980) (Chapter 1). Minimally invasive surgery (i.e. arthroscopy) is generally preferred to open joint surgery except where there is clear evidence of advanced degenerative joint disease.

The literature on TMD, JHS and EDS reports various surgical interventions. Shortening of the temporalis tendon by scarification (Gould 1978), implant of articular eminence attached to the zygoma (Howe et al 1978) and the application of plastic bolting (Schmoker et al 1979) have all been applied to restrict the hypermobility of the mandibular condyle. The later approach involved 28 patients and the subjective patients' report revealed success.

McDonald and Pogrel (1996) described two cases of EDS cases presenting with TMDs and their subsequent surgical management. In the first case, an exploration of the right joint of a 49-year-old Caucasian female revealed a severe degenerative displaced disc, degenerative condyle and enlargement of the joint space with fibrotic changes.

This was relined (glenoid fossa) with a myofascial temporalis flap. The left joint showed joint dislocation with no fibrotic or condylar degenerative changes and was managed by disc repositioning. In the second case, a 31-year-old Caucasian female was shown to have displacement and degeneration of the disc with condylar degeneration and osteophyte formation on the right side during surgical exploration. The only abnormalities identified on the left side were disc displacement and perforation. Here the management included condylar recontouring and excision of the discs followed by reconstruction with temporalis myofascial flaps.

Use of a muscle flap has been shown to result in the condyle developing a smooth cortical margin and functional improvement (Pogrel & Kaban 1990).

Rossi and Kappel (2006) reported that temporalis muscle osteofascial flap represents a potential treatment modality in the management of advanced degenerative joint changes and myofascial pain in EDS patients. In their report, a 40-year-old Caucasian female had a series of interventions to her right TMJ, including: splint therapy and conservative orthodontic management, arthroscopy and arthrolysis, injections and manipulation, and implantation of a permanent epidural morphine pump. She remained symptom-free for two and a half years.

Medra and Mahrous (2008) succeeded in providing TMJ stability in a group of 60 patients (40 with chronic recurrent dislocation and 20 with hypermobility) by glenotemporal osteotomy with interpositional bone graft. Their cohort was followed up for a mean of 3 years with satisfactory results.

Common reported surgical complications following open TMJ surgery in this group of patients (hypermobility and EDS) include:

- poor control of haemorrhage
- haemarthrosis and haematoma formation
- vascular perforation
- wound dehiscence
- aneurysm and arteriovenous fistula.

This leads to an increase in morbidity and mortality (Sacks et al 1990, Rossi & Kappel 2006). Also reported are recurrent subluxation creating preauricular and infraorbital ecchymosis, and intense wave-like masseter myospasm of up to 12 hours (Létourneau et al 2001).

The reported cases of temporalis muscle osteofascial flap with bone-to-bone attachment and interosseous fixation as a functional replacement for articular disc showed an alleviation of the symptoms of TMDs with minimal complications (McDonald & Pogrel 1996, Rossi & Kappel 2006).

Surgical intervention and joint exploration in JHS has been rarely implemented (Goodman & Allison 1969, Fridrich et al 1990, Sacks et al 1990, McDonald & Pogrel 1996). At the University College London Hospital Head and Neck Centre, London, UK a cohort of 18 cases of EDS who presented with signs and symptoms of TMD, were assessed for surgical intevention. The most common presenting complaints were joint pain, hypermobility and subluxation. Assessment of the TMJ and its related muscles of mastication were employed by a 2D orthopantomograph and magnetic resonance imaging. Results were variable but subluxation and a few cases of degenerative arthropathy were highlighted. TMJ arthroscopy followed by an arthrocentesis was employed in all cases, as well as intra-articular morphine injections. Some patients required surgical removal of symptomatic teeth with intraoral debridement. The postoperative period was characterized by delayed healing and reports of severe postoperative pain, some patients reporting such severe excoriating pain that they required regular opiates. Follow-up over a period ranging from 1–7 years showed satisfactory outcome with resolution of symptoms.

One of the patients from the above series was a 26-year-old Caucasian female with EDS – hypermobility type. She presented with bilateral pain, clicking, and locking, and occasional dislocation of the left TMJ. She reported a series of major medical and musculoskeletal problems, including arthroscopy and lavage of the right hip, laminectomy for spinal stenosis, and small and large bowel resection with a diagnosis of sclerosing panniculitis. Further reported problems were cervical spondylosis, osteoarthritis of left knee, and an unstable third left metacarpophalangeal joint. Clinical examination of the oral and maxillofacial region revealed internal derangement of the left TMJ with clicking and pain in both joints. The patient also reported symptoms of pain, recurrent swelling and infection in right and left posterior mandible as well as the left posterior maxilla, which coincides with symptomatic third molars. Imaging revealed subluxation of the left TMJ. Subsequently she underwent bilateral arthroscopy and arthrocentesis with bilateral morphine injections; the three third molars were also surgically removed. Arthroscopic examination revealed bilateral hyperaemia and adhesion formation within the joints capsule, with minor erosions of the condylar surface and early osteophyte formation. Postoperatively the patient was covered with analgesics, antimicrobials and steroids (dexamethasone). One-year follow-up revealed control of symptoms.

SUMMARY

Patients with JHS or EDS may present with various TMJ pathologies including painful myospasm, osteoarthrosis and other degenerative diseases, disc perforation, internal derangement and haemarthrosis. Care must be taken when managing those patients; surgical intervention should be the last choice with arthroscopy/arthrocentesis being the first intervention. Even then, this group is characterized by prolonged postoperative pain and while arthroscopy is usually performed as a day case (general anaesthesia), the authors advise a low threshold for admitting the patient for the first postoperative night at least.

References

Arneson MA, Hammerschmidt DE, Furcht LT, et al: A new form of Ehlers-Danlos syndrome. Fibronectin corrects defective platelet function, *JAMA* 11; 244(2):144–147, 1980.

Buckingham RB, Braun T, Harinstein DA, et al: Temporomandibular joint dysfunction syndrome: a close association with systemic joint laxity (the hypermobile joint syndrome), *Oral Surg Oral Med Oral Pathol* 72(5):514–519, 1991.

Fridrich KL, Fridrich HH, Kempf KK, et al: Dental implications in Ehlers-Danlos syndrome. A case report, *Oral Surg Oral Med Oral Pathol* 69(4):431–435, 1990.

Goodman RM, Allison ML: Chronic temporomandibular joint subluxation in Ehlers-Danlos syndrome: report of case, *J Oral Surg* 27(8):659–661, 1969.

Gould JF: Shortening of the temporalis tendon for hypermobility of the temporomandibular joint, *J Oral Surg* 36(10):781–783, 1978.

Harinstein D, Buckingham RB, Braun T, et al: Systemic joint laxity (the hypermobile joint syndrome) is associated with temporomandibular joint dysfunction, *Arthritis Rheum* 31(10):1259–1264, 1988.

Howe AG, Kent JN, Farrell CD, et al: Implant of articular eminence for recurrent dislocation of the temporomandibular joint, *J Oral Surg* 36(7):523–526, 1978.

Jerjes W, Upile T, Abbas S, et al: Muscle disorders and dentition-related aspects in temporomandibular disorders: controversies in the most commonly used treatment modalities, *Int Arch Med* 30(1):23, 2008.

Létourneau Y, Pérusse R, Buithieu H: Oral manifestations of Ehlers-Danlos syndrome, *J Can Dent Assoc* 67(6):330–334, 2001.

McDonald A, Pogrel MA: Ehlers-Danlos syndrome: an approach to surgical management of temporomandibular joint dysfunction in two cases, *J Oral Maxillofac Surg* 54(6):761–765, 1996.

Medra AM, Mahrous AM: Glenotemporal osteotomy and bone grafting in the management of chronic recurrent dislocation and hypermobility of the temporomandibular joint, *Br J Oral Maxillofac Surg* 46(2):119–122, 2008.

Pogrel MA, Kaban LB: The role of a temporalis fascia and muscle flap in temporomandibular joint surgery, *J Oral Maxillofac Surg* 48(1):14–19, 1990.

Rossi DC, Kappel DA: Temporalis muscle osteofascial flap reconstruction of a temporomandibular joint disk in an Ehlers-Danlos patient, *Plast Reconstr Surg* 117(3):40e–43e, 2006.

Sacks H, Zelig D, Schabes G: Recurrent temporomandibular joint subluxation and facial ecchymosis leading to diagnosis of Ehlers-Danlos syndrome: report of surgical management and review of the literature, *J Oral Maxillofac Surg* 48(6):641–647, 1990.

Schmoker R, Spiessl B, Trzeciak W: Plastic bolting device for the temporomandibular joint for treatment of hypermobility (Re-examination results of the first 28 cases), *SSO Schweiz Monatsschr Zahnheilkd* 89(3): 213–221, 1979.

Westling L: Temporomandibular joint dysfunction and systemic joint laxity, *Swed Dent J Suppl* 81:1–79, 1992.

12.8 The thoracolumbar spine

Kaye Walls

With contribution from Alan J Hakim

INTRODUCTION

Non-specific low back pain affects all ages and is thought to affect 70% of people in industrialized countries (Van Tulder et al 2006, Chou et al 2007). Many practitioner groups have endeavoured to put guidelines in place for the classification and management of this patient group (Richardson & Jull 2000, Comerford & Mottram 2001, Sahrmann 2002, O'Sullivan 2005).

The clinical presentation of individuals with joint hypermobility syndrome (JHS) may include symptoms of low back pain which can extend into the thoracic spine. This may be a result of trauma, or may be of insidious onset with no obvious cause. The diagnosis of instability in the lumbar or thoracic spine is controversial, because there are no clear criteria for diagnosis either clinically or radiologically (Nizard et al 2001, Leone 2007). It is only through careful questioning, examination and considered clinical reasoning that patients with spinal symptoms can be successfully managed.

CATEGORIZING BACK PAIN

It is important to remember that not all 'back pain' is musculoskeletal in origin; retroperitoneal, aortic and pelvic pathologies should always be considered.

Non-specific pain is said to account for 80–85% of low back pain. Though a cause may not be clear, instability (see below) should be considered.

Classically, the duration of pain is used to describe 'acute' (duration < 6 weeks) and 'chronic' (> 12 weeks). Approximately 25% of the adult population report acute pain within any 3 month period, and 5–7.5% a severe episode > 1 day within the previous year, with a peak presentation age of 35–50 years. Over 90% will recover within 6 weeks (hence the definition threshold). Approximately 12% of the population are disabled to one degree or another by chronic low back pain (Van Tulder et al 2006, Chou et al 2007).

Neuropathic pain accounts for at least one third of acute and chronic low back pain. It is a composite set of symptoms including burning, 'electric shock', and paraesthesia, well documented and assessed using the tool painDetect® (Freynhagen et al 2006).

Back pain symptoms are also classified as 'Red Flag' i.e. potentially serious organic pathology, or 'Yellow Flag' i.e. related psychosocial concerns (Boxes 12.8.1 and 12.8.2).

Specific causes of low back pain are uncommon and account for less than 15% of all conditions. These include:

- symptomatic herniated disc (4%)
- compression fracture (4%)
- spinal stenosis (3%)
- cancer (0.7%)
- ankylosing spondylitis (0.3%)
- cauda equina syndrome (0.04%)
- spinal infection (0.01%).

BOX 12.8.1 'Red Flag' symptoms and history in back pain

- Age of onset < 20 years and > 55 years
- Recent Hx of trauma
- Pain constant, progressive, no relief with rest
- Thoracic pain
- PMHx malignancy
- Osteoporosis risk
- Infection risk
- Systemically unwell – weight loss/fever, etc.
- Neurological symptoms/including bladder function
- Structural deformity

BOX 12.8.2 'Yellow Flag' symptoms and history in back pain

- Belief that pain and activity are harmful
- 'Sickness behaviour', e.g. extended rest
- Low/negative mood
- Work environment (low support/satisfaction conflicting evidence for high pace/demand)
- Seeking treatments that seem excessive/ inappropriate
- Inappropriate expectations
- Lack of social support in private life (moderate evidence)
- Compensation claims

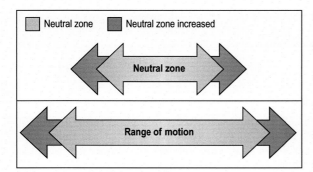

Fig. 12.8.1 The neutral zone *(after Panjabi 1992a)*

All these issues and diagnoses should be considered in the hypermobile patient. More often, however, no apparent pathology is found, yet the 'non-specific' pain may be a consequence of instability, which constitutes the discussion for the remainder of this chapter.

STABILITY OF THE SPINE

Spinal stability results from an interaction of structure and neuromuscular function. Panjabi (1992a) described the neutral zone, a part of physiological movement, as 'a small range of displacement near the joint's neutral position where minimal resistance is given by the osteoligamentous structures' (Fig. 12.8.1). This neutral zone may be increased in hypermobile patients due to collagen changes in connective tissue matrix proteins causing laxity of supporting structures. It may be further increased by injury, articular degeneration and weakness of the stabilizing musculature.

Panjabi (1992b) also described a model of spinal stability which is dependent on three subsystems that are functionally interrelated. They are:

- the passive subsystem (consisting of the facet joints, the intervertebral joints, the intervertebral discs, joint capsule and ligaments)
- the active subsystem (consisting of the muscles and tendons surrounding the joint)
- the control or neural and feedback subsystem (consisting of movement receptors in tendons, ligaments and muscles and the neural control centres).

The connective tissue laxity associated with JHS has the potential to affect each of these subsystems and adversely influence stability in the spine (Fig. 12.8.2).

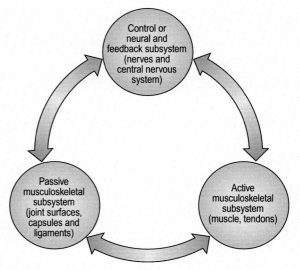

Fig. 12.8.2 Components contributing to joint stability *(after Panjabi 1992b)*

Ligamentous laxity often results in more 'give' in the spine of the hypermobile person, thus allowing them to demonstrate a greater range. In the assessment of spinal movement, knowledge of the normal range of movement throughout the spine and hips is essential. Generally, a spine is thought to be hypermobile if, during forward flexion, the palms can be placed on the floor with the knees straight (Chapter 1). However, this functional movement does not give information of the relative contributions made by the hip joints, lumbar and thoracic spine (Corben et al 2008).

The myofascial system of the thoracic and lumbar spine involves deep and superficial muscles as well as the fascial system. The deep postural muscles, such as multifidus and transversus abdominus, contract tonically to provide good neutral alignment, pre-activation or feedforward control of movement. The more superficial muscle system, which includes the oblique abdominals, latissimus dorsi and the gluteus maximus muscle, has phasic fibre recruitment characteristics to provide movement. Contraction of these large muscles puts the thoracolumbar and thoracodorsal fascia under tension which allows forces to be transmitted from trunk to lower limbs and trunk to upper limbs.

MOTOR CONTROL

The central and peripheral nervous system is the control system which responds to feedforward and feedback mechanisms, producing the static and dynamic stability required for normal function. Feedback mechanisms originate in the periphery from continuous sensory impulses, via receptors in muscles, tendons and joints. Information from the muscle spindles and golgi tendon organs ensures a constant monitoring of muscle length and tension. It serves to provide proprioception, detect movement and preset and regulate muscle stiffness (tone). Proprioceptive acuity is reduced in individuals with JHS (Mallik et al 1994, Hall et al 1995, Ferrell et al 2004) and often affects their ability to find lumbar neutral and maintain this during movement (Chapter 6.4).

Feedforward mechanisms ensure that the body is responsive to all input from the periphery and higher centres for function. These mechanisms ensure smooth, correctly timed movements with a resultant force that is adequate to control the amount of glide within the neutral zone. In the lumbar spine, the deep muscle system contracts milliseconds before peripheral movement occurs (Hodges & Richardson 1998). This is known as 'setting' of deep muscle, and implies a readiness for movement, which provides postural control. With chronic low back pain this feedforward mechanism is inhibited leading to a delay in deep muscle recruitment (Hodges & Richardson 1998). Hides et al (1994) suggest this may be due to inhibition via a long loop reflex, while Radebolde et al (2001) demonstrated that a deficiency in proprioception is a main cause of the delayed muscle response. Preuss and Fung (2005) hypothesize that acute low back pain during submaximal activities may be due to a temporary loss of stability at an intervertebral segment. This may cause transient segmental 'buckling' (i.e. the segment will briefly exceed its maximum safe range of motion) due to transient loss of co-ordination or control of one or more intersegmental muscles. Errors in neuromuscular control, that is feedforward and feedback modulation, are thought to be predisposing factors.

INSTABILITY OF THE LUMBAR SPINE

STRUCTURAL INSTABILITY

Young people who have inherent flexibility are drawn into activities such as ballet and gymnastics (Gannon & Bird 1999, McCormack et al 2004) which involve repeated loading of lumbar structures in extension. For hypermobile participants this may create a risk of stress fracture of the pars articularis causing spondylolysis, due to repetitive loading. Spondylolysis is a precursor to spondylolisthesis, which is a forward slippage of one vertebra on another. The occurrence rate of spondylolysis is thought to be as high as 47% in adolescent athletes with lumbar pain (Micheli & Wood 1995). There are, as yet, no data to support a link with JHS. Clinical examination should include single-leg lumbar extension test and standing extension stress test, which would increase pain on the ipsilateral side to the instability (Heck & Sparano 2000). If slippage has occurred, there may be a palpable step in the lower lumbar region, indicating forward movement of one vertebra on another. Any athlete who is less than 20 years of age, participates in a hyperextension sport, and has a positive extension test, warrants referral to a medical specialist to rule out spondylolysis. An oblique radiograph will confirm suspicion by the 'scotty dog' appearance of the pars defect.

FUNCTIONAL INSTABILITY

Instability not related to trauma is more difficult to recognize and consequently more difficult to manage. The diagnosis of lumbar instability is controversial in the absence of structural changes on X-ray. There are many different presentations and no clear criteria for diagnosis either clinically or radiologically (Nizard et al 2001, Leone 2007). Many authors have written describing assessment techniques and rehabilitation protocols for lumbar instability with chronic low back pain patients (Richardson & Jull 2000, Comerford & Mottram 2001, Sahrmann 2002, O'Sullivan 2000, 2005), although there is little or no reference to patients with joint hypermobility (JHM).

INSTABILITY OF THE THORACIC SPINE

MASQUERADERS

Thoracic pain can be benign in origin, but clinicians need to be alert when faced with isolated thoracic pain. Thoracic spinal pain is often caused by metastases, most commonly from the lung or breast (Greenhalgh & Selfe 2006). Most internal organs can refer to the spine and present as thoracic or lumbar pain (Grieve 2000). Patients with mechanical disc disorders of the thoracic spine comprise only 1.96% of all patients with mechanical low back pain (McKenzie 1990).

RELATIVE FLEXIBILITY

However, if the thoracic spine is habitually used in flexion, an extension dysfunction will occur. Relating to the concept of 'the path of least resistance' (Sahrmann 2002), any function requiring spinal extension is preferentially likely to occur in the more mobile segments above and below the stiff thoracic spine. The points of 'give' and potential overuse, are the mid cervical segments and the lumbar spine, at the levels of L4/5 and L5/S1, which are the most mobile lumbar segments. Clinical observation has shown that hypermobile patients often brace or stiffen their thoracic spine to provide stability, leading to overuse of other segments of the spine.

ROTATIONAL INSTABILITY

Research has shown that thoracic anatomical changes occur commonly within the general population (Wood et al 1995) and it is hypothesized that these changes predispose the patient to the development of instability of the thoracic spine. If changes occur in the disc, then rotational instability is thought to occur. Specific mobility testing of segmental spinal movements and of lateral translation at the costo-vertebral joints will detect this instability (Lee 1996).

RIB SUBLUXATION/DISLOCATION

Hypermobile patients may report popping or clunking in the thoracic spine, often after lifting a heavy weight or sometimes changing out of a rotated position, for example, getting up from lying on a couch after watching television. Pain may be localized over the costovertebral joints, be aggravated by spinal movements and with deep breathing, and may or may not radiate around the chest wall. Specific mobility testing at segmental level will confirm the diagnosis. Patients respond well initially to taping to relieve pain and support the area, followed by specific stabilization exercises for intervertebral muscles, especially multifidus.

DYSAUTONOMIA

The autonomic nervous system (ANS) is an important consideration when discussing the thoracic spine. The sympathetic trunk lies closely associated with the thoracic vertebrae and costovertebral joints and may be subject to compromise through direct and indirect trauma to the area, such as a rotational injury occurring during a road traffic accident. There is evidence that symptoms of dysautonomia are a prominent feature common to JHS, chronic fatigue syndrome and fibromyalgia (Tulloch & Phillips 2008) (Chapters 5 and 6.1).

PHYSIOTHERAPY ASSESSMENT

Clinical experience has shown that the key to managing these patients is a thorough assessment. Discussing and agreeing treatment goals that are specific, measurable, applicable, realistic and timed, is helpful in treatment planning and managing expectations. These goals should be activity-based and not pain-related, since the subjectivity and inconsistency of pain make it unhelpful in goal setting. Psychosocial factors must be addressed concurrently and, if necessary, a multidisciplinary approach should be taken (Chapter 8).

SUBJECTIVE

Sufficient time must be allowed to listen to the patient and hear the history of their presenting condition, any previous treatment and its effect. It is well documented that the severity of an individual's functional impairment is greatly affected by personality, anxiety and depression (Waddell 2004). Listening to the patient will give an indication of the extent to which they have developed coping strategies. If, after careful questioning, serious spinal pathology is suspected, the patient should be referred for a medical opinion. It is helpful to identify the presence of 'Yellow Flags' (Box 12.8.2), which are associated with a poor prognostic outcome (Kendall et al 1997).

Body chart

Mapping the area of pain is important. One must consider local structures which could generate these symptoms and other areas that could refer to this area, for example, the cervical spine (C3–7) can refer to the scapula. Hypermobile patients often report that they feel unstable. Commonly they describe their back pain symptoms as 'recurrent, constant, catching, locking or giving way' (Cook et al 2006). Noting the intensity, depth, spread and relationship of symptoms is also helpful.

Behaviour of symptoms

Questions about aggravating and easing factors will give insight into postures and activities which are a problem. Sitting is frequently difficult, with low or prolonged sitting provoking spinal pain as it encourages spinal flexion. If sitting at work is a problem, a discussion around how workplace ergonomics can be improved is useful. An increase in pain with prolonged standing may indicate weakness of the deep postural muscles and poor control of hyperextension at the knees.

OBJECTIVE

Objective examination should involve a global assessment of general function to assess postural alignment, to see how the patient moves and changes position, and the efficiency of global proprioception, co-ordination and balance. Commonly, patients move quickly to compensate for poor proprioception and this deficit is only detected when the patient is asked to walk slowly, or backwards, or with the eyes closed.

Observation

When observing relaxed stance, the hypermobile patient will often 'hang at the end of range' of many joints and present with anterior pelvic tilt, increased lumbar lordosis, increased thoracic kyphosis, forward head on neck posture, hyperextended knees and pronated feet. This may be described as a kyphosis-lordosis or sway back posture where there is anterior pelvic tilt and relative hip flexion. This is a deviation from the proposed model of 'ideal alignment' (Kendall et al 1993). It has been postulated that this is an attempt to gain more stability through resting at the end of range of hypermobile joints (Keer 2003) (Chapter 9), and thought to be due to muscle deconditioning, poor joint proprioception and poor body awareness.

Movement analysis

It is essential to look at the whole spine for relative flexibility, that is, areas of stiffness, areas of 'give', and compensations at other joints. Hypermobile

patients often demonstrate abnormal spinal motion during active sagittal plane movements (flexion or extension), with or without an arc of pain. The emphasis is on abnormal movement rather then a restricted range of movement. It is often possible to see an 'instability jog' during one or more movements, particularly in flexion and on returning to neutral from flexion or side flexion (Pope et al 1992). An instability jog is a sudden movement shift or 'rippling' of the muscles during active movement, indicating an unstable segment. With instability there is often an inability to return to neutral from the fully flexed position without flexing the knees or 'walking' the hands up the legs. This demonstrates a lack of segmental control, which is primarily the function of the deep muscle system. Sometimes, simply teaching a patient to recruit the deep transversus abdominus muscle and repeating the movement while holding this contraction produces a favourable change in symptoms, which helps to confirm the hypothesis. There may also be pivoting or hinging with movement (Fig. 12.8.3), or muscle guarding or

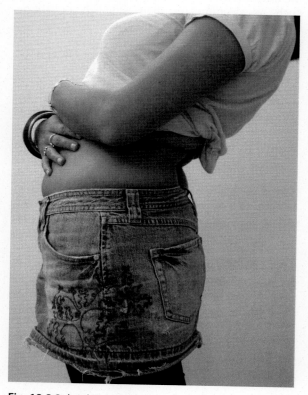

Fig. 12.8.3 Lumbar spine segmental hinging

spasm (Cook et al 2006). Dynamic palpation of spinous process gapping during flexion may help to identify hypermobility at segmental level. Accessory palpation of individual joints detects an abnormal compliance, indicating loss of stiffness or increased neutral zone at one segment (Schneider 2000). This can be addressed by retraining the deep multifidus muscle at that level (Richardson & Jull 2000) which will also address the dysfunction which occurs following an acute episode of pain (Hides 1994).

TREATMENT PRINCIPLES

Developing a good rapport with the patient is essential from the beginning. Education about the effects of joint hypermobility helps the patient to understand joint protection principles as they relate to their spine. This must start with general postural awareness and teaching the individual to find and maintain a 'spinal neutral' position in sitting and standing. This principle is extended to include advice about other unhelpful postures, such as sleeping on their stomach or sitting slumped. These measures often ease some of their acute pain immediately. Manual therapy may be of value to modulate pain if appropriately applied (Geisser et al 2005, Nijs & Van Houdenhove 2009), to mobilize stiff joints and release soft tissue restrictions. In addition, on the basis of a case study, Tulloch and Phillips (2008) propose that physiotherapy can influence ANS symptoms in an individual with CFS and JHS.

Motor control retraining starts immediately with recruitment of the deep stability muscles (transversus abdominis, multifidis, pelvic floor), in an antigravity position such as crook lying. Training of the deep abdominal muscles in isolation from other trunk muscles has been shown to improve the timing and activation of the trained muscles (Hall et al 2007). The importance of contracting at a low level and sustaining a contraction must be stressed in order to improve muscle endurance.

Progression to static control in different positions is the next stage of retraining, followed by dynamic stability under low load and progressing on to gradually increasing the load. Retraining of feedforward mechanisms is achieved by providing proprioceptive input at every level of motor retraining, such as tactile stimulation, visual stimulation (use of mirrors), and providing an unstable surface, such as using air cushions, balance boards and the Swiss ball. This, together with closed kinetic chain exercises, progressing to unilateral from bilateral will challenge proprioception further (Ferrell et al 2004).

Varying the load and speed of activity will also facilitate feedforward processing.

Late-stage motor retraining requires many repetitions in different functional situations, relevant to the individual, such as walking, climbing stairs and sitting at a desk at school or work. Fatigue is often a problem, so it is important not to overload the patient with too many home exercises. An ergonomic assessment of the workplace may also be needed.

EMPHASIS ON FUNCTION

It has been our clinical observation that hypermobile patients experiencing long-standing, widespread, chronic pain may need a more functional approach to treatment. This involves an emphasis on functional goals and pacing of activities. Education about chronic pain mechanisms helps the patient to understand and work with a level of pain in order to build up their level of activity. Advice on how to cope with flare-ups of pain can be reassuring and allows the patient to be more self-sufficient. This patient group are challenging to treat and often require a multidisciplinary approach.

SUMMARY

Patients with JHS affecting the thoracolumbar region often present a complex clinical picture. For the therapist a good background knowledge of the condition, of spinal anatomy and stabilizing mechanisms, combined with a thorough assessment is vital in the management of these patients. Sound clinical reasoning and effective communication skills are essential to help the patient understand their condition, and stay motivated to comply with exercise which should become an everyday part of their life. The ultimate goal for these patients is to foster self-management. For a proportion of these patients physiotherapy alone is insufficient, and referral to a multidisciplinary team is more appropriate.

References

Chou R, Amir Q, Snow V, et al: Diagnosis and Treatment of Low Back Pain: A Joint Clinical Practice Guideline from the American College of Physicians and the American Pain Society, *Ann Intern Med* 147(7):478–491, 2007.

Comerford MJ, Mottram SL: Functional stability re-training: principles and strategies for managing mechanical dysfunction, *Man Ther* 6(1):3–14, 2001.

Cook C, Brismee JM, Sizer PS: Subjective and objective descriptors of clinical lumbar spine instability: A Delphi study, *Man Ther* 11(1):11–21, 2006.

Corben T, Lewis J, Petty N: Contribution of lumbar spine and hip movement during the palms to floor test in individuals with diagnosed hypermobility syndrome, *Physiother Theory Pract* 24:1–12, 2008.

Ferrell WR, Tennant N, Sturrock RD, et al: Amelioration of symptoms by enhancement of proprioception in patients with joint hypermobility syndrome, *Arthritis Rheum* 50(11):3323–3328, 2004.

Freynhagen R, Baron R, Gockel U, et al: painDETECT: a new screening questionnaire to identify neuropathic components in patients with back pain, *Curr Med Res Opin* 22(10):1911–1920, 2006.

Gannon LM, Bird HA: The quantification of joint laxity in dancers and gymnasts, *J Sports Sci* 17:743–750, 1999.

Geisser ME, Wiggert EA, Haig AJ, et al: A randomized controlled trial of manual therapy and specific adjuvant exercise for chronic low back pain, *Clin J Pain* 21(6):463–470, 2005.

Greenhalgh S, Selfe J: *Red flags: A guide to identifying serious pathology of the spine*, Edinburgh, 2006, Churchill Livingstone.

Grieve GP: The Masqueraders. In Boyling JD, Palstanga N, editors: *Grieve's Modern Manual Therapy*, ed 2, Edinburgh, 2000, Churchill Livingstone, pp 841–856.

Hall MG, Ferrell WR, Sturrock RD: The effect of hypermobility on knee joint proprioception, *Br J Rheumatol* 34:121–125, 1995.

Hall L, Tsao H, Macdonald D, et al: Immediate effects of co-contraction training on motor control of the trunk muscles in people with recurrent low back pain, *J Electromyogr Kinesiol* Nov 26, 2007. (Epub ahead of print).

Heck JF, Sparano JM: A classification system for the assessment of lumbar pain in athletes, *Journal of Athletic Training* 35(2):204–211, 2000.

Hides J, Stokes MJ, Saide M, et al: Evidence of lumbar multifidis muscle wasting ipsilateral to symptoms in patients with acute/subacute low back pain, *Spine* 19(2):165–172, 1994.

Hodges PW, Richardson CA: Delayed postural contraction of transverses abdominis in low back pain associated with movement of the lower limbs, *Journal of Spinal Disorders Technology* 11:46–56, 1998.

Keer R: Physiotherapy assessment of the hypermobile adult. In Keer R, Grahame R, editors: *Hypermobility Syndrome: Recognition and Management for Physiotherapists*, Edinburgh, 2003, Butterworth Heinemann, pp 67–86.

Kendall FP, McCreary EK, Provance PG: *Muscles testing and Function*, ed 4, USA, 1993, Williams and Wilkins.

Kendall NAS, Linton SJ, Main C: Guide to assessing psychosocial yellow flags in acute low back pain: Risk factors for long term disability and work loss, Wellington, 1997, Accident Rehabilitation and Compensation Insurance Corporation of New Zealand and the National Health Committee.

Lee DG: Rotational instability of the mid-thoracic spine: assessment and management, *Man Ther* 1(5):234–241, 1996.

Leone A: Lumbar vertebral instability: a review, *Radiology* 245(1):62–77, 2007.

McCormack M, Briggs J, Hakim A, et al: A study of joint laxity and the impact of the Benign Joint Hypermobility Syndrome in student and professional ballet dancers, *J Rheumatol* 31(1):173–178, 2004.

McKenzie R: *The cervical and thoracic spine, Mechanical Diagnosis and Therapy*, Waikanae, 1990, Spinal Publications.

Mallik AK, Ferrell WR, McDonald AG, et al: Impaired proprioceptive acuity at the proximal interphalangeal joint in patients with hypermobility syndrome, *Br J Rheumatol* 33:631–637, 1994.

Micheli IJ, Wood R: Back pain in young athletes: Significant differences from adults in causes and patterns, *Archives of Pediatric Adolescent Medicine* 149:15–18, 1995.

Nijs J, Van Houdenhove B: From acute musculoskeletal pain to chronic widespread pain and fibromyalgia: Application of pain neurophysiology in manual therapy, *Man Ther* 14:3–12, 2009.

Nizard RS, Wybier M, Laredo JD: Radiologic assessment of lumbar intervertebral instability and degenerative spondylolisthesis, *Radiol Clin North Am* 39(1):55–71, 2001.

O'Sullivan P: Lumbar segmental 'instability': clinical presentation and specific stabilizing exercise management, *Man Ther* 5:2–12, 2000.

O'Sullivan P: Diagnosis and classification of chronic low back pain disorders: Maladaptive movement and motor control impairments as underlying mechanism, *Man Ther* 10:242–255, 2005.

Panjabi MM: The stabilizing system of the spine. Part I Function, dysfunction, adaption and enhancement, *J Spinal Disord* 5(4):383–389, 1992a.

Panjabi MM: The stabilizing system of the spine. Part II Neutral zone and instability hypothesis, *J Spinal Disord* 5(4):390–397, 1992b.

Pope MH, Frymoyer JW, Krag MH: Diagnosing instability, *Clinical Orthopaedic Related Research* 279:60–67, 1992.

Preuss R, Fung J: Can acute low back pain result from segmental buckling during sub-maximal activities? A review of the current literature, *Man Ther* 10:14–20, 2005.

Radebolde A, Cholewicki J, Polzhofer GK, et al: Impaired postural control of the lumbar spine is associated with delayed muscle response times in patients with chronic idiopathic low back pain, *Spine* 26(7):724–730, 2001.

Rasmussen-Barr E, Nilsson-Wikmar L, Arvidsson I: Stabilizing training compared with manual treatment in sub-acute and chronic low back pain, *Man Ther* 8(4):233–241, 2003.

Richardson CA, Jull GA: Concepts of assessment and rehabilitation for active lumbar stability. In Boyling JD, Palastanga N, editors: *Grieve's Modern Manual Therapy*, ed 2, London, 2000, Churchill Livingstone, pp 705–720.

Sahrmann SA: *Diagnosis and Treatment of Movement Impairment Syndromes*, USA, 2002, Mosby.

Schneider G: Lumbar instability. In Boyling JD, Palstanga N, editors: *Grieve's Modern Manual Therapy*, ed 2, London, 2000, Churchill Livingstone, pp 441–451.

Tulloch E, Phillips C: Chronic fatigue syndrome: a possible role of mechanical treatment? A case study, *Physical Therapy Reviews* 13:111–118, 2008.

van Tulder M, Becker A, Bekkering T, et al: European guidelines for the management of acute nonspecific low back pain in primary care, *Eur Spine J* 15:S169–S191, 2006.

Waddell G: *The Back Pain Revolution*, ed 2, Edinburgh, 2004, Churchill Livingstone.

Wood KB, Garvey TA, Gundry C, et al: Magnetic resonance imaging of the thoracic spine, *J Bone Joint Surg* 77A(11):1631–1637, 1995.

Chapter 13

Principles of rehabilitation and considerations for sport, performance and fitness

Jane Simmonds

INTRODUCTION

It is now widely accepted that for most individuals, well-designed exercise programmes and participation in appropriate physical activity not only reduce the risk of ill health, but are also an effective tool for improving the health of asymptomatic and symptomatic individuals (Bird et al 1998, Woolf-May 2006).

There is increasing evidence to support the beneficial effects of exercise in the management of individuals with joint hypermobility syndrome (JHS). Kerr et al (2000) report a good response to a daily monitored and modified exercise programme in children, and Shoen et al (1982) and Ferrell et al (2004), reported similar beneficial effects in adults. In their case studies, Simmonds and Keer (2008) and Hinton (1986), report favourable outcomes using carefully prescribed exercise as a primary intervention along with behaviour modification and lifestyle advice in both adults and adolescents.

The management of JHS can be complicated. Not only is there the challenge of improving static and dynamic joint stability and exercise tolerance, but also the associated problems of chronic pain and fatigue. Furthermore, joint hypermobility (JHM) is associated with fibromyalgia (FM) in adults and children (Chapter 5) (Goldman 1991, Gedalia et al 1993, Acasuso-Diaz & Collantes-Estevez 1998, Ofluoglu et al 2006, Sendur et al 2007).

Nevertheless, exercise plays a significant role in reducing symptoms. In the study by Goldman (1991), between 79% and 85% of the hypermobile patients diagnosed with FM displayed significant symptomatic improvements after performing a regular exercise programme. Although Cherpel and Marks (1999) cite criticisms of the study design, they make the comment that it is one of the few published papers demonstrating the effects of exercise on individuals with JHM and FM and its potential for modifying the course of the syndrome. In addition, Busch et al (2008) report 'gold' level evidence for beneficial effects of supervised aerobic exercise training on physical capacity and FM symptoms, in their impressive systematic review of 34 studies. The research also suggests that strength training may be beneficial for some FM symptoms.

Physical therapies that have not taken account of the presence of JHM or JHS may either be non-beneficial or detrimental (Hakim & Ashton 2005).

This chapter will discuss the application of the fundamental principles of exercise physiology and training, in the context of the tissue changes associated with deconditioning (a common finding in both FM and JHS), in developing comprehensive rehabilitation and fitness conditioning programmes for individuals with JHS. The issues related to injury risk, screening and management strategies pertaining to sport and performance participation will be addressed.

THE PRINCIPLES OF REHABILITATION, HEALTH AND FITNESS

PHYSICAL FITNESS

Rehabilitation and fitness reconditioning programmes are dynamic systems of prescribed exercise and activities aimed at reversing and preventing the

© 2010 Elsevier Ltd.
DOI: 10.1016/B978-0-7020-3005-5.00026-4

deleterious effects of injury, disease and inactivity. They aim to restore the individual to their full health and physical fitness potential. The definition of health has been updated as not just being a disease-free state, but has been extended to include the physical, mental, social, emotional and spiritual state of the individual on a continuum from near death to optimal functioning (Bird et al 1998).

Physical fitness has been described by Lamb (1984) as 'the capacity of the individual to successfully meet the present and potential physical challenges of life and comprises of elements, such as flexibility, strength, anaerobic power, speed, and aerobic endurance'. Other parameters of balance, skill and co-ordination, speed and muscular endurance may also be added to give an even more comprehensive definition.

Research has repeatedly demonstrated that regular participation in appropriate physical activity or exercise benefits all members of the population, regardless of age, gender or whether they suffer from recognized medical conditions or not (Bird et al 1998, Dishman et al 2006, Woolf-May 2006). The benefits of exercise are listed in Box 13.1.

EXERCISE PRESCRIPTION

When designing exercise programmes for rehabilitation purposes the term exercise prescription

---

BOX 13.1	The benefits of exercise

- Improved quality of life
- Reduced risk of cardiovascular disease
- Reduced risk of obesity and type II diabetes
- Reduced risk of colon and breast cancer
- Reduced risk of osteoporosis
- Reduced risk of developing neurological conditions such as Alzheimer's and Parkinson's disease
- Improved mental health
- Improved emotional and psychological health
- Improved ability to cope with the demands of life
- Reduced severity of particular diseases and disorders
- Minimized effects of ageing
- Improved physical capacity
- Assists the socialization process
- Assists the growth and development of children and adolescents

---

is commonly used. This implies making an assessment, planning and advocating exercises tailored to meet an individual's needs. For the practitioner this means having a good understanding of the adaptive changes in body systems, particularly the cardiovascular and neuromusculoskeletal systems, in deconditioned states and during the reconditioning process. Additionally, it requires the therapist to have an understanding of the principles of exercise physiology and training.

In the author's experience, individuals with JHS often present for physiotherapy with multiple joint instabilities and in a deconditioned state. This is usually as a result of recurrent injury, pain and long-term postural misuse. Deconditioning and development of symptoms is often also associated with lifestyle or physical activity changes, for example a sudden increase or decrease in physical activity, following childbirth, moving from school to university or university to a sedentary job.

Joint instability has been suggested as the underlying cause of microtrauma and subsequent joint and muscle pain in children with JHS (Gedalia et al 1993). It may be further postulated that it is responsible for at least some of the pain experienced in the adult JHS population. Joint stability is determined by the efficient functioning of the neuromusculoskeletal system. Deficiency in any part of this system, resulting from inflammatory disease, trauma or neural impairment, compromises stability (Kerr et al 2000). Panjabi's model of spinal stability (Panjabi 1992a, 1992b) explores the interrelation between passive and dynamic joint stabilizers and the neutral zone and provides us with a good biomechanical model for understanding spinal and joint stability (Chapter 12.8). This theory, in combination with our growing understanding of the effects of pain on muscle inhibition, motor control and subtle neurophysiological abnormalities, often associated with JHS (Ferrell et al 2007) (Chapter 6.4), helps us to understand the susceptibility to instability, which individuals with generalized tissue laxity and JHS experience.

Understanding the neuromusculoskeletal adaptive changes to immobilization and reduced physical activity, in relationship to joint stability, is then of particular clinical significance in the management of JHM and JHS.

TISSUE RESPONSE TO IMMOBILIZATION AND REDUCED PHYSICAL ACTIVITY

CONNECTIVE TISSUE

The effects of immobilization on connective tissue have been studied extensively. Animal studies on rabbit knees by Akeson et al (1980) showed changes in collagen, glycosaminoglycans (GAG) and water content. It was also observed that the connective tissue when immobilized appeared 'woody', rather than glistening and this was believed to be due to water loss. Theories regarding the pathomechanics of joint contracture suggest that the loss of water and GAG increased the space between the collagen fibres, thereby altering the amount of free movement between fibres. This lack of movement made the tissue less elastic, less plastic and more brittle; the implication being that capsular structures, including ligaments, would fail at lower loads after periods of immobilization.

Ligaments

In addition to the effect of immobilization on connective tissue, specific changes in ligaments as a result of immobilization have been well documented. Ligaments, like bone, remodel as a response to mechanical stress. The effects of immobilization on knee joint ligaments have been widely researched and it is now well established in the literature that the amount of time the ligament is immobilized is much shorter than the amount of remobilization time necessary for the ligament to reach its full pre-immobilization strength. The ligaments become stronger and stiffer when subject to load. A study on the anterior cruciate ligaments of rats revealed that inactivity and rest resulted in weaker, less-compliant tissue (Cabaud et al 1980). Again, early animal studies performed on dogs and primates suggest that the alterations in the mechanical properties of ligaments are a result of increased osteoclastic activity at the bone–ligament junction rather than actual ligament atrophy (Laros 1971, Noyes et al 1974). These alterations lead to a decrease in tensile strength and reduce the ability of ligaments to provide joint stability.

Bone

Equilibrium of bone absorption and accretion are maintained by weight-bearing, muscular contraction, adequate nutrition and hormonal status. The rate of bone cell turnover decreases after 10–15 days of immobilization. Loss of bone density is evidenced by a loss of the normal trabeculae pattern. The mechanical properties of bone, including elastic resistance and hardness, steadily decline with increased duration of immobilization (Burdeaux & Huychinson 1953, Landry & Fleisch 1964, Hardt 1972). By 12 weeks of immobilization, bone hardness is reduced by 55–60% of normal. Most of these losses are recoverable by muscle contraction and weight bearing in a comparable period of time (Steinberg 1980). However, they will be influenced by adequate nutrition and hormonal status. Bed rest studies and space research have increased our understanding of the effects of loading on bone metabolism. Reduced physical activity prevents the normal mechanical load signals that act to maintain bone balance, resulting in increased bone resorption and insufficient bone formation. Temporary bed rest has been shown to result in bone loss averaging 1% per week (Donaldson et al 1970, LeBlanc et al 1990). Bone loss is proportional to the relative changes in loading with greater percentage of loss. A greater percentage of bone loss is seen in the lower limbs than upper limbs when physical activity is reduced.

Muscle

The effects of immobilization and inactivity on muscle have been thoroughly investigated and reported in the literature. Changes include the following; a decrease in fibre size, changes in sarcomere alignment and configuration, and reduced muscle mass (MacDougall et al 1977, Booth 1987, Harrelson 1998). Mitochondria are also reduced in number, size and function and together with the histochemical changes that occur with immobilization, result in a reduction in the oxidative capacity of muscle (Booth & Kelso 1973, MacDougall 1977, Booth 1987). This increases the fatigability of muscles and reduces muscle endurance, which has been shown to occur as early as 7 days post immobilization (Rifenberick & Max 1974).

Disuse atrophy occurs in both fast-twitch (type I) and slow-twitch (type II) muscle fibres, but it is generally accepted that there is greater degeneration in slow-twitch fibres (Harrelson 1998). The rate of muscle atrophy is greatest in the first 5–7 days of the immobilization period, after which the rate of loss slows significantly (Booth 1987).

Muscle atrophy resulting from immobilization appears to be selective. Like bone, muscle loss is proportional to function. For example, muscle associated with postural joint stability (vastus medialis obliquus (VMO) and hip abductors) appears to atrophy at a faster rate than muscle with a more global stabilizing function, and is commonly seen in the deconditioned JHS population. Muscles also atrophy as a result of reflex inhibition due to injury, pain and fear of pain, which are often significant factors in this client group, as well as inflammation (Harrelson 1998), which is less common.

Nerve

Central and peripheral nervous system changes including a reduction in the production of neurotrophic enzymes and reduced dendritic branches in the motor cortex (Chapter 3), reduced dopamine release and/or loss of dopamine receptors in the brain have been observed in association with reduced physical activity (Dishman et al 2006). These changes may result in an alteration in muscle fibre recruitment patterns and timing, leading to altered movement patterns and reduction in co-ordination and skill. Empirical data, however, suggest that there is a neural reflex causing muscle atrophy resulting from joint damage and immobilization (Engles 1994, Harrelson 1998).

CLINICAL IMPLICATIONS OF IMMOBILIZATION

Bone that has become osteopenic or osteoporotic as a result of immobilization is less able to bear weight or withstand the normal forces of compression, tension and shear. Due care must be taken when remobilizing (using manual techniques and exercise), particularly in vulnerable groups: the elderly, post-menopausal women and individuals who have been taking long-term steroids. Individuals with JHS may also be considered a risk group as there is evidence to show that low bone density is associated with Ehlers-Danlos syndrome (EDS) hypermobility type (formerly type III) and JHS (Mishra et al 1996, Nijs et al 2000). It can be

postulated that in the case of JHS, reduced activity due to pain or following injury may confer a significant risk for developing osteoporosis, particularly in post-menopausal women. Osteoporosis is a very large public health burden (WHO 2003) and the prevalence and cost associated with managing the disease are expected to escalate, therefore addressing the issue of bone health early in a person's life is very important.

Immobilization and inactivity of muscles results in weakness due to loss of muscle mass. Additionally, muscle stiffness occurs with the laying down of irregular cross-linked connective tissue. Postural slow-twitch muscle fibres crossing one joint tend to atrophy the fastest (Engles 1994). This will be evidenced in activities requiring sustained or repeated muscle contraction, i.e. standing, sitting and walking. Such changes also contribute to joint instability, a common feature in JHS. Rehabilitation should therefore focus initially on developing the endurance capacity and strength of the local postural antigravity muscles.

It has been suggested that abnormality of collagen synthesis is the pathogenic root of JHS (Child 1986). If this already fragile connective tissue is further compromised in terms of strength and stiffness as a result of immobilization, inactivity and deconditioning, it could have a major impact on joint stability for individuals with JHM. Changes in the muscle and connective tissues, in addition to alterations of neurodynamic function that occur as a result of de-conditioning and immobilization, may provide some explanation of the observation in clinical practice of individuals with JHS who have become inactive because of pain or injury often displaying considerable joint instability, reduced muscle strength, endurance, poor proprioception and vulnerability to injury.

TISSUE RESPONSE TO REMOBILIZATION, EXERCISE AND PHYSICAL ACTIVITY

Most studies investigating the response of bone and soft tissues to mobilization have primarily studied normal subjects. Muscles begin to regenerate within 3–5 days of the start of a reconditioning programme (Cooper 1972, Zarins 1982). Within the first week, muscle weight increases. Witzmann et al (1982) report that muscle strength can be regained by 6 weeks of exercise, however, normal muscle weight may not be fully achieved until

3 months. Early strength gains are attributed to neurological recruitment pattern changes while longer-term strength gains are observed later when adaptation of tissue has taken place (Sale 1988).

Recovery of bone, nerve and connective tissue occurs at a much slower rate than muscle, due to differences in vascularity. A healing ligament may take between 6 months and 3 years to recover fully, depending on the severity of the injury and length of time it has been immobilized (Tipton et al 1990). Thus, although applying the overload principle to connective tissues in the recovery phase is necessary, it needs to be undertaken with caution. Moderate-frequency, low-intensity endurance exercises have been shown to have a beneficial effect on the mechanical properties of ligaments. It has been suggested that such exercises result in increased collagen production, hypertrophy and realignment of fibre bundles, rendering them stiffer and able to tolerate heavier loads (Woo et al 1982). This claim is supported by the work of Cabaud et al (1980) and Williams et al (1988). Non-weight-bearing isometric exercises, although helpful, are not a substitute for weight-bearing. Future research investigating the tissue response of collagen-defective tissue to exercise will be important in understanding and prescribing exercises for individuals with JHM and connective tissue fragility.

APPLIED PRINCIPLES OF REHABILITATION AND TRAINING

It is important to have a holistic view when designing rehabilitation and fitness programmes for hypermobile individuals. Physiological (Chapter 6), psychological and sociological factors (Chapter 8) need to be considered and addressed. The programme should include well-paced and monitored training to improve (Chapter 9):

- proprioception, kinaesthetic sense, co-ordination, static and dynamic balance
- core/local stability muscle endurance and strength
- global muscle strength and endurance
- controlled flexibility
- cardiovascular and functional capacity fitness
- relaxation and breathing.

It is essential for rehabilitation professionals to have an understanding of motor learning theory and be able to apply these principles to individuals

recovering from injury and when reconditioning. It is beyond the scope of this chapter to provide an in-depth overview of motor learning, but the reader is directed to two well-known models which have been proposed. Fitts and Posner (1967) present a three-stage model consisting of a cognitive, associative and autonomous stage and a two-stage model was developed by Gentile in 1972 and further enhanced in 1986. In this model the learner moves from 'getting the idea' to 'fixation and diversification' in the second stage.

The important principles for the rehabilitator to take from these models are that new movements and exercises take time to assimilate and should be carefully and systematically introduced and taught to the individual. Furthermore, the amount and type of practice and feedback needs to suit the individual's learning style. This is important to all patients and clients, however, it is especially important for individuals with JHS, where sensory input may be altered, for individuals with co-ordination deficits and also for those who are fearful.

Understanding and applying the theories and principles of motivation, behaviour change and self-efficacy are also key elements to successful rehabilitation outcomes. Developing shared goals has been shown to assist with adherence and concordance with exercise programmes and making longer-term lifestyle changes. Self-efficacy, the self-belief that an individual has regarding his or her ability to complete certain tasks and to achieve particular outcomes (Bandura 2000) is also important to success. Therefore a person with low self-efficacy will require a more supportive approach than someone who is more confident that they will succeed.

The reader is recommended to review and consider the work of Bandura (2000) in relation to understanding and applying theories of self-efficacy and behaviour change in rehabilitation. Similarly, the work of Di Clementi & Valasquez (2002), and Prochaska & Norcross (2001), in relation to motivational interviewing and stages of change, provides insight and useful practical information when needing to address issues such as lifestyle modification and physical activity behaviour change. Facilitating change is complex; understanding the process involved is an important part of the rehabilitation of individuals with long-term conditions, in order to help them identify and overcome barriers to change.

Visualization techniques may be taught to help promote relaxation, reduce pain and aid recovery.

There is now evidence to suggest that visualization techniques can be used to gain strength (Burford 2008). Furthermore, advice on diet, adequate rest and pacing is also important. The importance of rest should not be underestimated, because, it is only during deep sleep that the muscles fully relax. When sleep is disturbed, muscles fatigue (Ali 2001). Exercise classes and the use of music may also assist motivation and compliance.

PRINCIPLES OF EXERCISE PHYSIOLOGY AND TRAINING

Knowledge and application of the principles of exercise physiology and training are essential in designing effective rehabilitation programmes. These principles were originally developed by exercise physiologists to provide effective guidelines for athletic and sports training. They have been adapted and used by those involved with rehabilitation to optimize recovery after injury, disease and immobilization.

The classic texts by Rasche and Burke (1977) and Katch et al (2006) discuss the principles in detail. Harrelson and Leaver-Dunn (1998) include an excellent section on the principles of training in relation to sports rehabilitation. There follows a summary and discussion of the main principles and how they may be applied to rehabilitation in JHS and JHM.

Readiness principle

This can be understood to be the preparedness of an individual to undertake an exercise programme. The principle originally applied to athletes recommencing fitness training after acute injury or lay-off, but may also be applied to the rehabilitation situation. For example, in clinical practice, it is often necessary for a patient with JHS to have their pain moderated first, by medication and/or other therapeutic means, before being able to undertake a programme of exercise. It is equally important that the patient feels psychologically prepared and committed before commencing the programme.

Principles of self–efficacy and motivation

The readiness principle is closely associated with self-efficacy and motivation. The higher the self-efficacy rating the more likelihood there is of a positive outcome (Bandura 2000). Previous experience of exercise and physical activity plays an important role in an individual's beliefs. For example, if an individual has been successful in rehabilitation following previous injuries or bouts of pain, they will have a greater belief in their own ability to achieve a good outcome. Conversely, if individuals have had very negative or painful experiences of physical activity or exercise either at school in physical education or in physiotherapy, they are likely to have lower levels of self-efficacy and are less likely to comply, adhere and be successful with a programme of exercise. Where self-efficacy is low, rehabilitators need to spend more time educating and assisting in addressing barriers to exercise and change and provide positive feedback regarding accomplishments, even if very small.

Overload and progression principles

Beneficial human performance adaptations occur as a response to stress applied at levels beyond a certain threshold, but within certain limits of tolerance and safety (Katch et al 2006). Low levels of stress to which the body has already adapted are not sufficient to induce a further training response. In the useful range, i.e. where the stress is above the threshold, an adequate training response may cause some disruption of tissue and change in biomechanical balance. During the period between bouts of exercise, repair and restoration occur, after which an adaptation takes place in the tissue, raising the individual's stress threshold to a higher level. Because of the underlying defective collagen in the connective tissue of the hypermobile individual, it is important to be prudent when prescribing exercise, particularly with reference to increasing the number of repetitions and resistance. Stress is required to achieve strength or endurance gains, but if the threshold of a hypermobile individual is stressed beyond a certain limit, by too much and too early, there may be danger of symptom exacerbation and injury.

Specificity

Exercise, be it aimed at improving cardiovascular function, proprioception, or strength, needs to be targeted at specific systems and activities. For example, if one of the aims of a programme is to improve cardiovascular endurance, then the prescribed exercise needs to involve the large muscle groups and be performed for a minimum of two to three minutes in order to stimulate cardiac function and the aerobic energy system. Furthermore, if long distance running is an objective, then training the endurance capacity and functional actions of the muscle groups involved in running is also required. The exercise should be as closely related to the specific activity as possible. Therefore it is better to train on a bicycle, as opposed to a treadmill, if bicycling is the target activity.

Strength development in particular is known to be highly specific (Katch et al 2006). Strength can be divided into three discrete groups:

- dynamic strength, which is the ability to move or support the weight of the body repeatedly over a given period of time
- static strength, which is the ability to exert a maximum force continuously for a brief period of time
- explosive strength, which is the ability to exert maximum energy in one short burst (Rasch & Burke 1977).

In the case of JHM, both dynamic and static strength development are important for the development of joint stability. Therefore, when planning a programme of exercise specific types of strength training need to be considered.

Explosive strength applies particularly to sporting situations and should be specifically trained for should it be required, such as performing leaps in ballet, kicking in football or a sprint start in a 100-metre running event.

Intensity and frequency

Training needs to be sufficiently spaced to allow tissue growth, nutritional replenishment and biochemical resynthesis to take place. However, it needs to be frequent enough to stimulate neurophysiological change (Katch et al 2006). There are implications here for the JHS patient, as clinically, the author has found that recovery time after exercise is slow and the training response is reduced. This may be due to a multitude of reasons, such as lactic acid build-up and reduced oxidative functioning of the muscles, altered neuromuscular mechanisms, altered collagen synthesis and metabolic changes.

Issues of intensity and frequency are very important when designing exercise programmes for individuals with JHS, particularly those who suffer

from fatigue and more chronic and widespread pain. It is important to determine a baseline level of activity and facilitate the individual to pace the activity so that exercise is not too exhausting. In the author's experience careful spacing of exercise, physical activity and adequate rest is crucially important. Further investigation into this area is clearly required.

DESIGNING EXERCISE PROGRAMMES FOR JHS

ASSESSMENT

The problem-solving approach is the logical method for tackling the challenges of designing rehabilitation programmes. The assessment, including reliable and valid outcome measures, is crucial for identifying and prioritizing the problems to be addressed and evaluating the efficacy of the programme. Symptom irritability is frequently high in JHS and FM and often leads to an exacerbation of pain later. Questioning with regard to this is important and the objective assessment may need to be performed over several visits.

Subjective assessment

The subjective examination includes collecting information regarding age, race, gender, working status, stress levels and a current and past medical and family history. Of particular importance are questions or completion of questionnaires relating to current and past physical activity tolerance and preferred modes of exercise and physical activity. It is important to ask detailed questions relating to functional ability on good and bad days. This is helpful in determining the baseline functional level for the programme. An evaluation of current pain levels using a simple visual analogue scale (zero to ten) can be used. Alternatively, the short McGill Pain Questionnaire (Melzack 1987), or the SF36 short form questionnaire can be helpful.

Objective assessment and outcome measures

The objective assessment consists of documentable physical findings that the physiotherapist discovers through observation, inspection, palpation, muscle, joint and neurophysiological testing (Chapters 9, 10 and 11). In addition, when developing an exercise or fitness programme an assessment of cardiovascular function is required. It is important where possible to use reliable and valid outcome measures so that progress can be monitored.

Observation

The evaluation of posture, both dynamic and static, is of particular importance, as the impact of several hypermobile joints on the kinetic chain is substantial. Posture and gait analysis may be examined by direct observation or by photographic and video documentation, which provide excellent visual feedback systems for patient education and monitoring progress.

Functional active range of motion, muscle and nerve testing

Assessment of the quality and range of movement should be undertaken, observing both the recruitment and timing of muscle contractions. These elements affect static and dynamic joint stability, both of which are frequently impaired when individuals are requested to perform activities without locking their joints.

The assessment of the individual's ability to sustain static joint position and postures is crucially important and is largely determined by the degree of ligament laxity, muscle tone, static strength, proprioceptive ability and endurance capability of the muscles (Harrelson 1998). Specific static and dynamic muscle testing of core trunk stability muscles and other global and peripheral muscle groups should be assessed in functional positions as discussed in Chapter 9. For example, testing the ability to sustain a neutral knee joint position in standing can be useful in gauging functional isometric strength and endurance, particularly in a hypermobile individual who may have adopted the habit of 'hanging on their ligaments'.

Evaluation of the neural system structures may be necessary and includes testing mobility of the nervous system (Butler 2000) dermatome sensation, deep tendon reflexes and motor function.

Proprioception, kinaesthesia and co-ordination

The subject of proprioception deserves special attention when discussing the rehabilitation of hypermobile individuals. The component of neuromuscular control necessary for joint stability is very important in a rehabilitation programme (Harrelson & Leaver-Dunn 1998) and particularly so in the JHS population, where there are known deficits (Chapter 6.4).

Subjective and objective evaluations of proprioception, kinaesthesia and co-ordination can be assessed using a battery of tests, although clinical proprioceptive and kinaesthetic testing validation is still in its infancy. Balance exercises are most commonly used as subjective testing procedures for the lower limb and trunk proprioception, such as subjective observations of postural sway (Romberg's test), one-legged standing (stork test) and tandem Romberg's test (placement of one foot in front of the other, heel to toe) (Guskiewicz & Perrin 1996).

Functional capacity, cardiovascular and morphological measures

An assessment would not be complete without an evaluation of cardiovascular function or at least functional capacity. As discussed earlier in this chapter, a comprehensive rehabilitation plan should include global aerobic fitness measures. Baseline measures of blood pressure and resting heart rate need to be taken routinely. In the author's experience, low blood pressure is a frequent clinical finding in JHS. This has been associated with autonomic dysfunction in patients with JHS (Gazit et al 2003) (Chapter 6.1). Low blood pressure resulting in dizziness should be investigated and monitored before advocating any strenuous exercise. Any suggestion of cardiac or respiratory problems from the medical history should be thoroughly explored, because mitral valve pathologies may occasionally be associated with vascular type EDS and Marfan syndrome (Chapter 1). Postural tachycardia is also frequently found to be associated with the condition and should be investigated if suspected. Asthma and wheezing have also been found to be associated with JHS (Morgan et al 2007), so breathing exercises and education advice regarding use of inhalers should be addressed as necessary.

Cardiovascular function, functional capacity and walking ability can be assessed using a number of tests. The choice of test will depend on age, current disability and health. For older, less-able individuals, the 3-minute walk test as described by Worsford & Simpson (2001) may be used. The 10-metre increment shuttle walk test as described by MacSween et al (2001) is a useful baseline indicator of aerobic capacity.

For the fitter individual, the 3- or 5-minute step test, 6–12-minute walk test, Physical Work Capacity (PWC) 170 bike test and treadmill gas exchange tests can be utilized. The American College of Sports Medicine (2005) has produced good resources for exercise testing guidelines.

Body weight, girth measurements, height and percentage body fat may also be measured and documented to complete the morphological clinical picture.

ANALYSIS AND DEVELOPMENT OF THE REHABILITATION PROGRAMME

Following the examination and identification of a specific problems list, the rehabilitation programme can be designed. At this point it is a good idea for the physiotherapist and patient to develop shared and realistic short-, medium- and long-term goals. These goals may include strength and endurance gains, personal independence, weight loss, return to sport and return to work. It is also important at this point to spend time educating the patient about the nature of the condition, the rationale behind the approach to rehabilitation and the need for compliance to exercise, pacing of activities, modification of lifestyle, self-responsibility and joint care.

EARLY REHABILITATION

It is recommended that rehabilitation in the very early stage focuses on improving body awareness, proprioception and proximal joint stability. Muscle strengthening and endurance exercises may include isometric and joint proprioception exercises in pain-free positions, gradually progressing to functional positions. Exercise should be carefully monitored and paced to avoid flare up of symptoms and early failure (Moseley 2003). Swiss ball and hydrotherapy can be particularly useful, especially when dealing with patients where protective muscle spasm is an issue. It is important, particularly in the early stages, that exercises given to the patient, either during a therapy session or as home exercises, are pain-free. Clear instructions using the individual's preferred learning style and regular positive feedback help with skill acquisition, adherence and motivation. A distinction needs to be drawn between training pain and painful symptom exacerbation. This may mean modifying even the most simple exercise to ensure that it is being performed correctly and is appropriate for the individual's stage of rehabilitation. Where possible, recruitment of stability muscles, once learnt, can be encouraged during daily activities, such as walking, sit-to-stand, stairs and housework. Manual guidance, joint approximation techniques including PNF and rhythmic stabilization and the use of tape to facilitate proprioception (Callaghan et al 2002) may be helpful, although prudence is required where skin is fragile and sensitive.

MIDDLE STAGE

Once a reasonable level of proximal stability has been achieved, individuals should be encouraged to continue to improve their strength, endurance, balance and co-ordination and to engage in more regular physical activity. Graded exercises using theraband, aimed at improving both concentric and eccentric strength and endurance, are recommended along with the use of mirrors to enhance proprioception (Fig. 13.1). Controlled, supported stretching may be prescribed for tight tissues and clinical experience suggests that individuals with JHS frequently find stretching relieves sensations of stiffness and discomfort. Prudence is, however, recommended with stretching, since the hypermobile joints and more pliable muscles will have a tendency to stretch before the tighter tissues and may therefore lead to further muscle imbalance and aggravation of symptoms.

Achievable goals should continue to be discussed, agreed and monitored. The programme of rehabilitation reconditioning needs to be integrated and should address the three primary systems that influence normal movement: the cardiorespiratory, musculoskeletal and neurological systems. Cardiovascular training is an important component of the rehabilitation and reconditioning programmes. Importantly for JHS sufferers, cardiovascular training has been shown to help modulate pain, improve functional capacity and prevent a host of co-morbidities developing (Woolf-May 2006). Furthermore, there is conclusive evidence that it is beneficial for reducing the symptoms of FM (Busch et al 2008). Finding the aerobic exercise that an individual enjoys is very important as this will aid compliance. The Borg perceived exertion scale is a useful and valid tool for monitoring intensity

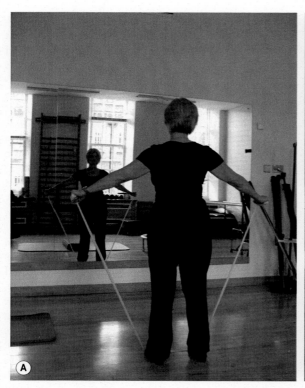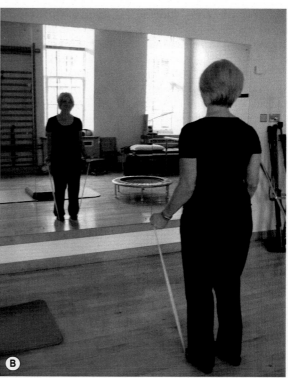

Fig. 13.1 Closed kinetic chain exercises using theraband and mirrors facilitate proprioception and motor unit recruitment: (a) shoulder abduction, (b) elbow flexion

of exercise (Borg 1982). Physical activity diaries, pedometers, accelerometers and heart rate variability monitors can all be used to help motivate and attain health-promoting, physical activity goals.

FINAL STAGES OF REHABILITATION AND FITNESS PROGRAMMES

Towards the later stages of rehabilitation, cardiovascular exercise can be increased to levels of between 60% and 80% of maximum heart rate. Attention to dynamic posture should continue to be emphasized. Use of light weights (Fig. 13.2), exercise bands and gym equipment can be used to improve strength, power and endurance. Climbing, an activity which requires the use of both the upper and lower limb stabilizers, has been found anecdotally to be helpful in improving dynamic core stability and integrated co-ordination. Nordic Poles and more advanced theraband activities can help to advance core strength and

dynamic stability. Vleeming's sling theory may support this suggestion (Lee & Vleeming 1998).

The time frame for rehabilitation of individuals varies according to the severity of the condition, level of deconditioning and commitment to the programme. Frequently, individuals with JHS need to be supervised and monitored for between 6 months and 2 years.

Maintenance of physical fitness and prevention of ill health through regular safe sport and physical activity is considered paramount for continued self-management of JHS. Individuals should be encouraged to develop a life-long commitment to physical activity and to remain fit through activities which are focused on neuromusculoskeletal control. Recommended activities therefore include recreational swimming, walking (with and without poles), Pilates, Tai Chi, Chi Gung, some forms of yoga and dance. Whatever form of sport or physical activity is adopted after the therapy intervention, it should be enjoyable, pain-free and relevant to the individual.

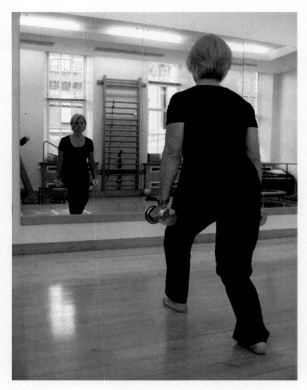

Fig. 13.2 Lunges using light weights in the final stages of rehabilitation

AQUATIC AND HYDROTHERAPY

Hydrotherapy and exercising in water is an effective and popular exercise medium for individuals with JHS. The combination of buoyancy, support and warmth makes it a very conducive arena for exercise. As well as being a medium for achieving physical goals, hydrotherapy has added psychological and social benefits (Skinner & Thomson 1993, Petajan 1996). The reduction in sympathetic activity that occurs as a result of buoyancy may alter tone, diminish pain and spasm and achieve relaxation. Sensory stimulus provided by turbulence can increase body awareness (Mano et al 1985, Hurley & Turner 1991, Fuller 1998). The three-dimensional resistive environment, combined with the viscosity of the water, aids kinaesthetic sense and improves the synchronization of motor unit contractions through the whole range of joint movement (Fuller 1998).

Bad Ragaz techniques as described by Davis & Harrison (1988), rhythmic stabilizations, isometrics,

slow walking and carefully controlled active exercises using open and closed chain movements are particularly helpful for developing core stability in the early and middle stages of rehabilitation. Exercises can be progressed using turbulence, webbed gloves and weights to increase resistance. Core stability, proprioception and balance can be further developed and progressed by reducing and/or modifying the base of support, for example, moving from arm exercises with a wide base of support to a narrow base (Fig. 13.3).

Once effective trunk and proximal stability have been achieved, deep water walking and running with the aid of a buoyancy vest can be used to improve co-ordination and cardiovascular fitness. This form of aerobic exercise training is particularly popular with injured athletes, those needing to lose weight, individuals with chronic low back pain and JHS sufferers, because they are often able to exercise for longer without exacerbation of symptoms. Water immersion has the added advantage of improving the circulation of blood to working muscles, which enhances oxygen supply and aids the removal of carbon dioxide and lactic acid (Fuller 1998). It is also a potent diuretic, natriuretic and kalluretic which may explain some of the perceived benefits (Grahame et al 1978).

Deep water running should not be undertaken in over-heated hydrotherapy pools because of the risk of hyperthermia and may be commenced with

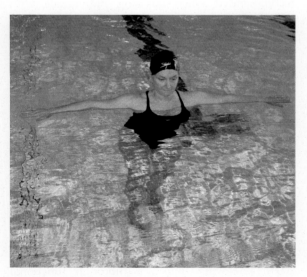

Fig. 13.3 Hydrotherapy is a useful medium for improving core stability, proprioception and balance

as little as 5 minutes. Speed and distance can then be gradually increased as tolerated, applying the principles of overload training as used for cardiovascular training.

HYPERMOBILITY, SPORT AND PERFORMANCE

Flexibility is an important physical fitness parameter in sport and in the performing arts. The combination of flexibility, neuromuscular control, dynamic co-ordination and rhythm are essential for most sporting and athletic performances. In particular, gymnastics, ballet and dance, playing of musical instruments, circus performance and diving require a high degree of flexibility. Grahame and Jenkins (1972) suggest that JHM may be viewed as an asset in ballet.

The relationship between generalized JHM, JHS and increased injury risk is not conclusive, but there is mounting evidence to suggest that JHM is an intrinsic injury risk factor in many sports and performance activities including: American football (Nicholas 1970), high-school athletics (Grana & Moretz 1978), gymnastics (Kirby et al 1981), basketball (Gray et al 1985), female soccer (Soderman et al 2001), professional ballet (Klemp & Learmouth 1984, McCormack et al 2004), male rugby (Stewart & Burden 2004) and junior netball (Smith et al 2005). Therefore a degree of caution is recommended when advising individuals with JHS in relation to sport and performance participation. Where appropriate, advice regarding correct-fitting footwear and the use of orthotics (to correct pes planus and lower limb alignment) is recommended.

Hypermobility and tissue laxity incur other risks related to tissue fragility including easy bruising, poor wound healing and hernias (Chapter 2). Sports physiotherapists, sports therapists, sport rehabilitators and trainers need to be aware of these clinical implications with regard to tissue healing. Interestingly, in a recent small study of professional soccer players in the UK, hypermobile individuals missed more training sessions and games when injured than their less-flexible counterparts, suggesting that recovery rate is slower for these individuals (Collinge & Simmonds 2009). Following injury, a thorough functional rehabilitation programme should be instituted with gradual return to training and match play. Education regarding joint care and tissue protection is recommended for coaches, parents and players.

Physiotherapists are encouraged to work closely with coaches, trainers, physical education teachers and fitness instructors in order to help raise awareness of JHS, prevent injury and pain and to assist in prehabilitation, rehabilitation and long-term management. Screening for hypermobility and JHS is advisable for children, adolescents and adults who wish to participate in competitive sport and performance activities in order to establish potential risk. Specific exercises and education can be given to prevent injury. In some cases, people may be steered away from particular sports and towards safer activities. Individuals with marked joint hypermobility, JHS, EDS, or Marfan syndrome (Chapter 1) should be screened for cardiorespiratory abnormality before undertaking strenuous physical activity. The presence of JHS, joint hypermobility and tissue laxity, joint instability, muscle imbalance, poor alignment, age and gender of the individual, skill level, personality type and the demands of the sport or performance should all be considered when determining an individual's suitability for a particular activity and to assist in the planning of individual training regimens.

SUMMARY

In summary, JHS is a complex multisystemic disorder, in which the management and rehabilitation process can be challenging, for both physiotherapist and patient, but essential in order to achieve a good quality of life. The development of an appropriate rehabilitation programme requires careful and thorough assessment, the formulation of realistic and shared goals and is underpinned by sound physiological and psychological principles. Progress is often slow and may be hampered by setbacks, exacerbation of pain and psychological distress. However, a comprehensive rehabilitation programme with careful progression of exercises and functional activities can result in substantial improvements which allow a hypermobile individual to remain fit and active, enjoying sport and performance for the benefit of their joints and general health throughout life.

References

Acasuso-Diaz M, Collantes-Estevez E: Joint hypermobility in patients with fibromyalgia syndrome, *Arthritis Care Res* 11(1):39–42, 1998.

Akeson WH, Amiel D, Woo S: Immobility effects of synovial joints: the pathomechanics of joint contracture, *Biorheology* 17:95–110, 1980.

Ali M: *The Integrated Health Bible*, London, 2001, Vermillion, pp 158–169.

American College of Sports Medicine (ACSM):*Guidelines for Exercise Testing and Prescription*, ed 7. Philadelphia USA, 2005, Lippincott, Williams and Wilkins.

Bandura A: Health promotion from the perspective of social cognitive theory. In Norman P, Abraham C, Connor M, et al, editors: *Understanding and changing health beliefs: from health beliefs to self regulation*, Reading, 2000, Harward Academic Publishers, pp 299–339.

Bird SR, Smith A, James K: Exercise and physical activity: an overview of the benefits, *Exercise Benefits and Prescription*, London, 1998, Nelson Thornes, pp 1–15.

Booth FW, Kelso JR: Effects of hind limb immobilization on contractile and histochemical properties of skeletal muscle, *Pflugers Archives* 342:231–238, 1973.

Booth FW: Physiological and biochemical effect of immobilization on muscle, *Clinics of Orthopaedics & Research* 219:15–20, 1987.

Borg GAV: Psychophysical bases of perceived exertion, *Medicine & Science in Sport and Exercise* 1(5):377–381, 1982.

Burdeaux BD, Hutchinson WJ: Etiology of traumatic osteoporosis, *J Bone Joint Surg* 35:479–488, 1953.

Burford C: *The use of mental imagery to improve the performance of the craniocervical flexion test*,

International Federation of Manipulative Therapists (IFOMT) proceedings, Rotterdam, 2008, June, 8–13.

Busch A, Schachter CL, Overend TJ, et al: Exercise for fibromyalgia: a systematic review, *J Rheumatol* 35(6):1130–1144, 2008.

Buttler DS: *The Sensitive Nervous System*, Adelaide, Australia, 2000, Neuro Orthopaedic Institute (NOI) Publications.

Cabaud HE, Chatty A, Gildengorin V: Exercise effects on the strength of the rat anterior cruciate ligament, *Am J Sports Med* 8:79–86, 1980.

Callaghan MJ, Selfe J, Bagley PJ, et al: The effect of patella taping on knee joint proprioception, *Journal of Athletic training* 37(1):19–24, 2002.

Cherpel A, Marks R: The benign joint hypermobility syndrome, *New Zealand Journal of Physiotherapy* 27:9–22, 1999.

Child AH: Joint hypermobility syndrome: Inherited disorder of collagen synthesis, *J Rheumatol* 113(2):239–243, 1986.

Collinge R, Simmonds JV: Hypermobility, injury rate and rehabilitation in a professional football squad – a preliminary study, *Physical Therapy in Sport* 10(3):91–96, 2009.

Cooper RR: Alternatives during immobilization and regeneration of skeletal muscle in cats, *J Bone Joint Surg* 54:919–953, 1972.

Davis BC, Harrison AD: *Hydrotherapy in Practice*, Edinburgh, 1988, Churchill Livingstone.

Di Clementi CC, Valesquez M: Motivational interviewing and the stages of change. In Miller WR, Rollnick S, editors: *Motivational interviewing: Preparing people for change*, ed 2, New York, 2002, Guildford Publications, pp 201–215.

Dishman RK, Berthoud H, Booth FW, et al: Neurobiology of Exercise, *Obesity* 14(3):345–356, 2006.

Donaldson CL, Hulley SB, Vogel JM, et al: Effects of prolonged bed rest on bone mineral, *Metabolism* 19:1017–1084, 1970.

Engles M: Tissue Response. In Donetelli R, Wooden M, editors: *Orthopaedic Physical Medicine*, Edinburgh, 1994, Churchill Livingstone, pp 25–28.

Ferrell WR, Tennant N, Sturrock RD, et al: Amelioration of symptoms by enhancement of proprioception in patients with joint hypermobility syndrome, *Arthritis Rheum* 50:3323–3328, 2004.

Ferrell WR, Tennant N, Baxendale RH, et al: Musculoskeletal reflex function in the joint hypermobility syndrome, *Arthritis Rheum* 57(7):1329–1333, 2007.

Fitts PM, Posner MI: *Human Performance (Basic concepts in psychology)*, London, 1967, Brooke Cole.

Fuller CS: Aquatic Rehabilitation. In Anderson JR, Harrelson GL, Wilkes KE, editors: *Physical Rehabilitation of the injured athlete*, ed 2, London, 1998, WB Saunders Company, pp 615–631.

Gazit Y, Nahir AM, Grahame R, et al: Dysautonomia in the joint hypermobility syndrome, *Am J Med* 115(1):33–40, 2003.

Gedalia A, Press J, Klein M, et al: Joint hypermobility and fibromyalgia in school children, *Ann Rheum Dis* 53:494–496, 1993.

Gentile AM: A working model of skill acquisition with application to learning, *National Association of Kinesiology and Physical Education in Higher Education* 17(1):3–23, 1972.

Goldman JA: Hypermobility and deconditioning: Important links to Fibromyalgia/Fibrositis, *South Med J* 84:1192–1196, 1991.

Grahame R, Jenkins JM: Joint Hypermobility - asset or liability? A study of joint mobility in ballet dancers, *Ann Rheum Dis* 31:109–111, 1972.

Grahame R, Hunt JN, Kitchen S, et al: The Diuretic, Natriuretic and Kaluretic Effects of Water Immersion, *Q J Med* 45:579, 1978.

Grana WA, Moretz JA: Ligament laxity in secondary school athletes, *J Am Med Assoc* JAMA 240:1975–1976, 1978.

Gray J, Taunton JE, McKenzie DC, et al: A survey of injuries to the anterior cruciate ligament of the knee in female basketball players, *Int J Sports Med* 6(6):314–316, 1985.

Guskiewicz KM, Perrin DH: Research and clinical applications of assessing balance, *J Sport Rehabil* 5:45–63, 1996.

Hakim AJ, Ashton S: Undiagnosed, Joint Hypermobility Syndrome patients have poorer outcome than peers following chronic back pain rehabilitation, *Rheumatology* 44(3 Suppl 1):#255, 2005.

Hardt AB: Early metabolic responses of bone to immobilization, *J Bone Joint Surg* 54:119–124, 1972.

Harrelson GL: Physiological factors of rehabilitation. In Andrews RJ, Harrelson GL, Wilk KE, editors: *Physical Rehabilitation of the Injured Athlete*, ed 2, London, 1998, W.B. Saunders Company, pp 13–37.

Harrelson GL, Leaver-Dunn D: Introduction to rehabilitation. In Andrews RJ, Harrelson GL, Wilk KE, editors: *Physical Rehabilitation of the Injured Athlete*, ed 2, London, 1998, W.B. Saunders Company, pp 175–217.

Hinton RY: Case Study: Rehabilitation of multiple joint instability associated with Ehlers-Danlos Syndrome, *J Orthop Sports Phys Ther* 84:193–198, 1986.

Hurley R, Turner C: Neurology and Aquatic Therapy, *Clinical Management* 11(1):26–29, 1991.

Katch W, Katch F, McCardle V: *Essentials of Physiology*, ed 3, Philadelphia, 2006, Lippincott Williams & Wilkins, pp 432–741.

Kerr A, Macmillan CE, Uttley W, et al: Physiotherapy for children with hypermobility syndrome, *Physiotherapy* 86(6):313–316, 2000.

Kirby RL, Simms C, Symington VJ, et al: Flexibility and musculoskeletal symptomatology in female gymnasts and age-matched controls, *Am J Sports Med* 9:160–164, 1981.

Klemp P, Learmouth ID: Hypermobility and injuries in a professional ballet company, *Br J Sport Med* 18:143–148, 1984.

Lamb DA: *Physiology of Exercise*, ed 1, London, 1984, MacMillan Press.

Landry M, Fleisch H: The influence of immobilization on bone formation as evaluated by osseous incorporation of tetracyclines, *Journal of Bone Joint Surgery* 46(7):764–771, 1964.

Laros GS, Tipton C, Cooper RR: Influence of physical activity on ligament insertions in the knees of dogs, *J Bone Joint Surg* 53:275–286, 1971.

LeBlanc AD, Schneider V, Evans HL, et al: Bone Mineral loss and recovery after 17 weeks of bed rest, *J Bone Min Res* 5(8):843–850, 1990.

Lee D, Vleeming A: Impaired load transfer through the pelvic girdle-a new model of altered neutral zone function. In *3rd Interdisciplinary World Congress on Low Back and Pelvic pain*, November 19–21, Austria, 1998, p 76.

MacCormack M, Grahame R, Briggs J: Joint laxity and the benign joint hypermobility syndrome in student and professional ballet dancers, *J Rheumatol* 31:173–178, 2004.

MacSween A, Brydson G, Creed G, et al: A Preliminary Validation of the 10-metre incremental shuttle walk test as a measure of aerobic capacity in women with rheumatoid arthritis, *Physiotherapy* 87(1):38–44, 2001.

MacDougall JD, Ward GR, Sale DG, et al: Effects of strength training and immobilization on human muscle fibres, *Eur J Appl Physiol* 43:700–703, 1977.

Mano T, Iwase S, Yamazaki Y, et al: Sympathetic nervous adjustments in man to simulated weightlessness induced by water immersion, *Journal of the University of Occupational and Environmental Health (UOEH)* 7:215–227, 1985.

Melzack R: The short McGill Pain Questionnaire, *Pain* 30:191–197, 1987.

Mishra MB, Ryan R, Atkinson P, et al: Extra-articular features of benign joint hypermobility syndrome, *Br J Rheumatol* 35:861–866, 1996.

Morgan AW, Pearson SB, Davies C, et al: Asthma and airways collapse in two heritable disorders of connective tissue, *Ann Rheum Dis* 66:169–174, 2007.

Moseley GL: A pain neuromatrix approach to patients with chronic pain, *Man Ther* 8(3):130–140, 2003.

Nicholas JA: Injuries to knee ligaments. Relationship to looseness and tightness in football players, *J Am Med Assoc* 212:2236–2239, 1970.

Nijs J, Van Essche E, De Munck M, et al: Ultrasound, axial and peripheral measurements in female patients with benign hypermobility syndrome, *Calcif Tissue Int* 67:37–40, 2000.

Noyes FR, Mangine RE, Barber S: Biomechanics of ligament failure. II. An analysis of immobilization, exercise and reconditioning effects in primates, *J Bone Joint Surg* 56:1406–1418, 1974.

Ofluoglu D, Gunduz OH, Kul-Panza E, et al: Hypermobilty in women with fibromyalgia syndrome, *Clin Rheumatol* 25(3):291–293, 2006.

Panjabi MM: The stabilizing system of the spine I. Function, dysfunction, Adaptation and enhancement, *J Spinal Disord* 5(4):383–389, 1992a.

Panjabi MM: The stabilizing system of the spine II. Neutral zone and instability hypothesis, Commentary, *J Spinal Disord* 5(4):390–397, 1992b.

Petajan JH, Gappmaier E, White AT, et al: Impact of aerobic training on fitness and quality of life in multiple sclerosis, *Ann Neurol* 39:432–441, 1996.

Prochaska JO, Norcross JC: Stages of Change, *Psychotherapy* 28:443–448, 2001.

Rasch PJ, Burke RK: *Kinesiology and Applied Anatomy*, ed 6, London, 1977, Lea & Febiger, pp 417–444.

Rifenberick DH, Max SR: Substrate utilization by disused rat skeletal muscles, *Am J Physiol* 226:295–297, 1974.

Sale DG: Neural adaptation to resistance training, *Med Sci Sports Exerc* 20 S:135–145, 1988.

Sendur OF, Gurer G, Taskis Bozbas G: The frequency of hypermobility and its relationship with clinical findings of fibromyalgia patients, *Clin Rheumatol* 26(4):485–487, 2007.

Shoen RP, Kirsner AB, Farber SJ, et al: The hypermobility syndrome, *Postgrad Med* 71(6):199–208, 1982.

Simmonds JV, Keer RJ: Hypermobility and hypermobility syndrome. Part 2: assessment and management illustrated via case studies, *Manual Therapy* 13(2):e1–e11, 2008.

Skinner AT, Thomson AM: *Duffield's Exercise in Water*, ed 3, London, 1993, Balliere Tindall pp 4 & 141.

Smith R, Damodaran AK, Swaminathan S, et al: Hypermobility and sports injuries in junior netball players, *Br J Sports Med* 39:628–631, 2005.

Soderman K, Alfredson H, Pietila T, et al: Risk factors for leg injuries in female soccer: a prospective investigation during one out-door season, *Knee Surg Sports Traumatol Arthrosc* 9:313–321, 2001.

Steinberg FU: *The immobilized patient: Functional Pathology and Management*, New York, 1980, Millen Press.

Stewart DR, Burden S: Does generalised ligamentous laxity increase seasonal incidence of injuries in male first division club rugby players? *Br J Sports Med* 38:457–460, 2004.

Tipton CM, James SL, Mergner W, et al: Influence of exercise on strength of medial collateral knee ligaments of dogs, *Am J Physiol* 218:894–902, 1970.

Williams PE, Catanese T, Lucey E, et al: The importance of stretch and contractile activity in the prevention of connective tissue accumulation in muscle, *J Anat* 158:109, 1988.

Witzmann FA, Kim DH, Fitts RH: Recovery time course in recovery function of fast and slow skeletal muscle after hind limb immobilization, *J Appl Physiol* 52:677–682, 1982.

Woo SL-Y, Gomez MA, Young-Kyun W, et al: Mechanical properties of tendons and ligaments II: the relationship of immobilization and exercise on tissue remodelling, *Biorhelogy* 19:397, 1982.

Woolf-May K: *Exercise Prescription: Physiological Foundations*, London, 2006, Churchill Livingstone, pp 1–5.

World Health Organisation (WHO): *Prevention and management of Osteoporosis – Geneva*, 2003. http://whqlibdoc.who.int/trs/WHO_TRS_921.pdf.

Worsford C, Simpson JM: Standardisation of a three-metre walking test for the elderly, *Physiotherapy* 87:25–132, 2001.

Zarins B: Soft tissue injury and repair: Biomechanical aspects, *Int J Sports Med* 3:19–25, 1982.

UK Support Groups and Further Reading

HYPERMOBILITY SYNDROMES

The Hypermobility Syndrome Association
P.O. Box 1122
Nailsea
Bristol
BS48 2YZ

www.hypermobility.org

EDS

Ehlers-Danlos Support Group
PO Box 337
Aldershot
Surrey
GU12 6WZ

www.ehlers-danlos.org

FIBROMYALGIA

Fibrolmyalgia Association UK
PO Box 206
Stourbridge
DY9 8YL

www.fibromyalgia-associationuk.org

MARFAN SYNDROME

Marfan Association UK
Rochester House,
5 Aldershot Road
Fleet
Hants
GU51 3NG

www.marfan-association.org.uk

Additional Reading:

Hypermobility Syndrome: Recognition and Management for Physiotherapists

Rosemary Keer, Rodney Grahame 2003
Butterworth Heinemann, London
ISBN 0 7506 5390 6

Issues and Management of Joint Hypermobility

Brad T Tinkle 2008
Left Paw Press, Greens Fork, IN, USA
ISBN 978-0-9818360-1-0

Hypermobility of Joints

Beighton P, Grahame R, Bird H 3rd ed. 1999
Springer Verlag, London
ISBN 1-85223-142-9

Fibromyalgia Syndrome

Leon Chaitow 2003
Churchill Livingstone, Edinburgh
ISBN 978-0443072192

Explain Pain

David S Butler, Lorimer Moseley 2003
NOI group Publications, Adelaide, Australia
ISBN 978-0-975091005

Painful Yarns: Metaphors and Stories to Help Understand the Biology of Pain

Lorimer Moseley 2007
Dancing Giraffe Press, Canberra, Australia
ISBN 978-0980358803

Chronic Fatigue Syndrome (The Facts)

Frankie Campling, Michael Sharpe 2nd Ed 2008
Oxford University Press, Oxford
ISBN 978-0199233168

Index

Note: Page numbers followed by *b* indicate boxes, *f* indicate figures and *t* indicate tables.